Powered by Nature

Also by Logan Christopher

Mental Muscle
The Master Keys to Strength and Fitness
Deceptive Strength
The Indestructible Body
Practicing Strength and Movement
The Ultimate Guide to Handstand Pushups
The Ultimate Guide to Pullups and Chin-ups
The Ultimate Guide to Bodyweight Squats and Pistols
The Ultimate Guide to Bodyweight Ab Exercises
The Ultimate Guide to Bodyweight Conditioning
Secrets of the Handstand
Learn How to Back Flip in 31 Days
Berzerker: Psyching Up for Strength and Sports
101 Simple Steps to Radiant Health
101 Advanced Steps to Radiant Health
Upgrade Your Breath
Upgrade Your Testosterone
Upgrade Your Growth Hormone
The Money System that Never Fails

POWERED

BY

NATURE

How Nature Improves Our Happiness, Health, and Performance

By Logan Christopher

DISCLAIMER

The health advice contained within this book is for educational purposes only and is not intended for medical purposes. The author and publisher of this book are not responsible in any manner whatsoever for the use, misuse or dis-use of the information presented here.

Powered by Nature: How Nature Improves Our Happiness, Health and Performance

ISBN: 978-1-7329321-0-4

Printed in the United States of America

Published by:

Legendary Strength

Santa Cruz, California

www.LegendaryStrength.com

DEDICATION

To my mother and Mother Earth

Table of Contents

PART 1

How this book came to be and how we humans got off track

1
Emissary of Nature

"In the Western world visionaries and mystics are a good deal less common than they used to be...In the currently fashionable picture of the universe there is no place for valid transcendental experience. Consequently, those who have had what they regard as valid transcendental experiences are looked upon with suspicion, as being either lunatics or swindlers. To be a mystic or a visionary is no longer credible."
– Aldous Huxley

I did not set out to write this book; I was called to write it. To properly understand what you have begun to read, you must understand where it came from. The story is only partially my own.

Back around the early 1990's, an indigenous people, the Achuar, had initiated contact with the outside world because they saw the destruction that was happening to their neighbors from the rubber and oil companies.

They feared the 'West' but did what they feared most because they knew having to interact with the West was inevitable. Their elders saw that by initiating contact with the right people, they could exert some control over the situation.

Their elders convened with a group of Westerners and spoke at length about what to do. An Achuar elder said this:

"If you're coming to help us you're wasting your time. If you're coming because you realize your salvation is tied into our own, then let us work together."

This message was the spark to create the charity organization Pachamama Alliance. When I heard what was said, shivers rippled through my body. The goal of the Pachamama Alliance isn't to merely preserve the rainforest and its peoples, although that is an important part of its role. Instead its aim is to change the "dream of the modern world"

2

so that destruction of the natural world isn't sought out in the first place.

I had never heard of the Pachamana Alliance until I met them by being a member in Maverick 1000. This is a private, invitation-only global network of top entrepreneurs and industry leaders created by Yanik Silver. Maverick 1000 has a purpose that is three-fold: personal and business growth, making an impact, and having fun and epic experiences.

I was in Seattle attending a Maverick event. We were working with the Pachamama Alliance, using our collective entrepreneurial skills to show how the charity could not just raise money through donations but could also expand through certain business-like operations. Perhaps most importantly, we discussed how to get their message of a sustainable and ecologically-sound future, into the heart of businesses.

Prior to this I had never heard of the Pachamama Alliance. What I did not know is that my introduction to the organization would end up becoming a pivotal point in my life.

I was invited to come along on the Founder's Journey to the Amazon rainforest in Ecuador with John Perkins and Lynne Twist, best-selling authors of *Confessions of an Economic Hitman* and *The Soul of Money*, respectively. I already had other events planned during the time of the trip, but the pull was strong. I knew that this was something that I simply had to do, so I canceled the other events and made it happen.

In the time before I left for the Amazon, I studied more about Pachamama and pored over their recommended reading materials. I was far from an activist. In growing my businesses, I was focused on what my team and I could accomplish to be profitable. We were doing good things and helping people, but I wasn't looking at the bigger collective picture, nor at the ripple of impacts that what we did would cause. Getting involved here began to open my eyes to a wider perspective.

For years, after watching my mother succumb to breast cancer, I was motivated to teach people how to be healthier naturally. And now, what became abundantly clear was that so much of human health is tied to environmental health. The plastics, pollution, and pesticides that disrupt our hormones, causing cancer, cause similar destruction in nature.

Finally, it was time for my Amazon journey. I flew into Quito, Ecuador. From there it was a couple more days of journeying by bus, truck, canoe, and more planes until we arrive deep in the heart of the rainforest. Spending time with the Achuar, those previously uncontacted people, showed me just how different cultures could be. At one point, standing in the rainforest, with the cacophony of chirping and buzzing from birds, frogs, and insects, I was almost moved to tears in gratitude for the experience. And I'm not normally a crier.

Elements of that journey are spread throughout this book. For now, I want to zero in on a particular part of it.

For years, I had heard about ayuhuasca, a psychoactive drink made from vines and bark used by indigenous peoples for thousands of years. From the very beginning I knew I wanted to experience it, but, if I was going to do it, I wanted to do it right.

Ayuhuasca is highly revered by the cultures in which it originates. Because of its capacity for transformation, its popularity spread far and wide—a fact both beneficial and detrimental. On the one hand, many Westerners seeking transformation, enlightenment, or healing sought out the medicine with various impacts. On the other hand, ayuhuasca is misused by others. The worst I've heard is that at the Peruvian airport you can see people holding signs offering ayuhuasca ceremonies. And some unscrupulous so-called shamans have then robbed and raped those seekers.

Anyone can claim to be a shaman. It's not a licensed profession. And how would anyone from the West know the legitimate from the not? (Many in the West would even doubt that a shaman could be legit.)

So, as I said, if I was going to experience ayuhuasca, I wanted to do it right—to work with a legitimate shaman who had been practicing for years and to do it in the place where ayuhuasca comes from. This isn't to say that a ceremony taking place in downtown San Francisco can't be good; I just wanted my experience to be as authentic as possible the first time. In my journey into the rainforest with the Pachamama Alliance, this opportunity was available.

I heard many amazing stories from different people. Ayuhuasca effects everyone differently. And these stories ranged from the harsh (purging from both ends all night) to amazing visions and talking with the spirit of ayuhuasca. Whatever was to happen, I thought I was ready for it. I was ready for my life to be changed in some way. In fact, life-changing visions are exactly what I desired and expected.

The day the ceremony was to take place we spent fasting. When you first meet your shaman and he's wearing an IBM shirt you have to laugh. These people live in their cultures fully, yet small things like this act as reminders of how our cultures interact and have intertwined. One way or another, the culture of globalization is growing strongly.

I was excited to learn that our shaman was the one who had originally spoken those words about our salvation being tied together, over 20 years ago, that had sent shivers across my body.

When we arrived at the shaman's village we set out on a long hike. During this journey, we took the time to sit individually in the forest and be with nature. Our destination was a sacred waterfall where we snuffed a liquid tobacco infusion and set our intentions for the night to come.

Returning to the village we waited until night fell. Ayuhuasca increases your photo sensitivity, even helping you to see in the dark, so it is not done during the day.

Finally, it was time. We sat in a circle around the shaman. The ayuhuasca had already been brewed and awaited us in a plastic soda bottle—another oddity in my mind, but I suppose they do make good carrying vessels able to be reused. One at a time we sat in front of the shaman as he chanted and whistled into each cup. When he was done he handed it to us and down the hatch the liquid went.

I had heard stories of how awful ayuhuasca tastes. Yet being used to some powerfully bitter and bad tasting herbs, like reishi and tongkat ali, I have to say it wasn't that bad. It was not an enjoyable taste, but not the worst thing ever.

After the whole group had drank, we were invited to go lie down on our palm leaves under the stars. These were laid out in a large semi-circle around the hut, with plenty of space between people. Ayuhuasca is not a social drug; instead, with it you're meant to engage in a personal journey.

I sat there and wondered. Was it starting to come on? My body felt...something. My eyes saw figures appearing in the clouds above. But that happens normally when we stare at clouds, right?

A short time later, each person was invited to drink a second cup if they chose. I did so, not sure if I'm really feeling it yet, and certainly not feeling the strong effects I desired.

Our group had about ten people taking the journey. We also had helpers that were not taking the ayuhuasca there to lend a hand to those who were. Off in the distance I could hear the others beginning to purge.

I wait. It seems everyone else is purging. I notice some nearby can't even walk and need to be almost carried to the shaman for his cleansing.

And I wait. Time is hard to tell waiting under the stars. My body still felt that strange something but I'm not seeing anything spectacular. No psychedelic trip of fractal imagery or anything like that. I can feel frustration begin to build up inside my body. Why isn't it working?

I am let down. I had come all this way, waiting years to do this, and it doesn't affect me. Anger rises, and I try to let it go. It's an odd thing to be jealous of people who are throwing up, but I was.

I get up and walk around. Most everyone else is partially paralyzed it seems. Finally, a little nausea comes on. I try to make myself throw up, but this is unsuccessful.

Maybe two hours has passed. Or three or four. I talk to one of the helpers and say let's do a third cup. Mind you, no one else had drunk a third cup. Everyone else just had one. And one other guy, twice my size, had stopped at two.

I sit down with the shaman once again. He begins his whistling. Suddenly I am overcome with incredible nausea. I pause for a moment, thinking can I hold this in? No. I turn to the helper, Daniel, and say I need to vomit. He points to a spot a few paces away and I stumble over and let it all out.

Well, at least that finally happened.

After I am finished there, I notice the shaman is still whistling into that cup. I wonder, what is the protocol at this point? I sit down in front of the shaman and soon enough he hands me the third cup. Down the hatch once again. It is much worse on the way out then the way in. That being said, purging and drinking back to back only amplifies ayahuasca's bitter taste.

I go back to my palm leaf. Part of me is filled with nervousness. A third cup? I have heard the visions come on strong after purging. Maybe I'm in for something very intense.

I wait for maybe another hour. During this time, I'm fascinated by the jaguar sounds the shaman is making. He's working on healing someone. The growl emanates from deep inside his throat, and always ends the same, with him spitting onto the ground. Over and over again.

Eventually, I figure the visionary experience is just not going to happen for me. My thinking is that, for whatever reason, my ayuhuasca journey was meant to be entirely somatic. I've certainly been feeling things throughout my body, and I purged. Perhaps the visions only would have gotten in the way of the medicine. My conscious mind wasn't to be entertained, and everything would take place in the unconscious.

Waiting, while full of anticipation, can be exhausting, so I head indoors. Indoors was the shaman's hut. Unlike most of the Achuar people, he did have walls on his house. This was a defensive measure, as at one point he was the target of an assassination attempt because someone had accused him of using his shamanic powers for evil.

Our "beds" are simply palm leaves on the ground, though here we have mosquito netting around. I drift off into uncomfortable sleep, waking up once to head outside and dry heave heavily, and waking a second time to finish the deed more fully.

I don't recall any dreams that night or morning though I'm sure they occurred. At daybreak, we begin to arise. We weren't supposed to talk about our journeys until later, but after that surreal night, what else are you going to talk about?

After breakfast, we reconvene in the shaman's hut for him to interpret our visions. The process is lengthy as we first speak in English, have it translated to Spanish, and finally to Achuar. And then the reverse. This process is a good teacher of patience.

One after another my group shares their visions and receives insights into them. When my turn comes, I share something much like you just read.

Although my story was quite short in comparison to the others, the shaman spends more time speaking than in the others. In a nutshell, he says that my expectations were too high and that I had somehow messed up the instructions at the waterfall the day earlier.

He also said that I had visions, powerful visions, that I just don't remember.

What he saw was the whole forest talking to me.

Plus, at some point (spiritually not physically) I came up to him, shook his hand and said I wanted to be friends.

Quite naturally, this changed my viewpoint on my journey, and I would continue to contemplate it for some time. Having grown up in the West, to be able to enter the mystical realm I have fought to shift some of the viewpoints I had simply culturally absorbed. Considering that ayuhuasca and visions are the shaman's realm, I believe it's suitable to take his viewpoint with at least equal weight to my own, if not more so.

The rest of the day was spent heading back to our home base in the Amazon at the Kapawi Lodge, then relaxing there. As we rejoin with the whole group we pass our experiences back and forth. The larger group has been broken up into three different smaller groups, each one working with a different shaman. And very much in need of it, we all go to bed early.

The next morning John Perkins leads us on a ceremony to help us integrate the journey. They say that taking ayuhuasca lasts a lifetime. Its effects can spread far and wide. Sometimes people even have delayed reactions. The shaman's interpretation was a helpful stepping stone, and it would require even more work to integrate the teaching.

John begins to rhythmically beat the drum. I close my eyes, relax, and enter what the shaman saw the previous night…

Bom, bom, bom. The forest is talking to me and I begin shapeshifting from tree to tree. The great Kapok tree. Massive palms of many varieties. The "walking trees" of the jungle.

Bom, bom, bom. The same words from the Achuar now spoken from the rainforest to me: "If you're coming to help us you're wasting your time. If you're coming because you realize your salvation is tied into our own, then let us work together."

Bom, bom, bom. Shaking the shaman's hands. A conversation ensues. Secret whispers I can't quite make out, but the weight of importance is there…

Bom, bom, bom. A mission. A calling. An initiation. The journey occurred exactly as it was meant to.

Bom, bom, bom. The words flash across my mind, as the trees say that

I am to be an…

"Emissary of Nature."

The drum journey comes to an end. Those of us that wish to are invited to share, and I do so. Several people later tell me that my story gave them goosebumps. I'm reminded of the suggestion I've often heard to "follow the goosebumps."

This short drum journey proved to be more amazing than my ayuhuasca experience, though, of course, one could not have happened without the other.

Message received. But then the question over the next few days became, "What the hell do I do with that?"

Shortly after returning home I was back out to another Maverick 1000 event. This one was Camp Maverick, in the Connecticut mountains. The tagline is "Summer Camp for Entrepreneurs," and that's exactly what it is.

A group of more than one hundred entrepreneurs from all fields get together to share knowledge and party. This looks like several business sessions during the day, then activities like archery dodgeball and slip-and-slide kickball in the afternoon and dressing up for "prom" at night. The fact that I won as prom queen, because I was dressed up as the Stephen King character Carrie sums it up pretty well. Great times!

One of the optional activities was water skiing—only my second time trying the sport. In my first attempt, I wasn't able to stand up successfully. This time I was determined to do so. And I was successful. Although none of my runs were very long, I was able to stand a few times.

"Just one more," I yelled to the driver of the boat. And once again I was up and going…until I wasn't. When I hit the water, one of the skis came off my foot and cracked me right in the forehead.

I was dazed. Still conscious, I wasn't sure of the damage. I thought my skull could be split open. I put my hand to my head but didn't find the blood I expected. The boat came around, I got on, and was taken ashore to medical. It was bleeding slightly but not too bad. I certainly felt the impact, but wouldn't say I was concussed, having experienced that misery before.

I like to think I have a thick skull as well as a strong neck, which is useful for absorbing impacts. I counted myself as lucky that the ski hit there and not my eyes or nose instead. A large lump did come up though.

The next day I was making a joke to a group of people about my third eye being activated because it was exactly in that spot. One of the people in that group was another shaman named Sheryl Netzky. Although I was joking, she replied, "Actually..." and offered to do some energy work on it.

I gladly accepted. I could feel something going on as she explained that sometimes a physical whack on the head like that is part of something spiritual. An awakening of sorts. I couldn't help but think back to the Amazon, not even a week prior, as she spoke.

When I returned home from camp I decided I would continue to work with Sheryl. It felt like the appropriate next step, the leading of this golden thread, the continuation of this story, and so I went with that feeling.

We set up a call to discuss what that would look like and, importantly, what I sought from it. Still on my mind in a big way was the idea of being an emissary of nature.

What was that to look like in my everyday life?

And so, as the sessions began, that path further unfolded. I began spending much more time in nature. I got back to communicating directly with plants. And after a bit of time I started to write this story and this book.

This calling wasn't completely new to me. I'd been preaching the benefits of nature to health for years. My herbal supplement company, Lost Empire Herbs, is all about this. I had communicated directly with plants many times, and not just the so-called psychedelic ones. Details on that to come later.

Yet here it wasn't about what "I" wanted or was doing. Nature itself was calling me to have us work together. We needed to be mutually beneficial allies.

Humans can't "save" nature. Nature can't "save" humans. Neither of these ideas work as they're created via the wrong perception. The fact is that humans are part of nature, however much we try to deny it and remove ourselves from ecology. But we can get back in alignment. We can work together in a true ecology that supports all.

It became clear that my mission was expanding. Nature was calling me to take the mantle, to be an emissary–a person on a special mission, usually as a diplomatic representative.

As an emissary, I needed to communicate how to live more in alignment with nature to the masses.

What you are reading now is the unfolding of this mission and the message of nature, using me as an emissary to deliver it. I don't claim to have all the answers, but as William Shakespeare wrote, "In nature's infinite book of secrecy a little I can read." On that note, let me share with you some of the secrets I have discovered…

2
My Health Journey

"Cancer, like insanity, seems to increase with the progress of civilization."
– Dr. Stanislaus Tanchou

"Foolish the doctor who despises the knowledge acquired by the ancients."
– Hippocrates

I told you that story so that I can tell you this one, adding more broad strokes to the picture of my life and how I got to where I am today to deliver this message to you.

I am a child of my generation. Aren't we all? As a kid, I more often played indoors on video games and the computer than outside. I can recall camping a grand total of two times in my youth. I grew up without much respect for nature. It's not that I didn't like it, just that I seldom gave it a thought. My parents didn't guide me in thinking much about nature at all. An average modern-day family, leading average, civilized lives.

My regular meals included Hot Pockets and Honey Nut Cheerios, scarcely a fruit or vegetable in sight. Literally, as a kid I only ate two fruits—strawberries and watermelon. Zero vegetables. Sure, they were in some of the things I ate. Those hot pockets did have tomato sauce in them, but that was far from the natural form (which I hated for its texture and taste).

It comes as a surprise to most people, when they see some of the amazing strength feats I've accomplished, to learn that I am not naturally strong or athletic. In fact, I am naturally the opposite, weak and unathletic. I was the proverbial 98 lb. weakling entering high school. Those processed foods and computer games didn't make me thrive physically. Even though I hit a growth spurt, shooting up to my current 6'2", I still weighed about

155 lbs. after my senior year.

During high school my mother was diagnosed with breast cancer. I was a bit young to realize all that was going on, wrapped up in my own problems and a crisis of identity at the time. She did the standard Western treatment of chemotherapy and radiation, and the cancer went into remission. Without much thought about it, that's how I thought cancer worked. After all, that was my experience with it at the time.

What I know now is that while standard treatment may kill the cancer, it further destroys the immune system. And in the standard Western model, no attention is paid to restoring health.

A study done by three oncologists and published in the journal *Clinical Oncology* found that chemotherapy was responsible for a whopping 2.3 percent increase in five-year survival rates in the United States.[1] And that was a high estimate! Yet this damaging treatment is the standard. I highly doubt they tell you that in the doctor's office.

It was shortly after high school that I began to get fit. At first, this was just to look and feel good, but soon enough I came to enjoy training for itself. Because it wasn't easy for me, I was always on the lookout for an edge. While I wouldn't do steroids, I was open to pretty much anything else.

I realized that nutrition was important. As I studied books, I began to drop my childish ways, learning to develop a taste for all those fruits and vegetables I had strongly avoided previously. What few people realize is how tastes are formed by our beliefs and are quite malleable.

The more I learned the more I realized that great health would set me up to perform at a peak level, not just in the gym, but in my work and everywhere else. I could recover faster. I could think more clearly. I wouldn't get sick with the common cold.

Nutrition, in turn, led to herbalism through the path of Chinese tonic herbs. I took cordyceps mushroom and saw how it helped in my endurance workouts. I was hooked.

The idea of radiant health appealed immediately to me. It's not just about curing but about preventing any problem from occurring. And I was focused on peak performance, on what I could accomplish, all along the way.

Nowadays, as part of one of my businesses, Legendary Strength, I've done some crazy feats of strength. These include pulling an 8,800 lb. fire truck by my hair, supporting half a ton on top of me in a wrestler's bridge position, juggling flaming kettlebells, ripping decks of cards in half, and much more. That's all viewable on YouTube. And to make it easier, a good place to see the highlights is at the following page on my website: www.legendarystrength.com/best-of/

As I was building my body and my own health, and working to become a personal trainer, as often happens, my mother's cancer came back after a few years.

Back on the chemo and radiation she went. This time she also went through a double mastectomy. Got to get rid of those dangerous breasts!

I watched as her health further deteriorated. It is horrible to hear your mother not able to put together words because of how the "chemo-brain" robbed her ability to think clearly. She self-medicated with wine, falling asleep on the couch many nights and days. I could see what was happening, but there wasn't much I could do about it. I did try to help, but she was stuck in her ways. And I was only beginning to learn how I could communicate these ideas to others. Still, she had gotten better before, so I naively assumed this would happen again.

Yet the treatments weren't enough. The cancer spread throughout her body. She suffered through a series of mini-strokes, or transient ischemic attacks. After she was admitted into the hospital, her hip snapped in half, the cancer having made it brittle.

There were nights when she would wake up not knowing where she was, and there was nothing that could be done to comfort her, except to put her on anti-psychotic medication. I trusted the doctors and nurses who said that was for the best, though now I realize it was more for their convenience then hers. Haldol makes more manageable patients.

My two brothers were serving in the military at that time. One was being discharged from the Army right around that time, after being stationed in Alaska for years. The other had more recently joined the Marines. When he asked for leave to see his dying mother, he was told no, but that he would get funeral leave. Not accepting that bullshit answer, he decided to go AWOL.

Eventually, we got her home from the hospital and in hospice care. As the youngest son, and never really seeing death before, I was ill prepared. Part of me still thought she'd get better. I didn't know anything about how to make hers a good passing.

This was easily the worst time in my life, yet it propelled me to learn how such things could be cured and avoided in the first place.

Having done much psychological self-work on those events, nowadays, I see her passing as the last gift she gave me. I realize this may sound like an odd thing to say, because few people seem to be able to get past grief, some even believing that it never goes away. What I know is that I would not be where I am today had that not happened, so I am thankful for the difficult experience. I am thankful for her sacrifice.

It propelled me far deeper into health.

It propelled me deeper into understanding the mind and how beliefs operate.

Soon enough I started teaching not just about strength but also about health. To this day, I see health as being important for each person on this planet, for these two reasons:

1) You can prevent and even cure disease
2) You can unlock your peak performance at whatever you're doing

As the saying goes, "if you don't have your health, you don't have much."

Over the years, the learning continued, and the deeper I went, the more I realized how doing things naturally is often best for your health. That is largely what I mean by being powered by nature.

I found out that cancer is, for the most part, a modern phenomenon, at least at the frequency we are seeing it today.

Even though the average person lives longer in the modern age, largely because of avoiding infectious disease, acute injury, and infant and childhood mortality, it is not because we are far healthier. The fact is, the average lifespan is only six years longer than the lifespan of someone living before 100 BC. [2] Think about that. For all our advanced technology, and how advanced we considered our healthcare to be, we've gotten six

15

years out of it.

But that's only looking at one aspect. While they may live a little longer, people today are less metabolically healthy than previous generations.

A large cohort study compared generational shifts in metabolic risk factors for cardiovascular disease. They concluded, "The more recently born generations are doing worse…that the prevalence of metabolic risk factors and the lifelong exposure to them have increased and probably will continue to increase." [3]

The authors of this study found that people are diagnosed with disease at ages that are 33 percent younger than their grandparents' ages. Some of this is likely from more diagnosing occurring overall, but part of it is because of people's worse health.

And while the average life span is a few years longer, fewer people, based on percentage, are living to 100 years of age. To me, lifespan isn't nearly as important as health span. Are you healthy throughout the years, not just getting by? Only if you answer yes to that question should you be focusing on living longer.

What if we could have some of the benefits of modern living, while still being aligned with nature and drawing health benefits from doing so?

I'm not saying we should go back to living in caves. There certainly are benefits to modern civilized living. But there are drawbacks too, that most people are not aware of.

This book is about those factors. Nature seems to be calling me continually, in an ever-evolving way. Being born a civilized human being, without any real connection to the natural world, has, I feel, uniquely positioned me to deliver this message.

I'm a modern man. I like technology. I work at a computer many hours each day, making my living from it. Yet because I focus on health not just for prevention or curing of problems, but also to perform at a peak level, I can show how nature can do the same for you.

This is what I have found, and I believe it can be true for you as well.

How would you like to reduce stress?

Think more clearly?

Sleep deeply without effort?

Be filled with abundant energy?

Maintain the ability to move pain free well into old age?

Have an incredible sex life?

Nature helps provide all these things, if you act in alignment with it. Furthermore, by aligning yourself with nature you can begin to unlock your super powers. As a kid, I was a big fan of superheroes in the comics, as indeed most boys are. I especially enjoyed the X-Men, and my namesake, Logan, aka Wolverine.

Ever since then I wanted to develop super human powers. While claws coming out of my hands wasn't likely, I found out I could develop super strength, to learn faster than most and acquire many skills. Plus, I'm working on building businesses to make money so that I'm rich like Batman, another favorite superhero of mine. And wealth definitely is a super power, whether used for good or evil. After all, the nearly invincible Superman's arch nemesis, Lex Luthor, is just a man.

There are many super powers. Some you may have innate talent in. Others you can begin with a weakness and turn into a strength, through diligent work.

Nature itself can become a super power for you. Or at least a powerful ally on this quest that is life. Over the coming pages I will show you how it is in your best interest to realize this and act on it.

3
Principle-Based Health

"As to methods there may be a million and then some, but principles are few. The man who grasps principles can successfully select his own methods. The man who tries methods, ignoring principles, is sure to have trouble."
– Emerson

We're in the information age. It's only accelerating in pace. Following the headlines on the news about the latest studies on health is enough to make your head spin as they are often contradictory. How can we possibly keep up with everything that is going on? Unless we read research articles full time, how do we know what is true about health?

Here is my answer. The latest research isn't where we should be looking. We are not missing a secret key that makes everything easy, that has yet to be revealed by those in lab coats.

Instead, it's all about coming back to principles.

The problem is that without a foundation of principles you can easily be swept up in the latest fad or sent into paralysis by analysis when two conflicting viewpoints occur.

But tactics and strategies can be flawed and take you far down the wrong path, if you never take a step back to find out if principles on which they're based are sound. How long and how many people based their eating, even without thinking about it, on the low-fat strategy, that "science" said was the answer? Hopefully, you're aware just how wrong that is, and if not, I'll cover it in detail later.

Principles are timeless. It doesn't matter if you're a person that existed 2000 years ago, today, or will exist 2000 years hence. Access to resources and information has dramatically changed in that time and will continue to do so. Still, the principles do not change.

Yuval Noah Harari, author of *Sapiens* and *Homo Deus*, wrote, "A need shaped thousands of generations ago continues to be felt subjectively even if it is no longer necessary for survival and reproduction in the present." While he was talking about psychological needs, his idea applies to everything. What we as a species grew up with is needed now. It's not just about survival and procreation but what is required to be healthy and happy.

Throughout this book there are several strategies and many tactics. All of these arise out of the four principles listed below.

The tactics and strategies are derived from my experience of over a decade in studying health. I did not have these when I set out on my journey, but have since distilled all the information and experiments I've studied and conducted down to the following:

1) The Human System is a Holistic Ecology
2) Alignment with Nature
3) Aim for Radiant Health
4) Direct Experience

Let's dive into what each of these mean to you and your health.

1) The Human System is a Holistic Ecology

"All of the concepts that ecologists use to describe the continental-scale ecosystems that we see through satellites also apply to ecosystems in our bodies that we peer at with microscopes. We can talk about the diversity of microbial species. We can draw food webs, where different organisms eat and feed each other. We can single out keystone microbes that exert a disproportionate influence on their environment—the equivalents of sea otters or wolves. We can treat disease-causing microbes—pathogens—as invasive creatures, like cane toads or fire ants. We can compare the gut of a person with inflammatory bowel disease to a dying coral reef or a fallow field: a battered ecosystem where the balance of organisms has gone awry...All zoology is really ecology."
– Ed Yong

Seeing the body as an ecology is a cutting edge scientific way of looking at things. It is also the traditional way of seeing things. Only in the last couple hundred years have we left this principle and gotten way off track.

"*Cogito ergo sum.*" This is the famous quote from René Descartes, though you may know it better as "I think, therefore I am." His other work included the idea of Cartesian dualism, the separation of body and mind. He wrote: "There is nothing in the concept of body that belongs to the mind; and nothing in that of mind that belongs to the body."

As this false idea was spread, the body was relegated to the realm of doctors and the mind to the realm of priests, and, later, psychiatrists.

Yet, we all know that this separation is simply not true. The simplest of experiments can showcase this. Think of biting into a lemon right now. Imagine it in full multi-sensory detail. If you haven't shut down your imaginative skills *(Stop day dreaming and get to work!)*, your saliva will begin to flow. If the mind and body were separate, this would not happen, because this is your mind, your thoughts, affecting your body. While imagining biting a lemon is a simple example, hundreds more are available.

I love to teach mental training to athletes. By guiding them in slight tweaks to how they internally visualize I can get people to become stronger, faster, or more flexible, instantly and sometimes dramatically. This only occurs because body and mind are intimately connected.

Think about the biggest problem you're having right now, and what happens? Your body tenses up, and your blood pressure goes up. Now think of relaxing in nature, not a care in the world, and you'll find that the opposite occurs.

This process is not unidirectional. What's happening in your body influences your thinking in gross and subtle ways. If you are in pain, go ahead and try thinking as clearly as if you were not.

But just seeing the mind and the body as split is only part of the problem in recognizing our holism.

"*Cogito ergo sum,*" by implication, also means if you do not think, you are not. Such is the reasoning that led Descartes and others to see animals as merely machines and perform live dissections on them. A dog's cry of pain was thought of no differently than the chimes of a clock. As Descartes said, "I do not recognize any difference between the machines made by craftsmen and various bodies that nature alone composes."

Over the years, this line of thinking has stripped aliveness from everything. Contrast this to the indigenous belief of animism, which is the belief that everything is animated with a life force. In science, life was removed from most things and relegated just to plants and animals. Descartes took it further so that, essentially, only humans were living. Now many claim that humans are nothing but robots without free will— that nothing in the universe is alive.

The funny thing is that Descartes had a visionary experience that led him to discover "the foundations of a marvelous science" and to see the mathematical system behind matter in the world.

Along with this came the idea that the human body was a machine. Any metaphor that we use to describe something guides our thinking regarding that thing. If a part of a machine isn't working, we replace it. And that's exactly what we have come to do in surgery, with advances in 3D printing extending the possibilities each year.

If we look only at parts we tend to miss the systems and how they work together. There's cholesterol in these atherosclerotic arteries, therefore cholesterol must be the problem, which means we should eat less cholesterol…except it doesn't work this way. Yet that non-systemic line of thinking led to people fearing eating fat, and to drug companies selling billions of dollars' worth of statins.

The mind became another machine, a more advanced one as our technology progressed, a computer that resides in the head. There are those who believe everything that happens—including our thoughts, feelings, and consciousness—can be described as mechanical brain activity. And this computer, of course, runs the rest of the machine, the robotic meat sack, that is the body.

Think about it now. Do you believe this? Likely, it was never implicitly taught to you, but this assumption lies behind so much that we absorb this belief, as if by osmosis.

Another metaphor offers a more complete picture and a more useful way of thinking about the entire human system. It is, in my opinion, not really a metaphor—it is reality—but we'll be using some metaphorical language to explain it.

The human system is an ecology. The origin of *ecology* is from the Greek *oikos*, meaning house. This is paired with *-logy,* which means a subject of study or interest. Thus, ecology is the study of the house. Since we can't escape living in our bodies, at least until we're no longer alive, this is an apt description.

A more modern definition of ecology is the branch of biology that deals with the relations of organisms to one another and to their physical surroundings. The key word in this definition is *relations*.

In the human system, every cell relates to one another. These cells come together, specialized in some task, and make up a whole that is greater than the individual. Different cells come together to become the liver. The liver works along with the other organs involved in digestion, in circulation, in energy production, and in the mind.

Every cell senses changes in the environment and then acts on those senses. That is how all living things work. Only so much can be learned when we extract cells and put them into a petri dish, as opposed to when they're at work in their natural ecology.

Simply replacing the part, the liver, only sometimes works. Organ replacement must be combined with immunosuppressive drugs or else the ecology rejects the outsider.

We can also see further ecological and systemic function by the fact that in organ replacements, especially the heart, the recipient sometimes takes on new thinking or habits. If the mind is purely in the brain, how do you explain this?

An article that looked at several of these cases found a foundry worker with a new heart began to enjoy classical music. Another woman with a heart transplant began to drink beer and eat chicken nuggets—habits of the man who died in a motorcycle accident, who donated his heart. Recurring nightmares of murder in a young girl who received a murdered girl's heart led to the apprehension of the criminal.[1]

While skeptics will say there are many people who receive transplants who don't take on new traits, or that the traits come about from other reasons, their protests don't explain these cases. In the Heart Field and

Heart Perception chapter, I'll be sharing research that shows just how much information the heart passes to the brain.

3D printing human organs may revolutionize medicine and save lives, but if it is not looked at in relation to the ecology, the tool will be fraught with difficulty. Will the organs contain the necessary neurology to connect with our own? Will those that receive these organs have robot dreams?

Beyond the relations of our cells and bodily systems, the most apparent aspect of the human ecology is that we're made up of more bacteria than human cells. While the often-quoted number of 10 trillion bacteria to 1 trillion human cells isn't completely accurate, it promotes this point. More recently the number has been revised to just a few trillion more bacteria cells than human cells overall. [2]

What are these bacteria doing? They are undertaking so many processes that the answers couldn't all be contained in this book. More roles for the different families and species of bacteria will be found as more research results are published.

Most well-known is the role of the microbiome in the gut. These bacteria play a huge part in our health as they help digest food, transform nutrients, promote elimination, and so much else. Plus, they make up a large part of our immune system. They're our first line of defense.

Antibiotics, which are like launching a nuclear bomb into your system, decimate the ecology. While there are circumstances that call for using antibiotics, as they can be lifesaving, our overuse of them has produced negatives for human health.

Furthermore, our human centric focus without thought for the larger ecology has caused the microbes to evolve to become resistant so that deadlier forms of bacteria exist which can't be stopped by the same weapons. Many biologists suggest that we're entering the post-antibiotic era. [3]

Then there is the skin, which is absolutely filled with bacteria. The fact is that we need a healthy ecology on our skin to support skin health, in turn supporting the rest of our health. Destroy the ecology, which many of our soaps, scrubs, and other skin care products do, and it's no wonder so many people have so many problems.

But bacteria aren't the only part of our ecology. We'll go far deeper into the subjects of bacteria, viruses, fungi, and even helpful parasites in a later chapter.

If you want to be healthy it's not just about taking care of yourself, because your "self" is more than you. You are more of a steward that needs to take care of the land, which is your body.

Support the ecology and the ecology will support you. Don't support the ecology and it will fall apart, as nature seeks to reclaim it.

This ecology, then, affects you in many ways for good or ill. A dysbiotic microbiome causes you to crave more of those things that feed it, further exacerbating the issue. Until the microbiome is brought back into a healthy ecology you will suffer symptoms. Because bacteria produce neurotransmitters and other chemical signaling molecules, they even affect your thoughts.

Considering our ecology exhibits mind control, don't you think it will be helpful to think ecologically for health and performance?

All of this is explored deeper in the chapter on Symbiosis. This is the first principle because it is crucial. That chapter may be the most important one of this book.

When we see how natural ecology works on the land, the interplay between different species, even all the different kingdoms of life, we can see parallels into our own existence.

Beyond thinking of the human body as a machine, we tend to demonize anything that isn't human. Animals are dangerous. Bacteria, viruses, and parasites are out to kill us. Don't eat plants and mushrooms because they're poisonous. Of course, some of this is certainly true, but in our overt fear we've lumped everything into these categories of danger, to our own detriment.

Just imagine a farmer who has animals that get sick. He decides to napalm his land to clear out the invaders. Then what? This metaphor is standard practice in what we do to our bodies by using antibiotics.

Now think of a farmer who has the same sick animals. Here he looks to the land, including the available food, water, shelter, and other factors and finds what is wrong. He tends to the animals. And upon correcting the underlying ecological issues the animals become healthy again.

I began this section with a quote from Ed Yong, who wrote *I Contain*

Multitudes. This book shows the importance of microbes all across the world in various symbiotic relationships with many animals. Later in this phenomenal book, Yong writes that dysbiosis is "not about individuals failing to repel pathogens, but about breakdowns in communication between different species—host and symbiont—that live together. It is disease, recast as an *ecological* problem. Healthy individuals are like virgin rainforests or lush grasslands or Kingman Reef. Sick individuals are like fallow fields or scum-covered lakes or the bleached reefs of Christmas Island—ecosystems in disarray."

Plus, when it's not just about you, you'll see how your ecology is tied into the greater ecology. You'll gain insight into how your internal environment is always interacting with the external environment chemically, electromagnetically, and in other ways.

Above all else this book is about ecology and how the line between "you" and "not you" is quite blurry. Therefore, holistic ecological thinking is the only way of thinking about our health that makes sense.

2) Alignment with Nature

"Life in all its fullness is this Mother Nature obeyed."
– Weston A. Price

As much as we try to rise above nature and be civilized humans, meaning "of the city," we can't escape the fact that we are natural beings. We came from nature and we'll return to nature in the end.

Regardless of whether you believe we evolved, were divinely appointed, or some combination of the two, it is clear we are part of nature.

Yes, we are different in certain ways than anything else. That is clear. But that doesn't mean we can escape this undeniable fact. At least as long as we are on this Earth, we are of this Earth.

This isn't to say that everything in nature is good for us. Arsenic is a naturally occurring metalloid, but ingesting it is not advised.

Just because something is natural doesn't necessarily make it good. And just because something is unnatural doesn't necessarily make it bad. That being said, a helpful rule of thumb is that if we can look to see what is in alignment with nature, and in alignment with our nature, we can tend to find better results.

Some would argue that death and disease are natural things. And they certainly are. Death is a natural part of life.

The whole rise of civilization seems to be to combat nature in an attempt to stop death. Immortality has always been sought, and always been promised in the future. The utopian scientific view, expounded by Ray Kurzweil and others, says that the opportunity for immortality may be as close as ten years away.

Yet, even if someday we can upload our consciousness to the web or use nanomachines to keep our cells eternally young, at some point our sun will explode or the universe itself will die. Death comes for everything. It is best to come to terms with this fact.

Goethe wrote, "The spectacle of Nature is always new, for she is always renewing the spectators. Life is her most exquisite invention; and death is her expert contrivance to get plenty of life."

Just because death is a reality, doesn't mean we can't have great health throughout life, even right up to that death. Our natural birthright is to be healthy, even radiantly so. Our natural birthright is to have abundant energy every day, at every age of our life. Why would nature create something that wasn't so? If it is not, the ecology is not in alignment. But by following natural laws we can bring it back in.

The standard image in the West of an elder is someone who shuffles around, takes handfuls of drugs each day, and has trouble remembering things. While this is a sad reality for many, it is by no means inevitable. There are countless examples of thriving elders well into old age. These are the ones who are taking care of their ecology and living in alignment with nature.

The best perception from which to look at living in alignment with nature is to see from where we came. We must go back to what our ancient ancestors did, before the advent of agriculture, as that is when everything changed.

Of course, every ancient culture has its superstitions and idiosyncrasies, just as is true for modern cultures too. All humans have flaws. But we can look at the broad strokes, especially those things that

26

are in common with all indigenous cultures throughout the world. Why indigenous peoples? Because these are the last vestiges of human beings living fully in alignment with nature and their surrounding ecology and environment.

Part of the difficulty is that there aren't very many people like this remaining in the world that haven't been assimilated in one degree or another to the spreading globalized Western culture. Assuming acute diseases or injuries don't take them out, many elders of indigenous peoples are thriving examples of health.

In the coming chapters, you'll learn that how we've always done things, up until the modern age, tend to be uniquely suited to our biology and psychology. Science is investigating this and finding often that ancient wisdom is true. (Duh! It's called wisdom for a reason.) This wisdom arose out of living in alignment with nature.

3) Aim for Radiant Health

"The doctor of the future will give no medication, but will interest his patients in the care of the human frame, diet, and in the cause and prevention of disease."
– Thomas Edison

My guess is that Edison would have thought his predication to be true by this century. Yet, what he forecasted is not what the doctors of the future gave my mother regarding cancer. And it doesn't look like the paradigm is changing. The promise is still better, more targeted medicine in the future. Sadly, in more cases than not, doctors are simply medication dealers. Edison didn't take into account how much money would drive healthcare in the future.

There must be a better way. And there is. It is for you to take responsibility for your own health, not give it away to your doctor.

I've noticed that the majority of people only become interested in health when it starts to be a problem. Then they work to fix those problems once they've begun.

Sounds like a good plan, right? While it certainly is better than doing nothing, this method comes with an inherent flaw. If you're only ever working to avoid problems, you'll never move towards an ideal.

Recall in my earlier story when I began learning about health to support my performance in my strength training practice. I wasn't trying to fix a problem but instead looked at how I could perform at 100 percent more often.

Thus, when I first heard about the idea of "Radiant Health" from Chinese tonic herbalist Ron Teeguarden, my attention was immediately grabbed. This is the man that first introduced me to the idea of "superior herbalism," which changed the trajectory of my life. The importance of this forgotten realm of natural living will be covered in the chapter on herbalism.

Radiant health is described as health beyond danger. It means your health is so good you don't get sick in the first place. It means your health is so good you'll be a high-performance human all the time, or at least the majority of the time. In his book *The Ancient Wisdom of Chinese Tonic Herbs*, Teeguarden shares a lesson that was emphasized by his teacher Sung Jin Park: "Protection is one of the primary characteristics of health." Later on, he writes, "Adaptability is the very measure by which an Oriental master would judge the true health of an individual."

Let me be clear. Lack of disease, of some sort of diagnosis, does not equal health. It's a part of it, but really only a mediocre level at best. Sadly, many people are walking around as if operating on fumes. What's worse is that they are unaware of how much more vibrantly healthy they could be. They falsely assume how it currently is, is how good it can be.

Nor is radiant health something you can only have when you're young. There may be more vitality with youth, or at least easier access to it, but the fact is you can be vital at any age. This is not out of step with natural laws. Sure, there may be a lot of sick and immobile elderly, but there are many who are exceptions to this rule. The question is, which group do you prefer to look at as your role models?

To me, going after radiant health gave me a goal to work toward. It provided a new benchmark besides lack of disease that I could strive for. I hope it does the same for you.

We may never fully reach radiant health as an ideal, but just aiming for it brings us up to a level of health that seeking to avoid problems never can and never will.

What does it take to do this? Part of this principle lies in the idea of doing more good and less bad for our health.

It's quite simple. To achieve radiant health, you need to move in two directions. You need to do more things that are good for your health, and you need to minimize the things that take away from your health.

Here's the rub. Health is not a black or white subject. We humans like to generalize things. It's a useful trait that allows us to get about in the world. However, overgeneralizing is often also problematic. The fact is that very few things can be categorized as purely good or bad, black or white. Instead, most things exist on a spectrum. This is certainly the case with health, as it is malleable and different from person to person or time to time.

Take peanuts as an example. For a person who is highly allergic to them, a matter of life and death, they are completely in the black.

But for those who aren't allergic are they good or bad? It depends on who you ask. Some would argue they're a great food. Other's would say the exact opposite. Who is right? They exist somewhere in the middle, depending on your body as well.

Of course, all peanuts are not equal either. Are we talking about organic or not organic? Heavily salted and roasted with rancid oils? Or a wilder version that's available? What are the soil conditions in which they're grown? Depending on all the answers to these questions how good or bad a peanut is for you moves into shades of grey.

Water is another great example. Is there a best water to drink? Does that make every other water bad? Once again, different water options exist along this spectrum. Heavily chlorinated, fluoridated, pharmaceutically contaminated, municipal tap water from many large cities would exist on the far end of the spectrum. Still, if you're dying of dehydration this is worth drinking!

Filtered, reverse-osmosis, well, distilled, and spring waters are other options. Some are better than others, and you'll see all kinds of arguments about what is best from different people. Don't worry, we will talk all about water in a later chapter, and I will be sharing my opinion about what is best because it fits in with the other principles we're discussing here.

There are some seemingly black things as well. Are trans fats a horrible option? The heavily processed, partially hydrogenated oils that were marketed as superior to butter sure are. But the fact is there are some natural trans fats, like CLA in dairy, which have some great benefits.[4] So, the over generalization that all trans fats are bad isn't quite as black as it seems at first either.

I say all of this to clearly demonstrate that good or bad, black or white, seldom exist in health. Instead you need to look at the spectrum.

For any area of health like your food, your water, your breathing, your movement—all the subjects of this book—you are doing a certain number of things and not doing other things. If we look at all of this together we can see where you are. From that vantage point, we simply need to start doing more good and less bad. Aiming toward radiant health is about following both pathways.

If you're just now realizing the importance of health and have fallen into the unhealthy standards that most people follow in in our modern age, because of how they're culturally enforced, then we can make a couple big but easy steps in the right direction.

If you're doing great already, we can look at small tweaks that further your aims. A small upgrade here and there may not make a huge impact by itself. But when you stack ten or twenty of them the overall effect can be huge. In either case, we do this until new habits take root. Then you do it all again. Doing more good and less bad is a never-ending journey, while aiming toward radiant health.

This is how I look at health. If you increase the good things you do that support and increase your health, you will be getting healthier. If you decrease the bad things that detract from your health, you'll also be getting healthier. This is very simple yet allows for complexity.

The great thing is that the 80/20 rule, also known as Pareto's principle, applies to health. What this means is that 20 percent of what we do is responsible for 80 percent of our health. This applies whether it's helpful practices or harmful. So, if we aim at these high-leverage activities we can achieve phenomenal results.

This means you don't have to be 100 percent perfect either. If you do the big things, you can cut loose and enjoy yourself the other 20 percent of the time. The thing is if you're constantly improving even that 20 percent becomes better than most people's 80 percent.

As you read through this book, think back to these principles. Ask yourself: what is the biggest thing I can start doing right now that will do more good for my health? What is the biggest thing I can stop doing right now that will do less harm to my health? Maybe you can just replace the bad thing with a better thing and you've accomplished both. Then you do it until it's a habit. Do it until you enjoy it and wouldn't want to go back to what you did before. I absolutely love all kinds of vegetables now even though years ago, I couldn't stand the taste or texture. To not eat vegetables daily for me would be problematic now.

At that point, you move onto the next thing. This way you keep expanding in an upward spiral of greatness.

4) Direct Experience

"Participatory holistic science is more than just an intellectual stance – it involves a radical shift in our fundamental perception of nature. The shift is primarily experiential rather than intellectual."
– Stephen Harding

The final principle of health is that you can only know things, truly know them, through direct experience.

While many studies are quoted and cited throughout this book, these are, at best, signposts. They point at what does and does not work well for a number of other people, or sometimes at what occurs in rats or in cells, when that is all that is available.

At its best, a study will inform you to make a decision; then you must do something for yourself and see if it works for you. The issue is that even if a study says that a particular practice or tool is effective at improving or negating something doesn't mean it will work for you. Nothing worth studying works for 100 percent of people 100 percent of the time.

Here's an example. Ashwagandha, a famous herbal root out of

Ayurvedic medicine, has been investigated for its role in lessening stress, as measured by the "stress hormone" cortisol in humans. In the study *"A Standardized Withania Somnifera Extract Significantly Reduces Stress-Related Parameters in Chronically Stressed Humans: A Double-Blind, Randomized, Placebo-Controlled Study"* 98 subjects completed the study. They were found, as a group to have a mean cortisol drop of 14.5 percent.[5]

But that number is an average. It's likely that no one in that group had that specific drop in cortisol. Some had lower. Some had higher. Some might have even received an increase in cortisol, and these people might have dropped out of the study because of it. Yet, when compared to placebo, it worked, at least in the majority of people, enough to give a statistically significant result.

Since this isn't the only study on ashwagandha and cortisol, we can pretty safely say that ashwagandha works for reducing stress. Still, this is a generalization. You, personally, may or may not get these benefits. How do you find out? There is really only one way. No amount of additional studies will tell you. You and only you can take ashwagandha and see how it works for you. You can measure it in testing. You can note it in how you feel. Either way, your direct experience will let you know.

There are other variables at play. Where does the ashwagandha come from, and how was it grown? How was it processed? Is a standardized extract even the best? What dosage do you take? When, how, and with what do you take it?

In the end, you must experiment and see if it works for you. For a variety of reasons, it may not work for you, despite science "proving" that it does work in general. And by you, that means your whole ecology, because the ashwagandha doesn't just affect you.

Of course, this is fraught with possible problems. As humans, we have amazing minds that can accomplish amazing things. One of those things happens to be self-delusion. That's why many things are tested against the placebo effect. Still, to put all the emphasis on what a piece of paper, which talks about scientists and subjects you have never met, says over your own experience is an oddity that our culture emphasizes (especially when you understand the problems of studying things, as explained in the next chapter!)

Direct experience is about something else. You may read this book. You may think it is exciting. You may applaud the information and think greatly of it. But if it doesn't get you out in nature doing the various things it describes, it is a failure.

The best way to learn from a book is by putting it down. This means acting on the ideas inside. Our culture elevates knowledge, often simply for knowledge's sake. The armchair theoretician is a classic example, someone who spouts second-hand knowledge and ideas, without any experience in what they are discussing.

This is why I journeyed to the Amazon to visit the Achuar. I wanted to experience indigenous people firsthand, not just read about them in books. Without that direct experience the information is ungrounded, even if it is true. It is not real knowledge. It is far from wisdom.

The first time you taste wild water…

The first time you feel serenity from being in a natural place…

The first time you get "high" from breathing exercises alone…

The first time your hunger goes away four days into a fast…

The first time you "hear" what a plant is communicating to you…

The first time you recognize yourself as a natural being connected to all of nature and feel it in your heart and bones…

Old paradigms fall away and something in you will shift. You will not be the same person again.

I know I wasn't. Despite early resistances to many of these exact experiences, I've come to do them and more. Throughout these pages, I will invite you to do these things too. Only through your experience will you begin to understand the difference they can make.

Inscribed at the oracle at Delphi is "*gnothi seauton*," which is translated as "know thyself." Only through direct experience can you truly accomplish that. This book, as virtually all how-to books do, aims to help you to accomplish that. However, instead of saying "this is the way," the book aims to point you to nature herself, for her to be your guide.

4
The Fall of Nature, The Rise of Scientism

"We count grains of sand at the sea shore and think we know the ocean deeps. Tremendous humility is an essential quality in any scientist, but it is in fact extremely rare to encounter. That hubris is going to be our undoing."
– Stephen Harrod Buhner

This book is written quite differently than most. I've come at it from two very different angles. The first, many people are going to be quite familiar with. Throughout this book, you'll find tons of the latest science, things you ought to be aware of but that have not reached the sphere of public consciousness. Much research is examined to show that what is written here is far from just my opinion. Listed for those who desire it is an extensive reference section found at the end, with the citations listed throughout this text.

I love science. I grew up thinking science was the answer to everything. It allows you to critically look at how things work. Yet in more recent years, I've become disillusioned that science will provide the answers to everything.

Our culture is led to believe that if something isn't "proven" by science then it's not true. But lack of evidence is not the same as evidence of lack. And, as you'll come to see, there are several problems with seeing the world strictly through this lens. It is a useful lens, but not the only one, and not necessarily even the best one.

What is commonly called "science" is fraught with major problems. Even at its best, science is a lagging indicator. Science comes about because of a hypothesis put forth by one or more people in the field. Then, experiments are done to find evidence that lends credit to this hypothesis.

If the experiments do not back up the hypothesis than a new hypothesis must be generated that better explains things.

Science never actually proves or disproves anything. Theories, and the experiments that back them, just build up evidence for how things work. These experiments take time, money, and people willing to do them. Thus, scientific evidence can lag far behind the ideas that guide them.

For example, I have lots of ideas about strength training, it being a field I am intimately familiar with through personal experience and teaching. Many of these ideas have never been used in a study, and some probably never will be. That doesn't mean they don't work. It simply means that science experiments lag behind the ideas of people in the field.

If you're the type of person that only looks for things that have been verified by science, then you'll be missing out on many things that do work. Besides, a double-blind placebo-controlled study was never conducted to prove that breathing air was good for you.

Furthermore, even once good-quality science has been done, it then takes, on average, seventeen years for that to be built into our clinical practices.[1] A doctor that doesn't follow the latest research in each field is going off what he was taught long ago in medical school, which is antiquated as new research is always coming out. That means standard medical practice is almost two decades behind research.

Those are the least of the problems. At worst, science is purposefully misled by big money and by its own belief in itself. Let's explore each of these ideas.

Theories All Get Overturned

A common saying is that at any given time 50 percent of our science is wrong. The problem is that we don't know which 50 percent. All you have to do is glimpse back at history to see that the facts of what is labelled by science as true on any given day are overturned at some point.

An atom was believed to be indestructible, but then it was discovered that they were made up of smaller parts. These were described with the plum pudding model of the atom, then Rutherford's model, Bohr's model, and nowadays we see the electron orbit as probability, with positions being determined only by conscious observation. What comes next?

If you think these kinds of things were just what happened in the past, that we have "real science" now, you're only fooling yourself. There are many things that are standard in science today, yet people on the cutting edge know them to be wrong.

The central dogma of molecular biology is the idea that, basically, information could only flow in one direction when it comes to DNA and RNA. Yes, it was actually called dogma—something that cannot be doubted—and this hypothesis led to the ideas that genes determined everything. This is something that our entire medical model has been largely based on.

However, this idea has been overturned in several ways.[2] The majority of scientists in the field know all about this. But many lay people know nothing about epigenetics though that is starting to spread into the masses. Rather than genes being the determiners of our fate, epigenetics shows that genes can be switched on or off, depending on a wide variety of factors. Still, the general public hasn't really heard about other gene swapping methods that occur in life such as horizontal gene transfer.

Sadly, many still think that genetics are the cause of cancer. When people get a preventative mastectomy because they have a cancer gene, as a famous actress did a few years back, it's because of what was once considered the holy grail of science. The truth is much more complex. While genetics play a role, an estimated 5 percent to 10 percent of cancers result from inherited mutation; even in those cases it is just one of many factors.[3]

We now know that things like sunlight, food, even your thoughts and movement all are factors in epigenetic expression. Put more simply, these things can change whether or not a cancer gene is turned on or off.

DNA is not the end-all be-all of life. It holds the codes for making amino acids and proteins. That is very important, sure, but that's it. The Human Genome Project promised to end disease. What it actually developed has been underwhelming. Still, some say the great results are just a few years away. This seems to be what scientists of failing theories always say. And I'm willing to bet they'll continue to say so.

After results came, the Director of the Chimpanzee Genome Project commented, "We cannot see in this why we are so different from chimpanzees."

Yes, genes and DNA are important, but they cannot and therefore never will explain everything about life. As Richard Milton put it, "Using the mechanistic, reductionist approach of Victorian science, biology has not so much explained life as explained it away." As you'll come to see in Part 3 of this book, much of the standard view of life in general has major problems.

But a lot of people, scientists and otherwise, still think that genes hold the answers to everything, despite much of the dogma being overturned.

Similarly, science thought that after puberty, the brain remained static, and then degenerated into old age. However, neuroplasticity was then discovered, and we learned that the brain could grow new cells at any age.

In the article "Neurogenesis in the Adult Brain: Death of a Dogma," (there's that word again) the author Charles Gross wrote, "For over 100 years a central assumption in the field of neuroscience has been that new neurons are not added to the adult mammalian brain. This perspective examines the origins of this dogma, its perseverance in the face of contradictory evidence, and its final collapse. The acceptance of adult neurogenesis may be part of a contemporary paradigm shift in our view of the plasticity and stability of the adult brain."[4]

Want a more recent example? The brain does not contain lymph vessels, which was puzzling because we didn't know how waste was removed from the brain. Except this was wrong. A recent study found that the brain does in fact have lymph drainage.[5] Walter J. Koroshetz, M.D., stated, "These results could fundamentally change the way we think about how the brain and immune system inter-relate." This has very important relevance for neurological disease. And for a long time, we just assumed lymph was not involved.

This is science. Theories get overturned based on new evidence. However, some hang around far longer than they should. Decades are common. Even a century, as mentioned above, a wrong theory can persist. Note, Gross wrote that the old idea persevered in the face of contradictory evidence. That is happening today in many different fields. Perhaps even most of them.

Thomas Kuhn explained this in his book, *The Structure of Scientific Revolutions*, back in 1962. Scientists share a set of perceptions or a paradigm, which then govern what sort of questions they ask, and thus, what experiments are done. Any anomalies that don't fit the paradigm are explained away. Eventually these anomalies build until the paradigm pops, and a new paradigm is set up. Those new paradigms then go through the same process.

In its ideal form, science is only interested in evidence. In practice, this does not occur. Instead, those who practice science develop beliefs in theories. Arthur Schopenhauer said, "All truth passes through three stages. First, it is ridiculed. Second, it is violently opposed. Third, it is accepted as being self-evident."

Scientists, seeing themselves as rational beings, as the "holders of truth," will both ridicule and violently oppose ideas and experiments that they believe to be wrong. Even if a theory is ultimately more accurate, even if the evidence is sound, this will occur.

Often, it takes a generation for new ideas to be fully accepted. Quantum physicist Max Planck said, "A scientific truth does not triumph by convincing its opponents and making them see the light, but rather because its opponents eventually die, and a new generation grows up that is familiar with it."

Much of the science found throughout this book is going through some phase of this massive issue, just like all science. Some of it is ridiculed. Some of it is violently opposed. Much of it, in time, will be accepted as self-evident.

In fact, there is a name for this known phenomenon. The "Semmelweis reflex" is the reflex-like tendency to reject new information and evidence that contradicts what is currently believed.

The name comes from the story of Dr. Ignaz Semmelweis. Even if you're not familiar with him, you are familiar with his work, in a sense. What he discovered is practiced every day in our age, but not in his.

He sought to find out why a large portion of patients in one obstetrics clinic at the Vienna General Hospital died from childbed fever, while the death rates were much lower at the second nearby clinic. After testing several theories that didn't pan out, he happened upon one, when a colleague cut himself while performing an autopsy and then died in a similar manner to the patients. His idea was that "cadaverous matter" got into the bloodstream and that this was happening to the female maternity patients as well. Doctors would routinely go from autopsies on dead bodies to the live births, in that first clinic. They did not do this same practice at the second clinic.

He found that the smell could be eliminated by washing the hands with a chlorine solution. Not knowing about bacteria at the time, it was unknown what matter could be transferred or why washing the hands changed what happened. Yet, when he instructed the doctors to do so, he found that the number of fever deaths dropped dramatically, even to zero at one point.

Unfortunately, his fellow doctors scorned the idea. It was ridiculed and violently opposed. They labeled it magical and superstitious. (Those same labels they give to many unconventional theories today.) They refused to wash their hands, and people continued to die in droves. Dr. Semmelweis lost his employment at the hospital and he moved to Hungary where he kept up his fight, yet the opposition continued. One opponent, Dr. Charles Meigs, an obstetrician in Philadelphia stated, "Doctors are gentlemen, and gentlemen's hands are clean." How's that for scientific reasoning?

Semmelweis continued to work to overturn this idea. But under the pressure, he started drinking. Eventually, his friends had him committed to an asylum, where he died of an infectious disease after the guards beat him for resisting.

This idea of washing the hands didn't catch on and become common practice for more than twenty years later, after Louis Pasteur popularized the germ theory of disease.

Once again, this is not just an old way that we've since overcome. The "Semmelweis reflex" is in effect in every area of science, up through today, and will continue to be.

There are also anomalies in every scientific field—things that either aren't explained or are simply explained away. An anomaly simply means that the prevailing theory is incomplete, at best, and completely wrong at worst.

William James described it as "Round about the accredited and orderly facts of every science there ever floats a sort of dust-cloud of exceptional observations, of occurrences minute and irregular and seldom met with, which it always proves more easy to ignore than to attend to... Anyone will renovate his science who will steadily look after the irregular phenomena, and when science is renewed, its new formulas often have more of the voice of the exceptions in them than of what were supposed to be the rules."

Did you know that much debate still takes place as to how water works? Yes, something as common and prevalent as water which makes up 70 percent of the earth and 70 percent of our bodies is surrounded in controversy. For years, there have been many anomalies that can't be explained about how water acts.

If we haven't figured out water, how much can you really trust science as having the answers to everything, in general? The good news is that there are some renegade scientists working on this, and it will be explored further in the chapter on water.

The Amorality of Science

Science can be also used for nefarious purposes. Thomas Huxley, known as Charles Darwin's bulldog for his strong support of the theory of evolution, observed that "No rational man, cognizant of the facts, believes that the Negro is the equal, still less the superior, of the white man." This sentiment was an echo of Darwin's own writings.

Stephen Harrod Buhner, a man you'll find me quoting a lot, as his teachings are instrumental to this book, writes, "At one time or another, using scientific rationale, women, blacks, Asians, and indigenous peoples all have been denied to be fully human or equal to white men."

At one time, these were inarguable "facts" of science...until they were overturned. As an ideal, science should only look at the truth, but in practice it is used to push agendas.

While I'd like to say that equality of race and gender in science is better today, though certainly not perfect, that doesn't mean other immoral agendas aren't being actively pushed.

How we looked at health hit a massive turning point in 1910 when the

Flexner Report was published.[6] This study, conducted by Abraham Flexner, on medical education in the United States, funded by the Carnegie Foundation, caused sweeping changes to the state of medicine. Half of the schools in the United States where closed or merged with others. Women and blacks were largely forced out of the profession, as it turned to be dominated by white males.

All other forms of healing, including osteopathic medicine, chiropractic medicine, eclectic medicine, phototherapy, naturopathy, and homeopathy were downplayed as quackery and not scientifically valid. In their place, a large focus was on so-called scientific and modern medicine, the use of a new industry, pharmaceuticals.

While a few good things undoubtedly came from this, this was a large part of how our state of medical care in the West got to where it is today. Even the mainstream media shows that this led to negative consequences. Dr. Thomas Duffy's "The Flexner Report – 100 Years Later," asked, "Did the Flexner Report overlook the ethos of medicine in its blind passion for science and education? What was the cost of our success, and who has borne that burden? Review of medical care in the last century documents that the trust and respect that were extended to the profession 50 years ago have been substantially eroded…Physicians have lost their authenticity as trusted healers…The $14 million SUPPORT study to understand and improve care for patients at the end of life found that more than 40 percent of families were unhappy with the fashion in which their loved ones were cared for as they died. The discontent with doctor's errors, doctor's silence, doctor's experimentation, and the crass monetary orientation of the profession is legion. The profession appears to be losing its soul at the same time its body is clothed in a luminous garment of scientific knowledge."[7]

Did you know that the word *doctor* comes from the Latin *docere*, which means "to teach?" And physician comes from *physickos*, meaning "nature" or "natural." Sadly, neither of those are occurring in the standard medical practice these days. When science told us the soul didn't exist, just because researchers couldn't cut up the body and find it, the idea of the soul was removed from the process of healing.

That doesn't even touch upon the fact that this agenda to hold onto the mantle of scientific medicine forced out and labeled as quackery all other forms of healing. It turns out that many other forms of healing are just as scientific, if not more so, if you look at the evidence.

Believing Your Beliefs

Another health example of misleading science, because it was accepted as incontrovertible fact for many years by the scientific community and the public at large, was that fat was the cause of weight gain and ill health.

Everybody knew a low-fat diet was the healthiest way to eat...except we were wrong. This has overwhelmingly been overturned; yet, even today, still so many people believe it.[8,9] The previous science, felt to be bulletproof, has been identified as full of holes. How did this happen? For the full story, I highly recommend reading Nina Teicholz's *The Big Fat Surprise*. You can also find a great summary in Dr. Joseph Mercola's *Fat for Fuel*, as well as in many other books. This case shows how things like lobbying, government, and scientists won't look outside what they "know to be true." These problems infect various scientific fields.

If you are not looking at some of the principles covered in the last chapter, there is likely lots of confusion. If your entire scientific paradigm is built on an idea, like that the body is a machine and nothing else, you can never figure it all out, if that paradigm is wrong.

At what point do you discount your own direct experience because of what "science" has told you? It happens every day. Despite people trying all kinds of low-fat diets and continually struggling, doctors and trainers will often blame the patient or client, accuse them of cheating, while keeping their hallowed theory intact.

Some of the scientifically minded aren't really scientific at all. If you come to believe your beliefs, you will not be open to outside information that conflicts with them. As human beings, we all do this. The fact is that it is very hard not to do. I am guilty of it myself, however much I try to be open to new ideas. It is part of human nature.

Yet, collectively, we feel like we have things figured out. This may just be another flaw in human thinking. An article that talked about the period around 1900 said, "Those were the days when the science of medicine in its infancy, and misguided notions of causes of disease ruled the day." I ask you: Is today really any different? Will a person from 2100 look back at our time and laugh at the doctors who recommended chemotherapy the way we snidely look at past doctors who recommended bloodletting? Will they chuckle as they say, "What were they thinking? Those people were so ignorant."

Dr. Joseph Mercola stated, "There are many examples in the history of medicine where routine use of pharmaceutical products and other medical interventions is accepted as the 'standard of care' for a period of time before they are found to be flat-out wrong and toxic to human health." Remember, after things are ridiculed and opposed, sometimes they're accepted as self-evident. At that point, the truth is obvious.

Once again, the ideal of science is that it only follows the evidence. But we never hit the ideal. A big problem is exacerbated because if the evidence leads you somewhere the grant money and your colleagues won't follow, you will be shunned and cast out, labeled a quack or pseudo-scientist, with your magical thinking and experiments that you must have done wrong. The Semmelweis reflex gets its power through group authority.

Rupert Sheldrake is a scientist who is fighting against these problems. One of his books, *Science Set Free*, details the problems that surround science. He writes, "I have spent all my adult life as a scientist, and I strongly believe in the importance of the scientific approach. Yet I have become increasingly convinced that the sciences have lost much of their vigor, vitality and curiosity. Dogmatic ideology, fear-based conformity and institutional inertia are inhibiting creativity."

If you're interested in science, this book is a must-read. In it, Sheldrake explores ten areas where the prevailing accepted science of today appears to be very wrong, where the counter-evidence is piling up, but it is discarded for a variety of political or economic reasons. It is ignored or explained away for non-scientific reasons.

Some of the scientific beliefs that are at the foundation of science today, but are wrong according to Sheldrake, that are appropriate for our discussion here include:

1. *Everything is essentially mechanical. Dogs, for example, are complex mechanisms, rather than living organisms with goals of their own. Even people are machines, "lumbering robots," in Richard Dawkin's vivid phrase, with brains that are like genetically programmed computers.*
2. *All matter is unconscious. It has no inner life or subjectivity or point of view. Even human consciousness is an illusion produced by the material activities of brains.*
3. *Nature is purposeless, and evolution has no goal or direction.*
4. *All biological inheritance is material, carried in the genetic material, DNA, and in other material structures.*
5. *Unexplained phenomena such as telepathy are illusory.*
6. *Mechanistic medicine is the only kind that really works.*

Sheldrake writes of the principle that underlies all of these, "Many scientists are unaware that materialism is an assumption: they simply think of it as science, or the scientific view of reality, or the scientific worldview. They are not actually taught about it, or given a chance to discuss it…For more than two hundred years, materialists have promised that science will eventually explain everything in terms of physics and chemistry. Science will prove that living organisms are complex machines, minds are nothing but brain activity and nature is purposeless. Believers are sustained by the faith that scientific discoveries will justify their beliefs. The philosopher of science Karl Popper called this stance 'promissory materialism' because it depends on issuing promissory notes for discoveries not yet made."

However much it would be denied, science is often taken on faith just as much as religions are. These ideas are treated as dogma, even those not so labeled. The root of the problem is that many people don't actually look at things scientifically. To do so would be to reserve judgment until after data has been gathered. Once again, this is very hard to do.

But many people are quick to label something as pseudoscience, even quackery, just because it doesn't fit their model of the world. Much of what is covered in this book has been labeled that by some. They turn a blind eye to the evidence that exists. They turn a blind eye to what can be perceived directly.

Sheldrake further writes, "Scientific dogmas create taboos, with the result that entire areas of research and inquiry are excluded from mainstream science and from regular sources of funding. The result is 'fringe' science, kept beyond the pale of orthodoxy by automatic skepticism."

Science has in many ways become a new religion. "Scientism" is described as the excessive belief in the power of scientific knowledge and techniques. Like many religions, there's even the promise of an ideal future, a kingdom of science, when our technology makes us immortal and god-like. Also apparent is an arrogance that comes with the belief that it's just a matter of time until science proves that its own viewpoint is correct.

Just as in the corrupt Catholic Church of years past, the scientific community embraces a self-preserving quality for the way things are done. The establishment reaps benefits in keeping things the way they are. And thus, things that threaten it will be put down in a number of ways.

The peer review process is supposed to protect against some of these issues, but in practice can just reinforce it. In 1997 Richard Smith, editor of the *British Medical Journal*, wrote, "The problem with peer review is that we have good evidence on its deficiencies and poor evidence on its benefits. We know that it is expensive, slow, prone to bias, open to abuse, possibly anti-innovatory, and unable to detect fraud. We also know that the published papers that emerge from the process are often grossly deficient."[10]

One example of this kind of thinking in a "scientific" government organization that was corrupt, is the American Medical Association Propaganda Department, created in 1906 to expose those they deemed as quacks. The department essentially extorted money from schools and people to provide the AMA Seal of Approval.

More recently, the AMA has been sued, and lost, for conspiracy and violating anti-trust laws. The AMA said it was unethical for doctors to associate with chiropractors, whom they called "unscientific cultists." In *Wilk vs. American Medical Association,* the judges found that the AMA had engaged in conspiracy "to contain and eliminate the chiropractic profession" and that the "AMA had entered into a long history of illegal behavior."[11]

That court ruling was in 1987. Do you think there's much difference today? The AMA receives funding from big pharmaceutical companies, including Merck and Pfizer.

If you don't think certain people, organizations, and governing bodies, are manipulating medical opinion on what is "scientific fact" when it comes to health and what is not, they've succeeded at what they set out to do.

The Problems with Studies

The gold standard of science is to do a well-controlled double-blind placebo trial, with enough participants to be statistically significant. This should then be replicated by other people in other studies, all showing similar results. This would be good evidence that something is true.

If that sounds like a lot of work, it is. And it's expensive too. Once again, this is why good science is a lagging indicator at best.

Because of the cost, typically only drug and medical device companies tend to be able to study something health-related. The companies have so much money that they can run multiple studies, often cherry-picking the data they want, to show that their new drug works.

Statistical manipulation is another dark side of science. The term *p-hacking* is used to describe the process of data mining to uncover patterns in data that will be statistically significant, even when they don't have to do with your hypothesis. Essentially, when you're paid to get a result, very often you will get that result.

Many pharmaceutical companies have been shown to produce fraudulent data and commit other crimes, including giving doctors kickbacks and promoting drugs for off-label purposes. GlaxoSmithKline was made to pay $3 billion in fines for the above illegal activities with drugs such as Paxil, Wellbutrin, and Avandia.[12]

Carmen Ortiz, the U.S. Attorney for the District of Massachusetts, in this court case stated, "This case demonstrates our continuing commitment to ensuring that the messages provided by drug manufacturers to physicians and patients are true and accurate and that decisions as to what drugs are prescribed to sick patients are based on best medical judgments, not false and misleading claims or improper financial inducements."

This is just one case of many that are on the public record. And these are just cases where the offending drug companies have been caught.

"It is no longer possible to believe much of the clinical research that is published, or to rely on the judgement of trusted physicians or authoritative medical guidelines. I take no pleasure in this conclusion, which I reached slowly and reluctantly over my two decades as an editor of *The New England Journal of Medicine*," wrote Marcia Angel, MD. If the person in charge of one of the leading journals says that the process is broken then that ought to tell you something.

"Most men only care for science", says Goethe, "So far as they get a living by it, and that they worship even error when it affords them a subsistence." He said that about two centuries ago. I wonder what he would say about it today.

Let's say there's a hypothetical study in which something is tested. Many people get results. This will include the people who receive the real intervention, whatever it is. This will also include people in the control group who only receive the placebo treatment. Both groups get some result. The thing is to look at the data and find if the intervention brings about a statistically significant greater result than just the placebo.

This is how studies are conducted, because the placebo effect is strong. The expectation that something will work triggers changes in our body. My favorite example of this has nothing to do with sugar pills, but sham surgeries, which are often found to work just as well as real surgery. Some examples include knee surgeries, artery ligation, and implantation of neural cells for Parkinson's disease.[13]

There are only a few of these surgeries studied like this because placebo-controlled studies on surgeries raise ethical concerns on the idea of "do no harm." But what about all the harm caused by not doing quality studies to find if things actually work and instead doing expensive, invasive, worthless surgeries?

Or what about the harm done by even properly prescribed medications, which are the third leading cause of death behind heart disease and cancer in the USA and Europe?[14]

Some people like to label all alternative medicine as quackery and unscientific. Yet if some of the most advanced surgeries aren't even more successful than a placebo, what does that say about conventional medicine? If properly prescribed medication is killing many people, what does that say about the state of our healthcare?

The placebo effect shows the power of the mind and the power of the body to heal. It also shows that something as scientifically advanced as surgery may not be quite as advanced as we're led to believe.

There are very often flaws in the experimental design. For instance, in a lot of health studies different macronutrients are analyzed to see bodily effects. One rat study compared a high-carbohydrate diet to a high-fat, or ketogenic, diet. The study specifically spells out that the chow diet was 60 percent carbohydrates, 17 percent fat and 23 percent protein, while the ketogenic diet was 80 percent fat, 15 percent protein and 5 percent carbohydrate. Nowhere in the entire study is mentioned what the food source of those macronutrients are.[15] The researchers falsely assume that the macronutrient ratios are all that matter.

The problem with this is that carbohydrates and fats aren't things but generalizations. Corn oil, which is often used in such studies, is not the same thing as butter or olive oil or lard. While they may be fats, not all fats are equal. The same is true of carbohydrates. Corn syrup is not the same as sucrose, fructose, potato, or wheat sugars.

There are also epidemiological studies, which are those that look at larger populations and where placebo controls are not done. Instead, something as vague as a questionnaire asking how much meat you eat per week is used to look at statistical correlation. And then using this to say that one thing causes another, although the media loves to jump on that, is fraught with issues.[16]

To prove this point, some fun websites illustrate various ridiculous correlations. Some of these include the age of Miss America being highly correlated with murders by steam, hot vapors, and hot objects, or the number of people drowned in a pool is correlated with the number of films in which Nicolas Cage appeared. (Damn you, Nick Cage!)

Epidemiological studies can be useful for pointing in certain directions, but an assumption of causation cannot be drawn—not scientifically at least, though people do it every day.

Even if one study shows some effect, that doesn't necessarily mean anything. John Ioannidis published the groundbreaking article *"Why Most Published Research Findings are False."*[17] In it he wrote, "There is increasing concern that in modern research, false findings may be the majority or even the vast majority of publishing research claims. However, this should not be surprising. It can be proven that most published research claims are false."

Industry Backed "Science"

Lastly, you have the issues between industry-sponsored research and independent studies. Ideally, it shouldn't matter who pays for the study, but because it is undertaken by humans, with prejudices and agendas, this is not the case.

For example, a review on the safety of the artificial sweetener aspartame found that 100 percent of the wholly or partly industry-funded studies found it to be safe. Meanwhile, 92 percent of independently funded studies found it had potential negative health effects.[18] Hmm, could a conflict of interest be driving these differing results?

The authors of this review wrote, "The glaring disparity in results from industry funded and independently funded research is clearly of considerable concern. [The writers of a positive review of aspartame] say that the public needs protection from 'misleading' websites warning of the hazards of aspartame. It seems that what the members of the public (and the medical profession) really need protecting from is editorials lacking in balance and objectivity."

The case of aspartame is not an isolated instance of this kind of science. Bioengineer Henry Lai researched issues with cell phone radiation. After doing so, Motorola worked to discredit his work and undermine his research. In a 2006 analysis he looked at industry-funded research versus that which was independently funded. In the industry-funded research only 30 percent found negative health effects, while 70 percent of those independently funded found such effects.[19]

Industries will lobby governments and pay scientists to back their science to show no ill effect. They hire PR companies to label independent science studies that show negative effects as "junk science." This term was coined specifically by industry experts to define things that stood against their aims and desires. Meanwhile "sound science" was research supporting their aims. In their original forms, these terms had nothing to do with the quality of the scientific research behind them.

What's worse is that these financial ties aren't always disclosed. In a sampling of studies in life-science and biomedical journals Sheldon Krimsky found about one-third of the papers had an author with financial interests involved (that could be determined) while none disclosed this.[20]

Everyone knows that the tobacco industry did this, fighting tooth and nail over decades to say their product wasn't dangerous. An executive of the cigarette company Brown & Williamson once wrote in a memo, "The Tobacco Institute has probably done a good job for us in the area of politics and as an industry we also seem to have done very well in turning out scientific information to counter the anti-smoking claims...Doubt is our product since it is the best means of competing with the 'body of fact' that exists in the minds of the general public. It is also the means of establishing a controversy."

Everyone now recognizes this was done by Big Tobacco. But they're far from the only ones. You only have to peruse history to find many other examples. A catalogue of these, and current practices, can be found inside *Trust Us, We're Experts!* by Sheldon Rampton and John Stauber. For example, "By 1960, 63 scientific papers on the subject of asbestosis had been done, 11 of which were sponsored by the asbestos industry, the other 52 coming from hospitals and medical schools. The 11 industry studies were unanimous in denying that asbestos caused lung cancer and minimizing the seriousness of asbestos—a position diametrically opposite to the conclusions reached in the nonindustry studies."

Rampton and Stauber's book shows the methods used by industries and the PR firms they hire to muddy the research around any issue. Another example is the lead that was previously in gasoline. "During 60 years that leaded gasoline was used in the United States, some 30 million *tons* of lead was released from automobile exhaust...Even today, however, the average North American carries between 100 and 500 times as much lead in his or her blood as our preindustrial ancestors." Any amount of lead is not good for you. And so-called science was used to slow the banning of this danger.

Everyone today knows that tobacco, asbestos, and lead are bad for you. It is self-evident. What fewer people know is that the exact same tactics are used today in the plastics, pesticide, GMO, and cell phone industries, as well as many more. Today these ideas are violently opposed. And twenty or fifty years from now, everyone will know that those are bad for you. It will be self-evident.

For instance, Tyrone Hayes Ph.D. at the University of California at Berkeley was hired by Syngenta to investigate the pesticide atrazine. He found that this pesticide could feminize frogs at concentrations 30 times lower than what is legally allowed in municipal water supplies in the United States. That was not the research this agribusiness elite wanted to hear, but Hayes still published it. Unsealed court documents showed that Syngenta then went on to hire a PR firm to discredit Hayes's research and his reputation.[21] Type in his name in a search engine and you'll find plenty of examples of this discrediting work.

At the time of this writing, atrazine is still legal in the United States, though more restrictions have been place. It has been banned in Europe since 2004.

Robert Proctor wrote, "Science has a face, a house, and a price; it is important to ask who is doing science, in what institutional context, and at what cost." Sadly, this is the reality we live in.

Enough to Turn You Off of Science

When you look at all of this, it might be enough to turn you off of science altogether. But that would be a shame. For all these flaws, science is still a powerful methodology that can be used for good.

It's just that the point of all this is that research results must be taken with a grain of salt, at least until it is investigated more thoroughly for all these issues. That means it is really difficult to get to the truth of the matter. Unless you're willing to dive deep into the details of studies with their technical jargon, you must remain wary. Unless this is part of your job you're not likely to find this a pleasant pastime.

Regardless of your beliefs on a subject, you can likely find science that backs up what you think. Think anything outside of conventional medicine is quackery? You can dig up plenty of research showing you're right. Know that alternative medicine works? Good news, there's lots of evidence that it does.

Whatever your viewpoint, you can find collaborating science. This shouldn't be how science is done, but unfortunately, it is the reality of the situation.

I've already pointed to several studies and as we go on I'll be sharing many more. These are included in the reference section of this book for those that would like to look deeper. And I'll be the first to admit that this data is selected. It must be. There's no way I could go through all science everywhere. Invariably, some of these studies I mention have flaws. In some cases, there are likely studies that say the exact opposite, but I either didn't come across these in my own research, or I eliminated them because of flaws I perceived.

My point is that what passes for science cannot be the only method we use when it comes to our health or otherwise. That is why we go back to principles. And that is why looking at science is not the only method used to create this book.

Besides, the roots of science are in sensory observation and the use of logic. This has been taken away from the common people because science these days is largely relegated to the microscopically small or the cosmically large. But it still can be done.

In *Rigor Mortis: How Sloppy Science Creates Worthless Cures, Crushes Hope and Wastes Billions*, Richard Harris discusses the issues facing scientists today. These include problems with reproducibility in studies, translating rat and mice research to humans, untrustworthy experiment design, dubious ingredients, poor lab technique, mishandled data analysis, the nature of getting published determining careers, funding, and much more. As you can see, we've only explored some of these issues here.

He writes, "Most of science is built on inference rather than direct observation. We can't see the atoms or molecules inside our bodies, and we can't truly explain the root cause of diseases. Science progresses by testing ideas indirectly, throwing out the ones that seem wrong, and building on those best supported by the facts at hand. Gradually, scientists build stories that do a better job of approximating the truth. But at any given moment, there are parallel narratives, sometimes sharply at odds with one another. Scientists rely on their own individual judgments to decide which stories come closer to the truth (absolute Truth is forever out of reach). Some stories that seem on the fringe today will become the accepted narrative some years from now. Indeed, it's the unexpected ideas that often propel science forward. Writers often don't say so clearly, but we too are in the business of weighing evidence and making judgment calls, assembling observations that bring us closer to the truth as we perceive it. It's a necessary element of storytelling. No doubt there will be those who see the world differently, who weigh a somewhat different set of facts and come to different conclusions. Since I explore the contingent nature of science in this book, it seems only fair to acknowledge that I'm making judgments as well, not revealing the objective Truth."

Ditto. While his book is mostly about research on conventional medical treatments and pharmaceutical medicine, I'm taking a different tact. And I'm also taking a different pathway, in addition to science, to get there.

5
An Old Way of Knowing

"I was most struck by the fact that the detailed knowledge of the plants and animals held by Indian elders was not considered valuable exactly because it was not book learning! It was as though our society's high regard for zoological or botanical 'facts' derived from lab experiments, books, and science films has invalidated knowledge learned by other means."
– Gary Paul Nabhan

"Scientific abstraction and fancy technologies are no substitutes for the wisdom that springs from knowing the world and its creatures in intimate, loving detail."
– Reed Noss

Science has gone down wrong paths because of its belief in itself. Science is corruptible in practice, even if not in its ideal. Science has created many of the problems we are currently dealing with.

Albert Einstein said, "We cannot solve our problems with the same level of thinking that created them." With that in mind, is more and better science really the answer to our woes? What if we had a different way of viewing the world that we can use?

Vaclav Havel, first President of the Czech Republic, wrote, "The relationship to the world that modern science fostered and shaped now appears to have exhausted its potential. It is increasingly clear that, strangely, the relationship is missing something. It fails to connect with the most intrinsic nature of reality, and with natural human experience. It is now more of a source of disintegration and doubt than a source of integration and meaning...Today, for instance, we may know immeasurably more about the universe than our ancestors did, and yet, it increasingly seems they knew something more essential about it than we

54

do, something that escapes us. The same thing is true of nature and of ourselves. The more thoroughly all our organs and their functions, their internal structure and the biochemical reactions that take place within them are described, the more we seem to fail to grasp the spirit, purpose and meaning of the system that they create together and that we experience as our unique 'self.'"

We need to find this missing thing. My belief is that it is largely our connection to nature, in a variety of different ways—all of which we'll be exploring.

That is why, although this book is rigorously backed by science, primarily it comes from direct perception of nature. You read my story of how this book came to be, from a calling from nature itself, working with shamans, not scientists. As an emissary of nature, my aim has been to bring this message directly from nature…and that's more directly than you might think.

How I've done that is described later. It hasn't been easy, but at times I felt I have tapped into something much deeper and grander than myself, and I have done my best to convey those ideas through the written word.

"As science itself develops, the mechanistic worldview is being progressively transcended. Nature is coming to life again within scientific theory. And as this process gathers momentum, it becomes increasingly difficult to justify the denial of the life of nature," writes Rupert Sheldrake, in *The Rebirth of Nature*, "Personal intuitive experiences of nature can no longer be kept in the sealed compartment of private life, dismissed as merely subjective, for they may indeed be revelations of living nature herself, just as they seem to be at the time. Mythic, animistic, and religious ways of thinking can no longer be kept at bay."

To step into this way of knowing, to get to the heart of the matter we must realize that we are not necessarily the peak of life. The peak of evolution. That the entire universe was not created just for humankind, so that one day we could play games on our iPhones.

Michael Crichton, the author of *Jurassic Park*, wrote "It is especially difficult for modern people to conceive that our modern, scientific age might not be an improvement over the pre-scientific period."

Think about that for a moment. Have you ever considered this as a possibility? Our culture strongly holds that it is the best culture in the world—the most advanced, most scientific. Our culture believes in itself.

But culture is a fascinating thing. Kurt Vonnegut Jr. wrote, "I didn't learn until I was in college about all the other cultures, and I should have learned that in the first grade. A first grader should understand that his or her culture isn't a rational invention; that there are thousands of other cultures and they all work pretty well; that all cultures function on faith rather than truth; that there are lots of alternatives to our own society."

This is one of the reasons that traveling abroad is highly recommended, so that you see the world from the viewpoint of different cultures. Even ancient cultures worked pretty well. In some ways, they worked far better than our own.

In a similar sentiment as Crichton, Henry David Thoreau wrote, "It would imply the regeneration of mankind if they were to become elevated enough to truly worship sticks and stones."

That implies getting back to nature, to realizing the amazingness of nature itself. With this book, I hope you come to worship sticks and stones, or at least clean, natural air, water, earth, sunshine, food, and microbes. Rebuild the connection. *Worship them.*

The left and right hemispheres of the brain, the masculine and the feminine, need to be balanced. Looking through a frame of reductionist science (heavily left-brained and masculine) can never properly explain the whole. While it is a useful tool, without a holistic viewpoint used to balance it, we can't learn everything.

The whole, except in math, is always greater than the sum of its parts. You cannot explain everything in the whole universe with just six quarks and four forces. When these things come together, more complex entities emerge: atoms, life, humans, planets, galaxies and the universe itself.

Buhner writes, from the perception of a plant, "Do you think it possible to dissect a human being, render it down into its constituent parts, feed them into a machine which measures such things and determine from that its ability to paint or create great music? No? Then why do you think that once you have done this with my body you know anything about me?"

If you want to learn from a plant, then learn from a plant. This is what I have done. The exciting part was when I received transmissions through this other way of knowing, through the direct perception of nature. Often times, then I looked up research on what I learned first-hand and found it there. In other cases, as I'll point out throughout this book I make predictions based on this, and the principles outlined earlier, on what future science will show us (the lagging indicator that it is).

Not all these words are mine. Beyond quoting other humans from which I've learned, words also come from the redwoods, the wild rose, artist's conk mushrooms, the Earth itself, the Sun, a fresh spring, and many other "voices."

I had to learn from nature how to directly observe nature itself. This process isn't taught in schools. Most of our learning these days comes from books and lectures rather than actual observation and practice. Yet nature teaches this kind of wisdom. The good news is that though it may be lost, it can be regained.

Why is it that we're disconnected from nature?

It's because we've disconnected ourselves. When you live in a natural ecology you experience it firsthand. When you don't, it's not so easy to understand.

The reasons there are thousands of different diets is because so many people have lost connections to the life of actual food. These concepts are debated because humans argue about things they often have zero experience with. I'm not talking about how you arrange your meals, but actually connecting to the life and ecology of your food.

Let me ask you, have you ever sat down and talked to nature? No? Then how do you know it doesn't talk back? Of course, plants don't have vocal cords, so the mechanism of communication is different, but just because we humans rely primarily on this method doesn't mean others don't exist.

Those immersed in scientism will say this is impossible because plants are scarcely living, just automatons acting out in a mechanical universe. They couldn't possibly be living, sensing, feeling, even thinking beings. In the chapter on the Life and Intelligence of Nature, you'll see what the latest science is actually revealing.

Speaking to this issue, Sheldrake wrote, "The knowledge and understanding of the naturalist is generally considered to be inferior to that of the professional scientist. But it seems to me that the opposite is true; the knowledge of the naturalist, which comes from intimate relationship with nature, is deeper and truer than the kind obtained by detached mechanistic analysis. Of course, ideally, the direct experience of the naturalist and the systematic investigations of the professional scientist can complement and illuminate each other…Direct experience is the only way to build up an understanding that is not only intellectual but intuitive and practical, involving the senses and the heart as well as the rational mind."

Humankind's condemnation of nature is a fascinating story. For the past ten thousand years, all recorded human history, we've known the struggle of rising above nature, becoming part of civilization. For a modern human living today in a civilized society, thinking of how we used to live as part of nature is incomprehensible.

The hidden belief behind our modern life is that we've gotten past nature. We've conquered it. In some ways, we certainly have. But because we cannot escape being from nature, whether we want to be or not, this comes at a cost.

I am not a luddite. I don't want to go back to how we used to live. I know that I don't have the skillset with which to do that, though I am beginning to learn. I stand indoors writing this book on a computer screen and make my living selling products and services worldwide with the Internet.

Strip away our modern food supply, transportation, energy, and housing. Could you survive? For how long? Most people wouldn't even know the first place to start.

Moving into the future, one thing is clear. All of us need to start living in closer alignment with nature, not against it. What I am here to reveal to you is just how much this will benefit your health and well-being personally. These methods are also ecologically sound, so it will not just benefit you. It will benefit all of Earth.

If this change in thinking does not happen, individuals will continue to suffer, our species will continue to suffer, as will other species and the Earth. And it will get worse. No technology can save something that is built on an unstable foundation, without correcting the foundation. I know people have always been saying the end is coming and so far, it has not come. But we need to keep our arrogance in check when we realize just how short a time frame, ecologically speaking, we humans have been doing what we've been doing.

Nature wants to bring us back into alignment. That is why she called me as she did. That is why she has called many others before me. That is why she called you and you're reading this. I do not mean this metaphorically. I mean this literally.

One of the fathers of Western medicine, Paracelsus, wrote, "Seeking for truth I considered within myself that if there were no teachers of medicine in this world, how would I set to learn the art? Not otherwise than in the great book of nature, written with the finger of God. I am accused and denounced for not having entered in at the right door of the art. But which is the right one? Galen, Avicenna, Mesue, Rhais, or honest nature? Through this last door I entered, and the light of nature, and no apothecary's lamp, directed me on my way."

In today's world, the right door would be medical school—something that Paracelsus helped found in a very roundabout way, despite also being an astrologer and alchemist, which are not recognized with the same level of authority. I did not enter through the Western medical door. Instead, like Paracelsus, I have strived to read from the great book of nature, and to show you how you can too.

Remember that I am just an emissary. Not the first, nor will I be the last. In part 1, I've done my best to make the case for why nature's message is necessary in this day and age. Over the next two parts, I do my best to deliver that message to you. Let me show you the best ways I know how to become better aligned with nature so we will all thrive....

PART 2

How we can better align ourselves with nature across 10 elements

6
Air

"The wind blows where it wishes, you hear its sound, but you do not know where it comes from or where it goes."
– John 3:8

"An organism that destroys its environment destroys itself."
– Gregory Bateson

W e start part two of this book with air, because it is a highly important element yet is often the least-considered aspect of our health and nature. This is for several reasons.

First, I call air the most important element because it is the one thing that you can survive without for only a few minutes. World record breath holders may extend the minutes into the double-digit range but surviving for minutes without air is nothing compared to the length of survival time without many of the other things we need to live. People can go more than a month, sometimes longer, without food. (Yet how many books are written about diet, as compared to breathing?) People have survived longer than a week without water.

Survival is possible in the long term without several of the other natural elements covered in this book. But that doesn't mean that the lack of sun or earthing, as examples, don't come without detrimental effects. That's because they are not just about survival. Still, air is necessary for every breath, and for that reason it is of top importance.

The second reason air is an important yet under considered element is that we all breathe unconsciously, meaning our body does it without our focused intent. Imagine if we had to consciously breathe all the time! Yet, because we all breathe, many people either don't think about it or think disdainfully about doing breathing exercises.

However, as a process that can be both consciously and unconsciously controlled, breathing is powerful. Ancient traditions assert that breath is the key to unlocking seemingly impossible abilities thought to be beyond our control.

The last, and perhaps most difficult reason is that we don't see the air. As the saying goes, "out of sight, out of mind." Yet, despite air's invisibility, its effects are quite large. Certain types of air can cause health effects in us, both positive and negative. We just don't notice them or see the cause-effect relationships that exist.

We'll start our discussion by diving into how bad much of the air we breathe is currently in our modern age. When I learned of these things I became angry, and you might become angry too. Our environment is being polluted in many ways that no one is revealing. I say we should become angry, and then use that energy to take positive action. I won't leave you with fear or anger about just how bad things are. We'll also cover what you can do about pollution. And there is plenty you can do.

How Polluted is the Air in Cities?

When I was a kid, I heard that living in a city is the equivalent of smoking a pack of cigarettes per day. That blew me away. Why would we allow things to become like that? But then life went on, and I promptly forgot about it.

Once again, since air isn't visible most people don't think of it. But it actually is visible in some places, just not right in your face. You can easily see the smog on the horizon when driving into Los Angeles. I strongly dislike going there because I can feel my body respond negatively inside the city, due, in part, to the air quality.

Beijing has a far worse reputation. People avoid the outdoors there, and the wealthy pay a lot of money for air purification systems. The market for these systems is poised to grow almost 20 percent, compounded year over year, because of this growing problem.

Just how bad is this air pollution for you?

Most people don't realize the level of threat from pollution. I don't hear doctors or the news telling people about it.

A review of many studies found that increases in particulate matter in the air, such as those that come from motorized traffic and especially those smaller than 2.5 micrometers in size, increased chances of dying from all causes by 6 percent. More specifically, cardiovascular mortality was up 11 percent.[1] While different particles create different medical effects, it is clear that these cause oxidation, stress, and inflammation throughout the body.

The ultimate issue is that living in a city with poor air quality is shaving years off resident's lives. That 6-percent increase in chance of death could similarly be translated to a 6-percent decrease in life span. That means an eighty-year-old would instead die at seventy-five because of this single factor of air they breathed.

Some people say they don't want to live long because they imagine the barely mobile and cognitively declined elderly that are unfortunately commonplace these days. Air pollution will drive disease that not only shortens life-span but lessens health during that time as well.

Although research on the negative impact of air pollution on health is still fairly new, fine particulate matter is implicated in various neurological disorders like Alzheimer's and dementia.[2] It is clear that many of those invisible particles in the air can not only enter the brain but also exhibit neurotoxicity.

Air pollution has also been shown to reduce cognition in children.[3] Anyone who wants a high-performance mind should take note. Air pollution doesn't just affect the young or the old but affects everyone.

Air pollution is widely associated with many problems during pregnancy, including low birth weight and various birth defects.[4] Studies have only scratched the surface on air pollution's long-term epigenetic effects from the mother to offspring. One study looked at heart malformations in the offspring based even on pre-conception exposure to pollution.[5]

The pollution problem is not just in our cities. While factories churn out polluted gases into the air, and heavy automobile traffic exacerbates the problem, at least the natural outdoor air flow is available to spread it thin. Air quality indoors may be even worse.

How Polluted is the Air Indoors?

Volatile organic compounds, or VOCs, are a group of organic compounds that easily become airborne. As a broad group, this includes many natural emissions, but the term is generally used to refer to off-gassing of chemicals in things such as carpet, paint, furniture, cleaning supplies, mattresses, air fresheners—basically everything inside buildings.

Because we spend more time indoors we receive an estimated 60 percent of our VOCs there. Many of these VOCs are known carcinogens, and contribute to asthma, respiratory disease, neurological disorders, and liver and kidney issues.[6]

In a condition called sick building syndrome (SBS), a building essentially makes people sick. Common symptoms include tiredness, difficulty concentrating, eye dryness, dry throat, and dizziness. What causes this? It's largely because of the indoor air quality. This includes high total VOCs as well as high carbon dioxide levels.[7] Humans breathe in oxygen and breathe out carbon dioxide. With no or improper air circulation, over time the ratio in the air changes to unhealthy levels, leading to what is commonly called stuffiness, which then contributes to these symptoms.

And the dangers aren't just in your home. You know that new-car smell? That may be one of the worst offenders. The fact that you can easily smell it means that tons of these molecules are entering your body. Toulene, benzene, formaldehyde, and heavy metals are all present.

"We have all become guinea pigs in a vast and uncontrolled experiment. At this moment in history, the image conjured up by the word 'pollution' is just as properly an innocent rubber duck as it is a giant smokestack," wrote Rick Smith and Bruce Lourie in *Slow Death by Rubber Duck*. They continue, "Over the past few decades, pollution has changed dramatically in the following important ways: 1. It's now *global rather than local*. 2. It's moved from being *highly visible to being invisible*. 3. In many cases its effects are now *chronic and long-term rather than acute and immediate*." Their book covers the dangers of phthalates and BPA (commonly found in plastics and more), Teflon, flame retardants, mercury, triclosan (an antibacterial chemical), 2,4-D (an herbicide), as well as other crop chemicals.

It is important to realize that many of these chemicals end up in dust and in the air that we breathe. This is, of course, on top of them accumulating in water, food, and inside our bodies. Sadly, switching to BPA-free bottles won't save you from BPA that has become airborne, from the many non–BPA-free plastic items around.[8] Your exposure may be lower, but it is not nonexistent.

Man-made chemicals are not the only harmful substances found in our air. Due to water damage and other causes, various toxic molds can be present in our homes. Fungi are known to release their own types of VOCs, some of which can be just as dangerous.[9]

Mold has long been known to be implicated in asthma, allergies and other respiratory issues.[10] But the effects can extend beyond those just the lungs. Such VOC's also have a connection to autoimmunity, where the causes aren't singular but are complex and multifaceted.

Issues with mold can be very hard to identify. Some people don't readily have symptoms. Others are rendered dysfunctional by it.

While large amounts of mold certainly are visible, it's often hiding inside walls, under the carpet, and in other places we don't see. And we definitely don't see what is airborne.

This may be the first time you've heard about the problem of mold, but awareness of it is growing. Dave Asprey, the man behind Bulletproof coffee, personally sees mold as a big problem because he is highly sensitive to it. He put together a documentary called *Moldy* to help people learn about the dangers.

I've personally had issues with mold. At the Lost Empire Herbs office, many of our employees were becoming sick often. I don't normally get sick, but I got a cough that I couldn't shake for almost a month! It was not your typical cold.

Then we noticed a patch of discolored area on the ceiling. We brought in the testers and sure enough there was plenty of mold there, including, but not limited to *Aspergillus, Penicillium, Chaetomium, Cladosporium, Fusarium, Stachybotrys,* and *Ulocladium.* The roof leaked, and this was the cause of the growth. Because mold is not easy to get rid of without replacing everything, we ended up having to move.

Around the same time my good friend had to rebuild his recently purchased home nearly from scratch because it was infected with mold. His young daughter had several issues that seemed to be either caused by or at least made much worse by the air in the house. Eradicating the mold involved gutting the house and therefore proved to be a very expensive and time-consuming process.

If you have had water damage in your house, there's a good chance that mold could be an active issue for you. Asprey states that 50 percent of the buildings in the United States have some water damage, and that the drywall used in construction absorbs moisture, creating an ideal environment for the mold to grow.

Remember, this book is about nature, and mold is natural. It's part of how things decompose. The problem is that the construction of our buildings allows mold growth to occur. More specifically, the issue is that we design things that we don't want to get broken down, yet that is how nature operates. Fungi are the great recyclers. In ancient times, if a lodging was affected by mold, we'd make another one and allow nature to reclaim the old. These days, when we need to save up for a lifetime to buy our home we don't want to move on so easily.

Bad-quality air, both indoors and out, will lead to shorter lifespans, more disease and cognitive decline—none of which you want. But now that we've covered all the bad parts of air quality, let's move onto the good parts, and what you can do to improve it.

Air Flow

Air is meant to circulate. And this is best done in a natural manner, rather than with air-conditioning machines. The wind blows, and air moves. So, for the most part you should make use of this natural method for cooling. Besides being outside as often as you can, when you are indoors you should keep the windows open when possible. Remember that air indoors is typically worse than air outdoors, largely because of the lack of air flow.

Screens can be used where bugs are a problem. If it is very cold in the area, perhaps you can open windows for short periods of time, like in the mornings. Exchange the stale air, the increased carbon dioxide, for fresh oxygen.

And even if you live in a city with less than the best quality air, likely keeping the windows open to circulate air is better than that same poor-quality air being stagnant.

The best place and time to open windows is in your bedroom while sleeping. Think about spending eight hours breathing the same air over and over again, especially at a point where your body is healing and repairing itself. It is much better to have fresh air during that time. And in this case, if it's cold, that's not so much a problem, as you can simply get under more blankets.

Even opening the window a small crack is better than having nothing open. Besides, having a colder temperature, within the range of 60 to 68 degrees Fahrenheit, or about 16 to 20 degrees Celsius, best supports sleep. This is because a decrease in core temperature induces sleep.[11]

Shinrin-yoku

Forest bathing is the English term for what the Japanese call *Shinrin-yoku*. Recent research in the East has begun to investigate these benefits heavily. These include reductions in stress, anger, anxiety, and depression, and better sleep. Hormonal changes have been noted in cortisol and adiponectin as well.[12] These are hormones of stress and metabolism, which govern, among other things, your ability to lose weight.

The benefits of forest bathing are driven by the quality of the air. In a forest, surrounded by trees, you'll be breathing in phytoncides or wood essential oils. These are also volatile organic compounds, but in this case, they're good for you. In fact, they seem to do the very opposite of many of our man-made pollutants, possessing anti-inflammatory, anti-cancerous and neuroprotective benefits.[13] Not only do these provide the benefits listed above but also have antibacterial and antifungal properties as well.

The word *phytoncide* was coined by Dr. Boris Tokin, a Russian biochemist. He found that a pinch of crushed spruce or pine needles could kill all the protozoa in a glass of water in less than a second. He also found that air in a young pine forest is virtually germ free because of these.[14] In short, they clean the air of both man-made and natural pollutants.

The great old-time wrestler Martin "Farmer" Burns stated that, "The morning air contains more vitality than at any other time of day." In my experience, and that of many others, this is true. But what makes it so?

Overnight the temperature drops. In the morning, you generally have a cooler temperature, but the sunlight starts to come out and the temperature begins to rise. Essential oils are extremely volatile substances, meaning that they easily become gas. This is why the smell of a plant with a strong scent, lots of essential oils, can take over a room. With the heat rising and the plants waking up from their slumber, these oils are released into the air, effectively cleaning the air with their antimicrobial properties. Hence the air is freshest in the morning. As noon approaches, the heat continues to rise and most of these molecules will further volatilize out of the area.

The second reason for morning freshness has to do with electricity and water. Moisture content, the dew, tends to build during the night, and similarly evaporates over the day as temperature increases. Water, being a dipolar molecule, has an electromagnetic effect on the air. This is why a forest, right after a rain storm, is also similarly fresh.

There are many reasons I love living close to the forest. The air quality is one of the many benefits. Even if you live in the city you'd want to find time to get out to nature when you can. A park is still going to deliver some of these benefits.

Being in nature you have a literal connection to plant life. You breathe in the oxygen they produce. They breathe in the carbon dioxide we produce. Contemplating this connection can be profound. Neither animal nor plant life could exist without the other. The web of life extends to the very air we all breathe. If we could perceive this dance of molecules it would give us an intimate look into how connected every living thing really is.

I doubt that forests are the only beneficial types of nature either, though a large amount of plant life certainly is a part of it. I'd bet that various bodies of water, deserts, and mountains would bring about similar benefits. Remember that air is always circulating outdoors, so even if trees and plants aren't all around, many of these benefits will still be there.

Getting outdoors in nature is best. Plus, this effect may be mimicked, at least in part, through the following method indoors to help clean up toxicity.

Bringing Nature Indoors

A diffusor is a device that allows you to evaporate any liquid through heat. Thus, you can use tree and plant essential oils to get a similar forest bathing effect indoors. You can also use any variety of other herbal essential oils for their effects. I keep one of these units running in my office while I do work. In fact, it's running right now, diffusing a pine essential oil while I write this.

Although technology can be useful, let's not skip the most basic detail. Plants create oxygen. They basically breathe the inverse of us, taking in our carbon dioxide and breathing out oxygen. And here's the good news. Plants do even more for the air, cleaning the area of various sorts of chemicals that our homes unfortunately are full of.

NASA conducted a study in 1989 to find ways to clean the air in space stations.[15] It was found that certain plants cleaned specific chemicals like benzene, formaldehyde, toluene, and ammonia. The common names of the plants are listed in the chart on the next page. A 'yes' indicates that the plant helps remove that chemical from the air. (This is not meant to say that only these plants clean the air, or only these chemicals should be considered. This is just what has been researched.)

After finding this I ran down to my local gardening store and picked up several of these plants. Just a couple feet away from my desk as I write this is a large snake plant, also known as Mother-in-Law's Tongue. Not only do these clean the air very well but they require very little watering, making them great plants, even for those with the brownest of thumbs.

The truth is that pretty much all plants will be beneficial, though when it comes to cleaning the air, those listed on this page are probably a good place to start. I would also argue that living among plants will do more for us than produce oxygen and clean the air, but that's another topic we'll detail more later.

Plant	Benzene	Formaldehyde	Trichloroethylene	Xylene/Toulene	Ammonia
Dwarf date palm	No	Yes	No	Yes	No
Areca palm	No	Yes	No	Yes	No
Boston fern	No	Yes	No	Yes	No
Kimberly queen fern	No	Yes	No	Yes	No
English ivy	Yes	Yes	Yes	Yes	No
Lilyturf	No	Yes	No	Yes	Yes
Spider plant	No	Yes	No	Yes	No
Devil's ivy	Yes	Yes	No	Yes	No
Peace lily	Yes	Yes	Yes	Yes	Yes
Flamingo lily	No	Yes	No	Yes	Yes
Chinese evergreen	Yes	Yes	No	No	No
Bamboo palm	No	Yes	No	Yes	No
Broadleaf lady palm	No	Yes	No	Yes	Yes
Variegated snake plant	Yes	Yes	Yes	Yes	No
Heartleaf philodendron	No	Yes	No	No	No
Selloum philodendron	No	Yes	No	No	No
Elephant ear philodendron	No	Yes	No	No	No
Red-edged dracaena	Yes	Yes	Yes	Yes	No
Cornstalk dracaena	Yes	Yes	Yes	No	No
Weeping Fig	No	Yes	No	Yes	No
Barberton daisy	Yes	Yes	Yes	No	No
Florist's chrysanthemum	Yes	Yes	Yes	Yes	Yes
Rubber plant	No	Yes	No	No	No
Dendrobium orchids	No	No	No	Yes	No
Dumb canes	No	No	No	Yes	No
King of hearts	No	No	No	Yes	No
Moth orchids	No	No	No	Yes	No

NASA is not the only one to look into this. Further research has found that ferns, especially the Japanese royal fern, were the best at removing formaldehyde. Some plants, like Spanish moss and those in the bromeliad family have been found to clean up mercury vapor in the air.[16]

Shortly after reading about this research, I met a man named Collin Cavote. He had started a company called Biome that implements this research in a novel way by building wall-mounted plant displays. Further, he told me that it is not the leaves that cleanse the air but instead the bacteria on the roots. The Biome units do not use soil but instead keep the roots exposed for more air cleansing benefits. While the units are more expensive than your average air purifier, it seems a worthwhile expense for many businesses and in public places. I love this idea because it is technology that works in alignment with nature.

So, if we can't get to the forest every day for a dose of forest bathing, we can at least bring some of the forest to us in the form of plants and their essential oils. However, it is important to realize that this is just looking at the air aspect of being in nature. You will not be getting some of the other benefits by following only these steps. Still, it is worth doing, if you spend any time regularly inside.

Researcher Kamal Meattle, in his TED talk, discusses how he used plants to get healthier after the air in New Delhi made him ill. He discusses that having four shoulder-high Areca palms, six to eight waist-high Mother-in-Law's Tongues, and an unspecified number of money plants, can produce all the fresh air you personally would need.[17]

Their research showed that many people who stayed in their building in Delhi, full of these plants, would increase their blood oxygen level. Furthermore, research from the Central Pollution Control Board showed that this building showed far less of those earlier symptoms described with sick-building syndrome. Eye irritation was down by 52 percent, respiratory symptoms by 34 percent, headaches by 24 percent, lung impairment by 12 percent and asthma by 9 percent. At the same time productivity was up 20 percent.[18]

Just imagine enough plants to produce all the oxygen you breathe indoors. See this as something you can build up to over time, adding a plant or tree to your home or office here and there. Give them as gifts and tell people about the tangible benefits they bring. And any business owner with an office full of employees should investigate this thoroughly. The cost to buy plants should return several-fold in improved productivity.

More Air Cleaning Technology

Considering that many of the issues come from our man-made technologies, we can help fight this with nature, as well as with other technology.

Air purifiers help clear the air of many particles that aren't the best for your health. One of the things you'll want to look for in this device is a HEPA (high-efficiency particulate air) filter. To be classified as a HEPA filter the device must meet particular standards of removing 99.97 percent of airborne particles 0.3 micrometers in diameter.

The size of the unit is a large part of how much area it can cover. Smaller units work for small rooms, while you might need something bigger if it's the only one in your house. A good practice, if you only have one air purifier, is to move it around from room to room over time.

Upon searching I came across the fact that an airborne-particle physicist using $100000 worth of equipment set out to test the different air purifiers on the market. The Coway AP-1512HH Mighty Air Purifier appears to be the winner for the most effective and at the same time cost effective. It beat out units twice its size and twice the price.

Since then more units have come onto the market that appear to be quite good. One of the issues in knowing the quality of these is being able to measure things like VOCs and particle matter in the air. Being a new area of study, it is hard to say what is going to be best, but there are several air-quality testing options available.

When you realize the importance of air quality, especially in places where you spend a lot of time, like your home and workplace, then you'll want to take multiple steps to improve it. Get a bunch of plants. Get one or more air purifiers. Get a diffusor. And still escape to nature when you can. Stacking up many small steps brings results.

While we can get out to nature, and use technology, to improve the quality of the air in our external environments, we also need to pay attention to our internal environment.

Deep Breathing Exercises

The other aspect that many people need to work on is learning how to breathe properly and effectively. For whatever reason, many people get in the habit of not breathing in the best manner, and thus further lower their oxygen intake. Our atmosphere has less oxygen it in now than it had in the past, along with more carbon dioxide.[19] Therefore, we need to focus even more on properly oxygenating our bodies.

There are many different options on how to do breathing exercises. Any one of them is not necessarily better than any other. Instead each method has its purpose.

Regardless of the method, almost all of them include deep breathing, meaning deeper into your lungs and body. The breath should not be constricted to the upper chest. Instead with each deep breath, it should make the diaphragm move, which typically causes the belly to move in and out along with breathing. This deep, or belly, breathing is going to allow your whole body to stay better oxygenated as a habit, especially when you breathe like this regularly.

When I first began my fitness and health journey, I began to regularly practice deep breathing exercises. Over the years I've done many kinds, but the important thing to note is that they are still a regular part of my routine.

As mentioned earlier, breathing is something that we can do either consciously or unconsciously. When we take it over consciously it allows us to begin to control other, normally unconscious, aspects of our body. In this way, breath work is the gateway to seemingly super-human abilities.

Wim Hof is known as "the Iceman" for his incredible exploits including running a marathon above the Arctic circle wearing just a pair of shorts and shoes, as well as staying immersed in ice for 1 hour, 13 minutes, and 48 seconds. He has done a lot to bring breathing to the forefront as a powerful method for human health and performance.

Research conducted on him and his students shows that deep breathing can activate the innate immune system and the sympathetic nervous system.[20] Until this time, scientists thought this was beyond our control. (Looks like science was again wrong about something that mystics knew about for centuries.)

In this experiment, the subjects were injected with E. coli bacteria. This would normally involve a flu-like reaction with multiple symptoms. Indeed, it did do so in the control subjects. Sounds like a horrible study to volunteer for, doesn't it? But in Hof and his students, not much happened except for a slight rise in temperature.

Wim Hof's breathing method is quite simple. The breath is a focused fairly big inhale, but not completely full, then the exhale is just relaxed. I personally like to breathe in through the nose and out through the mouth on this, though Wim says either nose or mouth breathing works either way.

With the emphasis on the inhale you're getting more oxygen in your body, allowing the exhale to happen naturally. Keep repeating this for a recommended twenty to forty breaths and you may notice yourself getting lightheaded or feeling different effects across your body, because this breathing triggers the release of epinephrine.

After breathing like this for many breaths, and after exhaling, you'll hold your breath, until it begins to get uncomfortable. Then repeat the breathing followed by the breath hold again. Continue this cycle three to five times.

Wim's methods are worth exploring in more detail, and you can find his full online course, where he also discusses the benefits of cold exposure, at www.legendarystrength.com/go/wimhof/

Another great deep breathing exercise is box breathing. This is a specific form of cadenced breath. It is called box breathing because each leg of the breath, inhale, hold, exhale, hold, is the same length. Thus, if you drew it out in the number of seconds for each breath, and turning ninety degrees for each transition, the drawing would look like a box.

The starting point with box breathing is to do each leg for a count of four. Inhale for four seconds, hold for four seconds, exhale for four seconds, hold for four seconds, and repeat. Most people are not used to holding their breath after exhaling so that can be a little tricky at first, but, like anything, becomes easier with practice.

You can do this with a fairly natural inhale and exhale or you can aim to fully inhale and fully exhale within those four seconds. The former keeps it more relaxing while the latter makes it a stronger deep breathing exercise. By fully exhaling, the hold afterwards becomes tougher too.

While this is a great drill to do just sitting or standing, I find that I like it best while moving. Start by walking. Instead of counting seconds, you can count steps. Thus, you start with a four-step inhale, four-step hold, and so on.

In any of these different ways of doing box breathing, over time you work to increase the length of each leg. Expand to a six count, a ten count, and beyond. The hold after the exhale will always be the limiting factor. If you're using this more for relaxation or meditation, you'll want to keep it easily within your control. If you're aim is deep breathing and expanding your lung capacity though, work to extend that count.

For far more exercises and details about breath work, please see my book *Upgrade Your Breathing*. In it you'll find many more exercises, divided over seven different applications: deep breathing exercises, breathing for lung capacity, breathing for strength, breathing for endurance, breathing for relaxation, breathing for flexibility, and breathing for energy circulation. It's the most comprehensive resource on breathing exercises available.

Getting High on Deep Breathing

Hot on the alternative health scene is hyperbaric oxygen treatments, in which machines are used to expose the body to greater amounts of oxygen, under higher pressure. These are being used for treatments including with autistic children[21], various brain injuries[22], cancer treatment[23], and more. Research is still early in many of these areas, but results have been promising in many cases, typically in combination with other treatments.

It makes sense that hyperbaric oxygen treatment could affect a wide range of diseases in that it helps oxygen reach all your cells more efficiently. Lack of oxygen in the brain is going to affect a wide range of neurological disorders. The Nobel Prize laureate Otto Warburg found that cancer cells do not use oxygen to grow and, as such, do not thrive in oxygen rich environments. [24] Thus, forcing your body to absorb more oxygen should have a wide range of benefits and challenge many diseases.

I bring all of this up to ask a question. How many of these same benefits could be gained simply by deep breathing in nature?

I don't deny that this technology is useful, but it seems that it is, in a sense, mechanically enforcing deep breathing. Personally, I have not yet had the opportunity to try this technique. Still, an exciting idea to me is to combine deep-breathing exercises inside of a hyperbaric oxygen chamber. It's likely you could increase the benefits.

But let's go back to nature. Earlier we saw that by having lots of plants in a building, many people had better-oxygenated blood. Now imagine if you can be inside the forest, with far more plants and trees all absorbing carbon dioxide and sending out oxygen. Those trees and plants all act as air filters; the entire canopy with a massive surface area is larger than any filter you could buy. Add to this your own deep breathing to drive that air further into your lungs. Not only would you get more oxygen but also all the other benefits of nature.

Recently on a trip out to the forest I practiced deep breathing exercises for a few minutes straight. It put me into an altered state, where I felt euphoric. So many people do all kinds of things to reach altered states; some are better options than others. I absolutely recommend you give this one a try. It's simple and free.

In fact, Stanislav Grof was a top researcher on the therapeutic benefits of LSD. But when the drug was illegalized, he switched to using the breath, through a method he called holotropic breathing, to achieve many of the same effects in therapy. Your breath is more powerful than you might think.

Get out and breathe the best air you can find. While we can fill our houses with technology and plants to support it, and that is worth doing, they won't compare to being deeper in nature. While we can turn air into a doctor-recommended treatment, we do not need a prescription to do it on our own.

Get out and breathe deeply. Take in the oxygen. Take in the phytoncides, essential oils, beneficial VOCs—whatever you want to call them. Take these beneficial airborne molecules and make them a part of you. We tend to think of our bodies being made up of the food we eat and what we drink, but it is also made up of what we breathe, for better or worse.

I hope that, by reading through all of this, you will look at air not as something invisible without any effect but as something foundational.

Those chemicals, natural and unnatural, found in the air can either hurt you or help you. In fact, they are doing so with every single breath. The effects of any one breath aren't likely to make a noticeable difference. But how and what you breathe all day will. Compound this over years and it can have a very real effect on disease or the lack of it, and even on how long you live.

This isn't just to say that this will affect your health decades down the line either. It very much may make you more productive and happier today. One study looked at office workers and the air quality in different buildings. And this is worth quoting: "It has now been shown beyond reasonable doubt that poor indoor air quality in buildings can decrease productivity in addition to causing visitors to express dissatisfaction. The size of the effect on most aspects of office work performance appears to be as high as 6–9%."[25]

A 6 to 9 percent change in performance level. Earlier we saw a 20 percent improvement. This is significant and tangible. Not only could you increase productivity, but you'd feel better while doing it. Why don't you upgrade your own air environment and see the effects for yourself?

After being oxygenated the next step is to be hydrated...

7
Water

"Life is water dancing to the tune of solids."
– Albert Szent-Györgyi

"How many nights now has the stream told you: This is the way to deal with obstacles."
– Dale Pendell

The vast majority of Westernized humans have never tasted pure, fresh, wild, spring water. Until a few years ago, I was among them. This is so obvious, yet so hidden, that many people reading this aren't even sure of what I mean.

Aren't Crystal Geyser or Perrier both spring water? Yes, they are. But there is a difference between bottled water, housed in plastic bottles, that is treated with UV (and hopefully nothing more) sold in stores, and getting it fresh from the source.

But you can't drink from a creek or a river, you may be thinking. You'll catch something! While this may be true, it's not what I'm talking about either. Animals may die or defecate upstream making this water possibly poisonous. Bacteria or parasites in water can cause havoc.

From this idea, all of the water in nature has been categorized as unsafe. Only uncivilized people would drink something that wasn't mechanically or chemically treated to make it pure. Make no mistake, in certain cases, that is absolutely necessary and life-saving.

But again, that is not what I am talking about. Instead, fresh spring water is where water literally springs from the earth. There is no earlier part of the flow except where it is underground. Being underground there is little to no possibility of something causing problems upstream.

Still they'll tell you it's not for drinking. The fear of nature is always present in man's mind. They say it is not for drinking because it is uncontrolled. It is wild. But if you dare break their warning you'll be delighted with the best-tasting and healthiest water there is.

Knowing the travesties of what's in most tap water, many people argue about what the best water filter is. This is an argument worth having because there are huge differences. Chances are you have one, so take a look at your filter. Perhaps it's a tiny Brita unit. Maybe it's a larger countertop unit. Or even a whole-house filter. Look at the size. Here is does seem that bigger is better, though size is not the only important factor. All else being equal, the larger size means more opportunity for that filter to catch and collect harmful contaminants. Often several different materials, like sand, stones, and carbon, are used.

If you're feeling good about the size of your filter, now compare it to the size of a mountain. Which is bigger? Which would you like to have cleaning your water? Notice that those same filtering materials are there too, just in far greater supply.

Not only is it a great filter, but these underground aquifers from which springs originate have been around a long time. In some cases, that water hasn't seen the light of day for decades or even centuries. Imagine water that has never been exposed to nuclear fallout, from the 2055 bombs that have been detonated on our Earth, or the vast plastic and chemical pollution we have spread. This is naturally clean water, as opposed to mechanically cleaned, or stripped, water that reverse osmosis (RO) brings.

Let taste be your guide. Fresh spring water, when it is low in minerals, has a sweet taste to it. Because of this, these are called sweet springs, or sweet water. The fact is that RO water needs minerals added back in or else it doesn't taste right. It doesn't taste natural. No one would drink it, which is why calcium chloride or magnesium chloride are typically added.

The World Health Organization put out a report showing that demineralized water, especially that lacking magnesium, may be implicated in raised risk of cardiovascular disease.[1]

Of course, most of your mineralization is going to come from diet, not from water. But that doesn't mean minerals can't be obtained from water, or that they shouldn't be in there. Some people like to point out the differences between inorganic and organic minerals. But the fact is that the body is very much affected by the minerals in water. When they are dissolved, as in TDS or total dissolved solids, the body can make use of them. Drink salt water and you'll know that these inorganic minerals do make their way into your body.

What is Water?

Scientists are trying to explore the tiniest building blocks of matter like quarks, the furthest reaches of space and how to create machines that think like we do. Most would assume, with something as prevalent and important to life as water, that we'd have it all figured out. But this is not the case.

It might surprise you to find out that we don't know all that much about how water really works. Sure, we know that a water molecule is made up of two parts hydrogen and one-part oxygen. But the interactions, the relationships, that make up how these molecules function is actually a hotly debated subject and has been for decades.

This miraculous substance has some very strange properties, when compared to other matter. Here are a few of water's anomalies.

The fact that it becomes less voluminous when it freezes, unlike everything else, allows a lake to freeze without everything inside of it being killed. This ice is also slippery compared to every other solid material which produce more friction in solid form.

The further away from a sound you are, the less you can hear it because sound is transmitted by pressure waves in the air. All waves dissipate over distances, except a tsunami in the ocean can travel around the Earth, even several times, before it dissipates. How does that occur?

Water travels up all trees. A tree can send up 130 gallons of water per day up from the roots to its branches and leaves. Inside conifers, the vessels through which this water flows may be a tiny as 0.0008 inches in diameter. The common explanations of capillary action, transpiration, and osmosis are not sufficient to explain how it happens. So how does water fight gravity like this?

Warm water freezes faster than cold water. This is an experiment anyone with access to a freezer, water, and a timer can do. Yet, this apparently breaks the laws of thermodynamics, so how does it happen.?

A single cloud, made up of water vapor, can stand alone in the sky. Shouldn't the gas all spread to areas of lower density rather than clumping up like this?

On and on we could go, which goes to show that our common understanding of water is anything but complete. Even Albert Einstein was incorrect about water, his theory of Brownian motion not living up to experimental cases! Our theories on water are just plain wrong in many ways. There are too many anomalies to be explained away, yet that is what we've been doing for many years.

The importance of water is underpinned by the idea that our bodies are made up of more than two thirds of water. That's by volume. If you actually counted the molecules that make up you, you would find that 99 percent of them are water. Thus, having a more accurate theory of understanding water might be very important when it comes to health.

Gerald Pollack, the author of *The Fourth Phase of Water*, has shown how far we've gone down the wrong path, and conducted a whole series of experiments that show "new" properties of water and what these mean. He writes, "If the currently accepted orthodox principles of science cannot readily explain everyday observations, then I am prepared to declare that the emperor has no clothes: these principles might be inadequate."

The history of how water actually came to be the proverbial red-headed step-child of science is fascinating. It's just one more example of how far down the wrong path our science can go, in this case at least partially because of political reasons during the Cold War. Long story short, the discovery that water acted differently inside capillaries, was blamed on impurities in the water caused by sloppy Russian science. This despite the fact that impurities didn't adequately show why the water would act differently at all. And theories becoming institutionalized shows how hard it is to overcome what is generally accepted as true, however wrong they are, because of the skepticism from the rest of the scientific community. Those are the reasons that most people will be completely unaware of what follows.

I leave you to read Pollack's book for the complete story. For now, the basics of it, as the title suggests, is that there is a fourth phase of water, one that is in between liquid and solid. This liquid crystalline phase is called EZ water throughout his book, because of how it formed an "exclusion zone," where certain areas of water would exclude microspheres suspended in it. Pollack writes, "The differences are appreciable. EZ water is more viscous and more stable than bulk water; its molecular motions are more restricted; its light-absorption spectra differ in the UV-visible light range, as well as in the infrared range; and it has a higher refractive index. These multiple differences imply that EZ water fundamentally differs from bulk water. The EZ hardly resembles liquid water at all."

This fourth phase is in action inside of nature and inside our bodies as well. Pollack shows how this fourth phase explains how all the aforementioned anomalies work. While the implications of these new discoveries about water regarding health are largely unknown, it does show that we shouldn't live our lives by unexamined assumptions about even the basics.

What we do know is that EZ water forms naturally in interactions with certain surfaces and elements, especially by light and heat. It is expanded by vortex motions to fuel the buildup of the liquid crystal formation.

Early researchers such as Viktor Schauberger felt that vortexed water, especially from streams was more alive than water that was stagnant. Rudolph Steiner found similar results even earlier. Vortexed water is used in the process of biodynamic farming he created. Now we can begin to understand the principles behind what these luminaries said long ago.

Here is another experiment you can do yourself. By shaking water in a container in such a way as to create a vortex you can find that the temperature drops. But shouldn't friction make it hotter? Yes, until you realize that water uses this energy to create more order instead.

This changes how water interacts in our body. Rather than being inert matter, this EZ water has powerful implications for how electric charge is distributed. In short, the EZ phase gets a negative charge, an alkaline pH, while the bulk water, full of extra hydrogen, becomes positive and acidic. This charge separation is an integral part of how water flows inside living beings, both human and tree.

Movement is just one way this forms. Another method is through the absorption of specific light and infrared frequencies. Pollack writes,

"When water absorbs light, the absorbed energy builds structural order and drives charge separation. That stored potential energy is harvestable: charge separation can produce electrical current; and structural order can drive cellular work."

Keep that in mind when you get to the chapter on sunlight and its ability to charge your body in multiple ways.

Because our blood and lymph are narrow tubes, filled with substances that are mostly water, by having more of the inputs that charge this water, including the sun and the earth, the better everything will flow. And of course, drinking quality water of this nature is also essential.

Picture the water that flows into your home through the miles of piping from the municipal water supply. The water is sent here and there under pressure. The metal, a conduit for EMFs and other electrical pollution, charges the water in unknown ways because of it being underground with the difficulties in replacing it, and the sheer volume needed, full of rust, decay, cracks, and disrepair.

Contrast this to that spring flowing underground. The water coming upward deep from within the earth. Imagine it flowing naturally in the way that water wants to flow, charged not by linear pipes, but by natural curves among stone, crystals, and minerals.

The chemical format of water is H_2O. Besides this, there is the mineral matrix present, because water is a universal solvent there is virtually always stuff in it. But it is not just chemical. As a dipolar molecule, it relates to other molecules in specific ways and is affected by electromagnetic forces.

The idea of a hexagonal structure to water, where six molecules of water bind in the shape of a hexagon, has been derided in many scientific circles. However, that is exactly how water transforms into ice. And indeed, it appears to be the same structure in which EZ water builds up. Not only that but, while the individual water molecules are neutral, this lattice bears a negative electric charge.

One way this can be experienced is that when drinking water of this nature, it can be described as "wetter." You can feel the difference in drinking it. The chaotic tap water configuration can sit heavily in your stomach. The "wetter" water absorbs more quickly into your body.

Pollack then goes on to describe the action in the body this could produce. "Since nature rarely discards available potential energy, EZ charge may be used to drive diverse cellular processes ranging from chemical reactions all the way to fluid flows."

This may just be fundamental to how all life works. And most people don't know this phase of water exists!

Liquid crystalline water is the type of water your body actually uses. Pollack says the EZ battery may be the suppliers of much of nature's energy. If you get it from the outside or get the proper energy inputs that drive the EZ water creation, your body won't have to use its own energy to generate it to complete all those cellular functions.

Dehydration

Water is critically important to our health. Our bodies are 50 to 80 percent water by volume. The higher percentage tends to be when we are born, while the lower percentage tends to occur with aging. Thus, we can see that hydration is important for helping your body stay young.

The quantity of water you drink is often talked about. Drink your eight glasses a day. And it should be talked about, because most people simply do not drink enough. But what isn't talked about nearly as much is the quality of the water.

Hydration is one of the most important aspects of our health. Many people are chronically dehydrated causing issues such as pain, inflammation, heart disease, diabetes, cancer, and more. Dr. Batmanghelidj discusses this in his books, starting with *Your Body's Many Cries for Water*.

As a political prisoner, he had access to no medicine but still acted as doctor to other inmates. His prescription was what he did have available: water. You have pain? Drink a liter of water and lie down. You have cancer? Drink a liter of water and lie down. Doing this he saw many of his patients get better, which led him to the understanding of the importance of hydration.

He writes, "It is the solvent—the water content—that regulates all functions of the body, including the activity of all the solutes (the solids) that are dissolved in it. The disturbances in water metabolism of the body (the solvent metabolism) produce a variety of signals, indicating a 'system' disturbance in the particular functions associated with the water supply and its rationed regulation."

In short, that means our internal water supply affects everything. While a human may be able to go a bit longer than a week living without water, most everyone reading this will never be in danger of that. Instead it is having enough water to get by, but a nonoptimal amount, that is a root cause of chronic disease and pain.

Of course, dehydration is not the only cause of these things, just a foundational one. As we just saw the phase of the water matters too, along with the energy inputs that allow water to drive the metabolic processes.

With just a small drop in hydration, a loss of less than 1 percent of your body mass, brain function begins to decline, with drops in memory, concentration, and alertness.[2] With 2 percent loss, we see declines in physical performance, and in challenging physical events, like athletics, loss of 6–10 percent is not uncommon.[3]

Water is at the heart of every bodily system and operates within every cell. Your cardiovascular, thermoregulatory, metabolic and nervous systems will all decline. Its relatively easy to see these sorts of effects in acute dehydration.

But what about the chronic dehydration that most people are experiencing? Could this mean that most people are physically and mentally impaired all the time? In most of the places we've looked, we find that this kind of mild dehydration does indeed have to do with chronic disease including hypertension, strokes, and fatal heart disease.[4]

In a review of the impact of water, hydration, and health, Barry Popkin stated, "Beyond [the] circumstances of dehydration, we do not truly understand how hydration affects health and well-being, even the impact of water intakes on chronic diseases…We need to know more about the extent that water intake might be important for disease prevention and health promotion."[5]

We know surprisingly little in this area, mostly because for decades our entire foundation of water science has been wrong.

Pollack also writes that "Hydration can reduce friction by some hundred thousand times." When you think about your joints and movement, water being an important part of the makeup of joint capsules and the synovial fluid inside, this then becomes critically important for moving well and without pain.

Once again, the thing that most people don't realize is that it is not just about the quantity of water you drink. Yes, most people could stand to drink more water. But equally important, perhaps even more so, is the quality of that water. This is going to allow you to get hydrated on a cellular level better than water that the body doesn't easily absorb. Just like we saw with air, the water you drink may be helping or it may be hurting you.

When I first drank fresh spring water I could feel my cells seemingly release the water they had been holding onto for who knows how long, swapping it out for this new fresh high-quality water. I could feel hydration on a cellular level like I had never felt before. It was a tangible difference that stuck in my mind.

Just about any clean water is better than no water. But quality, natural, wild water is far superior to what most of us live on.

Municipal Water

Let's look at the municipal tap-water supply. At the water treatment plant where the sewage flows in, piss, shit, toilet paper, pharmaceuticals, birth control, chemotherapy drugs, heavy metals, and more—all flushed from many humans—comes in. It is filtered. Yet no filter can remove everything (except perhaps one the size of a mountain).

This discharge is separated off and concentrated down into thick sludge. Surprisingly, this sludge is then sold as fertilizer! This is often called sewage sludge or bio-solids. The EPA deems this safe, stating, "the use of these materials in the production of crops for human consumption when practiced in accordance with existing federal guidelines and regulations, presents negligible risk to the consumer, to crop production and to the environment."

Do you believe that? Think of all those pharmaceuticals that require doctor's prescriptions, where you need to take specific dosages to get the benefits. Imagine all of these drugs being evacuated from people all across a city and concentrated down. Do you want your food grown with this? One thing we know for sure is that this is a good way to concentrate dangerous heavy metals.[6] That's not all. Triclosan (an antibiotic), PCBs, flame retardants, steroids, hormones, and asbestos have all been found in bio sludge. Knowing that, would you want food grown in this crap? (Literally!) But that's getting off topic.

Back to the water, many processes are done to help remove all of this stuff. It is treated with chemicals like chlorine to kill off any bacteria. Chlorine in water, and the by-products it produces, such as trihalomethanes and trichloroethylene, are linked to adverse birth outcomes.[7]

Depending on where you live, fluoride may be added, because the water you drink is supposed to help your teeth. Where does this fluoride come from? It's an industrial by-product from the chemical fertilizer industry.

Yes, fluoride may harden the teeth when applied topically, though that is no reason to add it to drinking water. Besides, teeth are not just discarded body tissue that should be hardened. They're living tissue. They need a proper ecology in the mouth, and in the whole body, to function properly. The way to accomplish this is not through chemical hardening.

Among other issues, fluoride impairs thyroid function. Until the 1970s, fluoride was prescribed to those that had hyperthyroid conditions. The opposite, hypothyroidism—diagnosed, undiagnosed, clinical, and subclinical—is pretty close to epidemic proportions in the United States. The National Research Council stated that "fluoride exposure in humans is associated with elevated TSH concentrations, increased goiter prevalence, and altered T4 and T3 concentrations."[8] The amounts of fluoride found in water have been shown to be sufficient to cause these effects in some people.

An article in *The Lancet* stated that fluoride also causes neurotoxicity.[9]

When the water is filter and treated, deemed ready, it is pumped back out. But not everything is removed. Parts per billion of many of these things still remain. Used toilet paper so small you won't notice it. Tiny amounts of drugs that everyone else is taking.

Our government agencies will tell you tiny amounts won't do anything to your health. There are no long-term studies to prove that claim. And while that may be true in isolation, what about the combination of these things which alter chemicals, in some cases making them more poisonous?

Your body can handle one part per billion of this here and there. The body is amazingly organized at running its detoxification systems. However, these things are coming not just from your water but also from your food and air. You're under constant bombardment. Do this day in and day out for years and is it any wonder cancer kills 20,000 people per day? Over time these pollutants will have very real effects on you.

Healing Springs

Water from a fresh spring also has stuff in it. There is a natural mineral matrix of total dissolved solids. Sweet waters have very low amounts of TDS (total dissolved solids). My local spring typically comes in around 50 parts per million, or ppm. These are dissolved minerals, not grit found at the bottom of the water glass. The minerals are suspended in solution through the water. Because water is a solvent it pulls things into it, whatever it comes in contact with.

Other springs are known as mineral springs. These may be rich in one or more minerals. And these minerals can have healthful effects.

Lithia springs are known for the trace mineral lithium. It's not just a drug for "crazy" people but a much-needed trace mineral used by every human body and known for its neuroprotective and mood-enhancing effects. In fact, lithium has been shown to promote longevity.[10] This natural mineral is typically found in some water and should also be readily available in the soil. Sadly, it is one of those minerals that has largely been depleted.

Chalybeate springs are rich in iron. Alum springs contain aluminum. Saline springs can be rich in calcium, magnesium, or sodium. Alkaline springs contain various alkalis. Soda springs contain the gas carbon dioxide. Yes, to the surprise of many, bubbly water occurs naturally.

Certain springs aren't meant for drinking but are great for bathing. Your skin is able to absorb and utilize certain minerals in abundant supply.

This is why a transdermal magnesium spray is the best way of getting magnesium into your body.[11] Sulfur-rich hot springs are an excellent example of this, sulfur being needed for skin and hair. What other minerals will your body absorb this way? And how many can we find in natural hot springs? In earlier periods we probably got a lot of these from being in natural bodies of water.

That's not to say that every spring is drinkable or bathable. Some are even radioactive, containing natural radium or uranium. But these are a tiny minority.

For centuries, different springs would earn reputations as healing springs. Was this all simply anecdotes and marketing by snake-oil salesmen? Or was there something to it, that we haven't fully investigated or understood?

Many people make a pilgrimage to Lourdes in France every year, where an apparition of the Virgin Mary appeared in 1858. Analysis of this holy water found nothing special, just typical amounts of minerals and trace minerals. While the spiritual effect of faith (or if you want to call it the placebo effect) may be part of the explanation, perhaps another part is that it is natural flowing spring water, that many people are not getting otherwise.

Even so, recent research conducted by the Institute of HeartMath found that adding small quantities of water from these sacred sites to normal tap water was able to modify the pH, conductivity, and redox potential, showing that something is occurring.[12]

The Seeds of Life

In tap water, chlorine is used to kill off possibly pathogenic bacteria. On one level, this is a smart thing to do. You don't know what things could be generating inside the water supply otherwise. Yet when we drink this, that chlorine continues to act as an antibiotic. Plus, there are the byproducts already mentioned that may be more harmful to you than the chlorine itself. While it may not hurt the human you, it is going to continue to kill bacteria, causing disruption in your microbiome. Fortunately, a good quality carbon filter can remove the rest of the chlorine.

Being able to treat water and make it drinkable is one of the things responsible for helping reduce the incidence of infectious disease that plagued generations past. In this way, it was tremendously useful. However, that doesn't mean it is ideal.

What if we want living water? Spring water is alive. It contains micro-algae. It is part of the natural web of life. Simply bottle up some water and store it for a few months in light and you'll notice the green begin to bloom.

This is why spring waters bottled on store shelves are treated with ultraviolet light to kill off anything inside, rather than chlorine. Humans wouldn't be so apt to buy bottles of green water at the store, and who knows how long those bottles may sit there.

Those micro-algae are harmless at worst. Perhaps someday we'll recognize they're actually beneficial. After all, how many people are paying for expensive spirulina, chlorella, and blue-green algae to take as supplements?

The concept of living water may sound funny to you. And that may be the case because you have only ever had dead water. How would you know the difference if you've never tasted it? Modern humans are so out of touch with the web of life that we do not recognize where drinkable water in nature comes from. Hundreds of years ago, and prior to that you could likely drink from a creek without much worry.

But humans used to know. Check out the number of places and things named after springs. Springfield is one of the most common city names. Spring Valley, Spring City, Springdale, Springville, Spring Grove are also popular. Colorado Springs, Palm Springs, Diamond Springs, and on and on the naming goes. A Spring Street exists in just about every city and town too. While many may be named because the name was popular, most often, if it goes back in time far enough, the name came from springs that use to be, or still are, in that area.

Daniel Vitalis is one of the leading authorities behind the "rewilding movement." By rewilding you're seeking to get back closer to how wild humans used to live and away from conventional methods. His ideas are very much in alignment with this book. What I've learned from him over the years, like on his popular podcast, has been instrumental in my thinking and writing.

Vitalis is also the man behind www.findaspring.com. On this website, you can look around the world and find springs close to you. While it is mostly used in the United States, with its rising popularity, more of the springs of the world are being mapped out.

Virtually everyone I know that has engaged in this practice of getting the best-quality water available is aware of this resource, and many got started going to springs with it. That's how I first started going to the headwaters in Mt. Shasta. That's how I located my local spring. Simply head to the website and look in your area.

Make it a fun journey the first time you do it. And be warned, sometimes the springs are tucked away and hard to find, even with a map and coordinates. Bring a bottle and drink up. If possible, bring lots of bottles and make this your regular supply of water for your home. Even if you have to make a couple hours journey the first time you do it, the experience is worth it.

Remember, that EZ water happens naturally at springs. So anytime you're there you should drink up. Be like a camel and stock up on the supply to fully nourish and hydrate your cells. As soon as you bottle the water, and let it sit, it will rapidly degenerate into bulk water. While it is still great water, it loses this special energetic something.

I would bet that a long-term study of people drinking from a good, fresh spring source would be healthier in pretty much every way, compared to just about any other form of water. Sadly, a study like this is not likely to be carried out anytime soon.

The In-Between Options

I recognize that if you've been drinking tap water your whole life, starting to go to a spring to drink it may be a big leap. Plus, not everyone has a spring near them. What do you do if that's the case? While fresh spring water is the best option and tap water in many big cities is the worst, there are many options between them. In this section, we'll explore some of those.

Many people like to drink distilled water. This heating and cooling process creates water that is devoid of minerals. Like reverse osmosis water, it doesn't taste the best.

Many people will say that this is the same thing as rain water. It is close but not quite the same. While it will be low in TDS, rain water still has a low count of minerals, which may be collected from the air, dust, and atmospheric gases. Unless it is acid rain, this should be fine to drink. But historically you can't rely on rain in most places as your drinking water. What if it doesn't rain for a month?

Reverse osmosis, also known as RO water, was mentioned earlier. Many whole-house filter systems use this. Besides the fact that this is an unnatural process, leaving the water tasting "off" without minerals added back in, it is extremely wasteful too. It typically takes three to four gallons of water to make one gallon of RO water.

Well water can be similar to spring water with just a slight difference. At a spring source, the water is ready to come up out of the ground and into the light. With a well you have to go get it. Just like every spring is not equal, neither are wells. Some may have too many minerals present and need some form of treatment. Still, for many people, a well is going to be the most suitable option. And with a good well it can be great.

Of course, depending on the extent of pollution in an area, chemicals can get into the ground water. This could pollute both wells and springs. Such is the state of the world we live in today.

Filtered water is going to be the most likely option for many people. However, recognize that all filters are far from equal. The size of the filter is one factor. What is in the filter is another. Certain filters remove fluoride. Many do not. Most will filter out chlorine by using activated charcoal.

Speaking of a filter, it is important to not just filter your drinking water but filter the water you bathe in too. While I can make sure I always have spring water to drink, I can't get a large enough supply for bathing. So, in my previous house, which was on the municipal water system, I made sure that my shower was outfitted with a filter. When it comes to chlorine, you're going to absorb more through your skin than you would in drinking the water. This is going to disrupt your skin microbiome. Plus, some of it will turn into a gas which will be inhaled.

Lastly, you can buy water. Buying bottled water is a recent thing. While there was some bottling occurring a few centuries ago, its modern carnation began in 1977, only forty years ago, with a successful ad campaign by Perrier. Now it is ubiquitous.

Basically, all of the options above are available at the store, and you should treat them as such. Spring water is the best option. While it will not be fresh, most of them are still good. Ideally, you'll want to get water that is in glass, not plastic. This way you can avoid the absorbed endocrine disrupting chemicals like BPA, BPS, phthalates and others found in the water from the plastic.[13] (In case you didn't know, many BPA-free bottles, since that chemical has recently taken the limelight, may still have other bisphenols which may be just as bad or even worse offenders than those with BPA!)

Some well waters are sold too. The popular Fiji water comes from a well. But most of what you find on the store shelves will be either filtered, distilled, or RO water that originally comes from municipal tap-water supplies. This is what the big soda companies sell you with Dasani or Aquafina, from Coca-Cola and Pepsi, respectively.

Making It Routine

What can you do to make your water healthier? It may be helpful to see how I have upgraded my water supply over the years. Regardless of what you're currently doing, there is likely a next step, and then a step after that. That is how I look at all these different areas of health and nature.

I used to drink straight from the tap. At some point, my family got a Brita water filter when those became popular. Sadly, while it may remove some chlorine these aren't going to help you with much else.

When I first started learning about water, at one point I was convinced that distilled water was the way to go. I got a small unit that distilled one gallon at a time. I never really liked this water, but I thought it was the best option. That unit eventually broke down, and I went back to the Brita or whatever was available.

It wasn't until years later that I learned about fresh spring water.

Unfortunately, I didn't do anything with that information for a while, not finding a nearby spring originally.

But then, when I was driving up to Oregon I decided to stop at Mt. Shasta and collect water there. This is some of the best tasting water I've ever had. So, every time I drove up that way I would stop there. It got so that I would bring about 25 gallons of water back home. And I would drink this all until I ran out.

For when I didn't have spring water, I got a larger countertop filter unit. Somewhere around this time, I also go my first shower filter.

Later, using www.findaspring.com, I found there was a spring close to where I live. Unfortunately, this flowed quite slowly so I only used it occasionally. I would go back and forth between having spring water and filtered water. The taste comparison and how I felt after drinking both was becoming more and more apparent to me.

Finally, I decided I would always have spring water at home. I made the decision and took the actions to do so. I kept the filter unit as backup, but I went many months without needing to bring it out, so I finally got rid of it, because I have stuck to my decision.

Although it would take over two hours to fill a five-gallon bottle at this spring, my wife or I would use that time to spend time in nature, getting the many other benefits discussed in this book, while collecting water. Recently, the drought got better in California, the water table rose, and this spring flows much faster. It now takes just over ten minutes to fill the same five-gallon bottle.

I still collect spring water for my drinking water to this day, even though I bought a house that has a good quality well on it. This is great water for bathing and washing things, but I make the effort to collect spring water to drink.

When I travel, and I do travel a fair amount, I stay relaxed about my water options. If I drive, I carry spring water with me. But that's not an option when I fly. Here, I always strive for the best, drinking Pellegrino, Crystal Geyser or Evian, and am willing to pay the premium price for it. But if there is nothing else available, I don't dehydrate myself because of it. I use plastic bottles when I have to.

A decade has passed since I first became interested in water. I didn't have this clear roadmap laid out in front of me, so realize that it may take some time to get the most natural and best water to support your health and performance. That being said, there's no reason you can't look up your nearest spring right now and head there today!

Water makes up the majority of your body. Isn't it time you start treating it with the respect and focus it deserves?

8
Movement

"It makes a wonderful difference if you find in the body an ally or an adversary."
– Goethe

"Exercise is movement, but movement is not all exercise."
– Katy Bowman

The human body is very adaptable in its ability to move, far greater in mobility and dexterity than other creatures on this planet. Just take a look at a circus performer, a gymnast, or a dancer and you'll see some of the endless variability in movement that is possible for us.

Yet, it's the lack of movement that is one of the roots of the chronic disease and degradation of the human body. In this area, the old maxim "use it or lose it" is very true.

An excellent book called *Move Your DNA*, by Katy Bowman, details why movement is not optional but is in fact necessary for far more than just getting around. She writes:

"The frequent consumption of varied movement is what drives essential physiological processes…Diet, stress, and environmental factors can all change the expression (or the physical outcome) of your DNA. But it is my professional opinion as a biomechanist that movement is what most humans are missing more than any other factor, and the bulk of the scientific community has dropped the ball. With respect to disease, the human's internal mechanical environment has been the least discussed environment of all – a staggering oversight when almost every cell in your body has specialized equipment *just to sense the mechanical environment*…Human diseases are repeatedly explained to us in terms of their chemical or genetic makeup; meanwhile, we've completely ignored the load profile that the function of our body depends upon."

These ideas have led to the new scientific field of mechanobiology—where biology and engineering meet. This groundbreaking idea is that movement itself alters genetic expression. Research has shown the cytoskeletal filaments transmit mechanical signals to components in the nucleus of cells, such as DNA.[1] The title of Bowman's book (move your DNA) is not a clever play on words, but actually how the body functions. Physical forces change cells and tissues, contributing to development, cell differentiation, physiology, and disease.

This was eye-opening to me. Even though I had professionally been engaged in exercise and movement for over a decade I had never quite realized the far-reaching effect it has on the body. Down to a cellular level, our bodies need certain types of movement to even function properly.

Contrary to popular opinion, it's not that you become less able to move as you age. Instead it's that the typical person spends less time moving, in an ever more limited way, and thus they lose the ability to move. If they had only continued to do what they previously did they'd be able to do the same. And if they worked on increasing what they could do, they would actually move better as they got older.

Not only would this allow the elderly to continue to move better, but since we know that movement affects DNA and disease, it would likely lower the risk of cancer, heart disease, and much more. In fact, as we'll come to see, better movement means less death from all causes.

Personally, I do all kinds of strange strength training and fitness feats like bending horseshoes and doing back flips. These aren't necessarily natural, at least in one sense of the word. But that's okay as it's something I enjoy doing, and specialization is something all of us humans do in the modern age.

While I've written many books on the subject of exercise, that is not what this book is about. You won't find kettlebells or feats of strength here. Instead, it is about natural human movements, and humans moving naturally.

Fitness can mean many things. The general idea is to be fit enough to go about your daily life, with a little extra fitness as room to spare. This applies to strength, flexibility, cardiovascular fitness, and more. While this idea may be great for someone who is engaged in a more natural lifestyle, the modern lifestyle is quite sedentary. We don't need much fitness to engage in our daily lives. Therefore, this definition does not work in practice.

A different definition of fitness is to be able to move as humans have always moved. The following list includes movements any human ought to be able to do:

- Walking, Running, and Sprinting
- Jumping and Landing
- Crawling
- Squatting
- Rolling
- Swimming
- Climbing and Brachiating
- Lifting and Picking Things Up
- Carrying and Dragging
- Fighting
- Balancing
- Mobilizing Each Joint Fully
- Resting Postures

Each of these should be easy enough for you to do, without struggle. Most important, they should be done without pain. Pain is a signal from the body, and if you have it chronically, something is off within the movements and structures of your body.

Why do people work out? Because they don't get this kind of movement in their everyday life, similar to supplementing vitamins or minerals in a deficient diet. In diet, it is ideal to get everything you need simply from what you eat. But with extra demands on the body because of environmental pollutants, and the fact that even good-quality food happens to have less of these micronutrients because of soil depletion, some supplementation is typically necessary when it comes to diet.

And so it is with movement too. We need to have some sort of formal training program to make up for the lack of what we do in our day. It acts to supplement our movement. That being said, a one-hour workout three times per week cannot make up for the sedentary lifestyle of the other 165 hours of that week.

As an article in *The American Journal of Medicine* put it, "The systematic displacement from a very physically active lifestyle in our natural outdoor environment to a sedentary, indoor lifestyle is at the root of many of the ubiquitous chronic diseases that are endemic in our culture. The intuitive solution is to simulate the indigenous human activity pattern to the extent that this is possible and practically achievable."[2]

The human body adapts to whatever it does to do things more efficiently. This includes things that we don't consider movement, like sitting. If you sit a lot, then your body becomes better at sitting. That's not necessarily a bad thing, except that for a body to be good at sitting it may not be so great at other things. The hip flexors tighten, and posture typically degrades.

A sedentary lifestyle adapts us to being more sedentary. The body becomes less able to move because those are the movements and positions practiced.

The popular tagline is that "sitting is the new smoking," because of its effects in increasing mortality, cardiovascular disease, obesity, metabolic disease, and more.[3]

But the fact is that simply standing there isn't the best thing for your health either. Around a century ago, because this caused blood flow issues, many factory workers were given chairs to work from. We seem to have forgotten this as many people jumped on the new bandwagon.

Bowman writes, "The position of sitting isn't problematic, it's the repetitive use of a single position that makes us ill."

You're not supposed to sit all day long. You're not supposed to stand all day long. What do you do then? The human body is meant to move— plenty and varied kinds of movement. Of course, that doesn't mean that you can't sit or stand at all, just that the more movement, overall, the better.

Gordon Hewes, an anthropologist, looked at how people rested in different postures across the world.[4] His findings support that it's not about any one magical position that should be used, but that you should use many different postures. Stand in different ways. Sit in different ways, and not just in chairs but on the ground as well, which opens up even more postures.

In fact, being able to get down and up from the floor, easily and without using extra support, is a predictor for dying from all causes. In one study, for every additional point on the sitting-rising test (SRT), which basically had to do with using less limbs for support while getting up, there was a 21% decrease in mortality. [5]

To put it another way, if you can only get off the floor by putting your hand on the floor or your knee to stand up, you're more likely to die than someone who can get up with just their legs.

A while back I wrote an article called "The Stand-Up Challenge." Based on the popularity I went on to develop this into an online video course. The aim was not just to stand up with little limb support but to "complexify" this movement even further. If it is good to be "normal" at getting up off the ground, what if you're above average or exceptional at it?

While some of what we discuss will best be fit into those formal workouts, other aspects must be incorporated into your daily life with frequency and consistency. Now, let's look at each one of these categories in a bit of detail.

Walking, Running, and Sprinting

This has always been our main mode of transportation, at least before the modern age. Our legs have significant amounts of the muscle mass in the body because they're needed to get us around all day long.

As a baby, one of the biggest steps for us is learning to walk. Once this skill is acquired we have freedom to move away from our mothers and explore the world on our own.

We're not limited to a single speed either. We can pick up the pace and start jogging. We can add a bit more until we are running. And going full speed, we are sprinting.

The ability to move fast is crucial in the wild. It can be used in both chasing prey as well as escaping from predators.

Increasing your ability to move fast and increasing your ability to run for extended periods of time are both useful. In the modern age of fitness, the latter is typically thought of as the epitome of fitness, best exemplified in a marathon.

Unfortunately, this is often done to the exclusion of other types of movement. And when it is done too much it can wear on the body.

It's also funny to think that we have created expensive machines to allow us to run in place, when we can simply move around to run. I'm not a big fan of treadmills, nor of other cardio machines. The gait, that is how you step, in the real world and on a treadmill, are different.[6] While they may be very similar, the difference is easily noticeable to anyone not acclimated to being on a treadmill. This makes sense as the ground does not move toward you while you remain in the same place within the real world.

One of the other issues with treadmills is that it screws with your visual and vestibular systems responsible for your balance.[7] Notice how you have to take a moment to reorient yourself after stepping off a treadmill. When we walk or run in the real-world things move past us as we move forward.

While the differences may be small, your body is going to adapt to those differences. While walking on a treadmill is likely better than not walking at all, why have an expensive piece of machinery when you can do it even better for free?

One of my favorite ways of training our locomotion is by doing hill sprints. Find a sloped surface that you can sprint up for about thirty seconds. This taxes your muscular and cardiovascular systems significantly. You'll get out of breath quicker than just about anything else. Walk down the hill and repeat. Do this just six or ten times, which takes about fifteen minutes, and you have finished your workout. This fits into what is called high-intensity interval training, or HIIT, which has been shown to be more effective, and better use of time, on several factors of health, then long, slow distance training.[8]

Because of the upward slope of the hill, as an added benefit, there is less impact on your joints. Plus, you'll be outside breathing fresh air.

Of course, do not jump into full hill sprints right away if you're not in shape. You can start with walking the hill, then jogging, and gradually make your way up to full sprints.

In my opinion, this is far more productive than running for an hour. If you enjoy doing that, that's fine, just recognize is that it is not the epitome of health. At the very least it doesn't touch on any of the thousands of other human movements that are required to move well. It gets you good at running, which your body adapts to, often at the cost of sacrificing other movements.

And just because sprinting is so great, doesn't mean we should forget about walking. Walking needs to be built into your daily routine. There is no way to be natural and healthy without regular walking. A general recommendation is 10,000 steps per day, which is about five miles.[9] Ideally, you'd want to do a couple hours of walking per day. This best stimulates the human body to function naturally.

Katy Bowman writes, "I am always surprised when people say they find walking boring. Walking defines us as a species. It is not a luxury. Not a bonus. It is *not optional*. Walking is a biological imperative, like eating and having sex. Which is why we should, as a species, see the inability to walk without pain for what it is—a huge, red, waving flag calling attention to the state of other parts and processes necessary to perpetuate our humanness."

Walking defines us as a species. Strong words, but true. We humans are the only ones that walk as we do. It is part of what makes humans human.

To boil it down, those that walk more, as compared to those that are sedentary, live longer, being less likely to die of all causes.[10] There we go again showing more and better movement means less death. Specific benefits include reducing risk of heart disease, improving lipid profiles and blood sugar levels, enhancing mental well-being, decreasing risk of osteoporosis, and more.

Another study showed that healthy adults who walked for 45 minutes, three times per week for a year, increased their hippocampus volume.[11] It made their brains bigger and stronger.

One of the main benefits of walking is that it stimulates our lymph flow. The lymph is a big part of our immune system and extends throughout our body. But unlike the circulatory system there is no pump to it. Instead, it is through movement that the lymph flows. Even just brief exercise dramatically increases lymph flow.[12]

Nor is it just the lymph that's affected. While we've been led to believe the heart pumps all of our blood, the fact is that this isn't true, at least not the full picture. Movement itself is also responsible for moving blood around your body. You need to move your body for blood, and the nutrition it brings, to get to all the cells in your body.[13]

Barefoot Movement

It's not enough to walk and sprint because there is an unnatural problem most of us are struck by, and that is wearing shoes.

Think about what happens if you break your arm and it has to be put in a cast for a month. All of the muscles atrophy. When the cast is removed, your arm is smaller than the non-casted one because of lack of use. While this may be necessary for a time for the bone to heal, it comes at a cost as the muscles waste away.

Now look at your foot in a shoe. Is this much different than a cast?

The bones aren't healing, but the muscles are wasting. Instead of a month that the cast may be on a broken bone, most of us have been wearing shoes throughout our lives and for many hours of each day. As such, all the musculature of the feet becomes weak with lack of use. The toe box squeezes in the toes stopping them from having their natural spread. This can even lead to issues such as hammertoe and bunions.

Furthermore, the majority of shoes have raised heels which shorten the calf muscles. I'm not just talking about women's pumps either. Few shoes are flat. Most have the heel raised from the rest of the foot. This changes the entire biomechanics of the rest of the body. By raising the heel, the angles of the ankle, the knee, and the hip all change. This further moves up the chain and affects your spine and shoulders too. Lots of shoes also raise up the toes which further changes the normal foot position.

This is one reason why many runners end up with knee or back pain. It is because of doing too much running in a position your body was never meant to move in. Almost all running shoes have thick heels which change your biomechanical position, allowing you to heel strike which can't be done the same when barefoot.

In a story, very similar to that of what Weston A. Price did for nutrition and dental health, podiatrist William Rossi travelled around the world looking at the feet of indigenous populations. He stated:

"In shoe-wearing societies a visibly faulty gait can often be corrected and made normal, but it can never be made natural as long as conventional shoes are worn. It is biomechanically impossible because of the forced alterations from the natural foot stance, postural alignment, body balance, equilibrium, body mechanics and weight distribution caused by shoes."[14]

Recently, a number of minimalist shoes have become available on the market. These are great in that you can begin to re-strengthen the feet. But be warned. If you've been running for miles in "regular" shoes and you try to do the same, you'll find out just how weak your feet and calves actually are. And if you push through it you can easily injure yourself.

You wouldn't expect that casted arm to come back to normal the next day. It may take a few months or even years to get it back to par with how it used to be. Be patient with the time it could take for adjusting back to what is natural.

For these reasons, and for the earthing benefits discussed in another chapter, I highly recommend you do any workout or movement practice barefoot when possible.

And when you're at home, please take off your shoes. Not to keep the carpet cleaner, but for your foot health.

Jumping and Landing

The legs can be used even more explosively than in sprinting by jumping. In nature, this is the method by which we can reach something higher or overcome certain obstacles.

I write jumping and landing because there are really two parts to this, the take off and the touchdown, and both are important.

This can be practiced in training as a high jump or a long jump. It can also be done repetitively as in jumping rope. As with all of our movements it can be combined with a number of others. For instance, running into a long jump, with a roll on the landing.

Watch kids play and you'll see them jumping all around in their games. If you want to move as well as kids, move like kids.

Crawling

Typically, crawling is the first locomotive movement we learn before walking. This is our original method of getting around. The unfortunate thing is that once we learn to walk, most of us forget about crawling and never come back to it. This is unfortunate because crawling has a number of benefits different from walking.

As an adult, we've found that practicing crawling can actually assist in coordinating the brain because of how it involves the vestibular system and proprioception of the body. Tim Anderson, creator of Original Strength, states that, "Crawling, like a baby, can help your body heal and make you stronger and more resilient." It utilizes more of our body than walking, and thus more of our neurology.

This is a great movement to do as part of a warmup before any other training to help awaken your coordination. Start with the normal knees-on-ground crawling.

And then we can make it more complex from there. We can crawl forward and backward. We can raise the knees off the ground and crawl that way. We can raise the hips up higher into what is often called a bear crawl. We can lower our whole body close to the ground and crawl like a lizard. These animal movements can be a fun way to work out that provide muscular, cardiovascular and DNA expression benefits.

If you're able to move around while close to the ground, you'll very likely be able to get up and down from the ground too. That means, by crawling, you'll live longer and healthier. No studies on this one, just an extrapolation that makes sense.

Squatting

Can you do a full squat?

By full squat I mean keeping the heels firmly planted on the floor and squatting all the way down until your thighs are resting on the calves. And

I do mean resting. Not only do you want the mobility to get into this position but holding it should be done with relative ease.

In my mind, there isn't any more basic of a human movement...that most humans cannot do.

In nature, the squat position is used for many things. It is used as a resting position where chairs aren't widely available. It is used to move low which may be used in hunting, and for all kinds of gathering as many plant foods are near to the ground. Before the toilet became pervasive, it was also how we all went to the bathroom.

The good news is that if you cannot do a full squat, through progressive training you can regain the ability. The easiest way to do this is to have an elevation you can comfortably squat to and work at. Then you gradually lower the elevation until you can squat all the way down. Like anything else, this could take weeks, months or even years, depending on how long it took you to lose this ability and for it to remain forgotten.

If you want to treat this as a workout, do a whole bunch of squats. Work up until you can do one hundred in a single set. This is a decent test of muscular and cardiovascular health, along with mobility and flexibility. I'd be willing to bet this could predict death rates too.

And in your daily life, because it's about moving throughout your day, do a few squats as breaks from sitting or standing. Why not do some right now?

Here's a challenge for you. Rest in the full squat position for five minutes straight. You can even do this while watching TV. But please work up to this challenge intelligently.

There are many other squat variations, and all are worth doing, but for simplicity's sake make sure you master the basic squat first. Then you can squat on your toes, or in various lunge positions with one leg further forward, backward, to the left or right. You can also use wider and narrower stances.

Also note that this is the best position for bowel movements too. As one study concluded, "the greater the hip flexion achieved by squatting, the straighter the rectoanal canal will be, and accordingly, less strain will be required for defecation."[15]

No, this doesn't mean you need to start using a hole in the ground outside. You can still use your toilet but pick up a Squatty Potty or replicate the squat position by raising your feet by using some other object while sitting on the porcelain throne.

Rolling

Rolling is another movement often done by toddlers and children, but then relegated to the past of our childhood when we grow up. This is unfortunate because rolling, in its many variations, mobilizes the spine and other joints of the body in ways not often used.

Being capable of rolling safely and effectively is also a useful survival skill. Should you need to dive from a speeding car or jump from a tall height, being able to absorb and redirect the impact through a properly done roll is essential for avoiding or limiting injury.

Even just your normal, average fall can be saved if you know how to redirect the impact forces through rolling. Plus, if you can roll it likely means you can get down and up from the floor with more ease. Thus, rolling equals a longer, healthier life too.

There are many types of rolls. In a comfortable environment, like on carpet or gymnastic flooring, you can roll directly over the spine both forward and back. When on harsher environments you want to traverse your spine as little as possible, so the rolls go from one shoulder to the opposite hip.

Like squatting, our ability to roll comes quite naturally, but if you don't use it you will lose it.

Swimming

Typically, swimming comes later in life than other land-based forms of locomotion. But if you live near large bodies of water, and spend time with people that swim, you're sure to pick up this skill.

In many ways, it is similar to walking, running, and sprinting in that there are different speeds you can achieve. You can simply tread water or dog-paddle at a slow pace. And if you learn the breast stroke and other forms of swimming you can begin to move much faster.

For many people, this is a preferred method of exercise. This works both the muscles and the cardiovascular components of the body. It can elevate mood. And in many people with diseases or injuries, the low-impact nature of it may be a better option than other forms of exercise.

Just being in contact with water, at varying temperatures, has also been shown to improve the immune system, help with pain, and positively affect several bodily systems.[16]

However, there is some bad news. Most people that engage in this movement do so in pools. While this may be the most ideal for ease of use in civilization, chlorinated water causes irritation of the skin, eyes, and more. Even if you don't notice it, your skin microbiome is sure too. Plus, the chlorine, and the by-products it creates, can damage your organs like your liver.[17]

More recently many pools use salt in order to keep clean. To be clear, these use a generator and still create chlorine by breaking off the sodium, but it is not added from the outside. Still, these are a better option than regular, chlorine-treated pools.

Of course, this being a book about nature, I recommend you swim in natural bodies of water when you can. Ironically, the best way to get earthed is through water, plus the transdermal absorption of minerals is available. And who knows what other health benefits being in the water brings?

Climbing and Brachiating

By land, sea, and air. We've covered moving on the ground. We've covered moving in the water. And while human beings can't fly without modern technology, we can move through the air. Several of our closest relatives in species, the primates, get about through the trees by climbing and brachiating.

You may not be familiar with this term. It comes from the Latin *brachium*, meaning arm. Specifically, it refers to locomotion, or movement, in which primates swing from tree limb to limb using just the arms. Human beings, descending from apes, still retain the possibilities for this type of movement.

So why should you engage in brachiation? Because, as humans we are made to brachiate. Let that statement sink in for a moment. This is a natural human movement; thus, to attain, regain, and progress in this ability allows us to function better, and more healthily. It changes our cells and our DNA.

Perhaps the importance can be understood better if we look at what the lack of brachiating may cause. Previously I mentioned what happens when people neglect to do other natural human movements like the rock-bottom squats, for example. Over time they lose the ability to do so. This contributes to problems. It seems everyone is getting knee and hip replacements because of lack of quality movement.

Specifically, the one joint that is primarily used in brachiation is the shoulder. The ball and socket joint is the most movable of any joint in the human body. With this range of motion also comes less stability, leading to the chance of many types of injuries and pain. How common are shoulder surgeries?

Thus, I ask, what if our lack of brachiation is a contributor to why so many people do not have healthy and strong shoulders? Here we have gravity pull the body down against the joint. This completely changes the loading pattern on the joint and likely plays a huge role in health.

While there are many different ways you can brachiate, simply swinging from one monkey bar to another is the main way most of us have done so at some point in the past. In addition to actual locomotion, we can add similar movements like hanging, pullups, and climbing into this group.

If we take this out into nature, all you need is a low-enough tree branch and you can begin to monkey around. Climbing trees is a lost art that can be a lot of fun. Rock climbing is a whole sport that many love.

Some human populations have physically adapted to being able to climb trees better, including far greater ranges of motion in ankle dorsiflexion.[18] Along with this there is some debate to how much time some of our ancient ancestors spent in trees. The human being the adaptable creature it is, it is likely some groups spent lots of time, and others did not.

Regardless of whether your closer ancestors did this, our very ancient ones certainly did. Thus, it is something that is healthfully expressed through movement in our bodies.

Lifting and Picking Things Up

You'll note that most of what we talk about here would fit into the category of what is known as bodyweight training. This is where your body's weight is the resistance versus lifting an outside weighted object. The way I see it, you should first and foremost know how to move your body, before adding outside things into the picture. If you can't control how your body moves, you have no business controlling another object.

As a reflex against the conventional training done in commercial gyms, bodyweight training has become significantly more popular in the last twenty years, in part because of the Internet and the spreading of knowledge on the subject. The fact is, just with bodyweight you can go very far in progressive training.

That being said, we do interact with other objects on a daily basis; thus, working to do that better is also important.

When it comes to something heavy all you have to do is lift it. How heavy it is will depend on whether you lift it just to hip level (as in a deadlift), up to the shoulders (as in a clean lift), or even overhead.

Barbells and dumbbells were invented to make the exercise of lifting easier. With a well-balanced object, any person can lift more weight. And with plate-loading bells, progression becomes much easier. These technological advances allowed weight lifting to become more specialized and widely available.

However, it all started with natural objects. Most notably lifting was done with stones and logs. Why? Because these heavy objects were what was available. We see the modern example of this in strongman competitions that involve atlas stones and the log clean and press.

Of course, these are specially made implements, standardized once again to be more easily lifted. But it all started with natural rocks and logs.

And if you go out into nature and lift actual logs and rocks you'll notice that there is something quite primal about it. For men, strength training is a way to tap into their masculine nature. There's not much that is more masculine than pitting your will and muscle against a large rock. Over history, many cultures had some sort of testing of strength using natural objects like these to move from boyhood to manhood.

That's not to say that women shouldn't engage in these movements, because they should. It's just that this is something that is built into masculinity.

Carrying and Dragging

Lifting something up and putting it down isn't the most useful of activities—great for testing your strength, but not often much else. More often than not, if you're going to pick something up, it has somewhere else you want it to be, and thus you'll be either carrying or dragging the object.

This would often be done for the purposes of building something. In hunting, the animal would need to be brought back to camp. In collecting water or plants, often a significant weight would be generated, and this too would need to be brought back to camp.

Since lifting is involved, as well as movement with the lifted object, this may be the most complete and functional single exercise you can do. We can carry things in a number of positions. Depending on which position you use, and the object itself, this can work every muscle in your body from your feet to your hands, as well as your cardiovascular system.

It can be replicated in a gym using dumbbells, kettlebells, barbells, and more. Some special objects like farmer's walk bars or the yoke are specifically for carrying. And it can also be done with objects found in nature.

Fighting

This is a combination of many different types of movement, typically the ability to move quickly and accurately. This would involve forms of striking with the hands and feet, as well as grappling. An addition would be the use of weapons. Unlike most other animals, we don't have great weapons built in, but we're awesome at creating and using tools, including those for fighting. Depending on the weapon this could include the skill of shooting or throwing.

Furthermore, this involves many different types of movement, so various forms of martial arts can be good long-term practices. They'll keep you moving, even if the rest of your lifestyle does not. Also, moving well in all other ways covered here helps us be fit for fighting and thus be better at it.

I won't belabor the point here but having a foundation of self-defense skills is useful for any human being to have, even if they never have actual use for it.

Balancing

Throughout all of the movement types covered some type of balance is involved. Put a rock overhead and try to walk with it and you'll know that it must be balanced, or it could potentially be dangerous. But, because it's so easy for us now, we might forget balance is used even just in standing. Watch a baby learning to walk and you'll see this is apparent.

Balance can be trained in a number of ways. When traversing nature, you might find you have to cross a fallen tree over a ravine. Good balance could mean the difference between life and death in such a situation. While I'm not suggesting you put yourself in harm's way like this, you can work balance the same way by walking across a fallen log on the ground.

This brings up another important aspect of nature. The earth is not flat in many places. Your position will shift with each step, as opposed to our perfectly flat and straight unnatural city paths. This challenges your body in making micro-adjustments, something we've not done often through our modern age. While the effects of this may be subtle, there are effects.

For these reasons, in many of my workouts, I want to be on natural uneven ground. It may not be as comfortable or easy, but it is more natural.

Another challenge that I feel any human being can work up to is balancing in a headstand. Often used in yoga, the headstand is a simple pose that also gives you the benefits of getting inverted. I'd be willing to bet the ability to do a headstand would correlate well with decreases in mortality too.

Mobilizing Each Joint Fully

This category isn't a type of movement pattern like many of the above. It isn't useful to get around or to move outside objects. But it is the foundation from which all of those things happen.

The human body has many joints, including the toes, ankles, knees, hips, every part of the spine (lumbar, thoracic, and cervical), jaw, scapula, shoulders, elbows, wrists and fingers. Joints are meant to move to a bigger or smaller degree, depending on the type of joint (ball and socket or hinge, for example).

Thus, to move well, every joint ought to be able to move through a full range of motion safely, easily, and with coordination. An extended range of motion is not required, but the full normal range. For some joints, like the elbow, most people have and maintain this without trying.

But for other joints, like the thoracic spine (mid-spine), many people become unable to articulate these vertebrae through lack of use. Go ahead and try to trace your sternum in a circular motion through the air using the mobility of the thoracic spine right now. Can you do it? This ability can be regained through specific practice if you can't.

And while all of the joints are meant to be mobile, they're also meant to be stable. This is where supporting your body's weight in different positions, like hanging or crawling on the ground, or with other objects, like a heavy stone, comes in. This is where strength comes into play. The joints need both mobility and stability to be healthy.

This not only allows us to move well and with strength, but if done properly, will keep us pain free and injury free. Freedom of movement is the natural state of a human, and if anything stops this, it can be restored through practice.

Resting Postures

Speaking of joint pain, another factor that is not often discussed is that of our soft and comfortable beds. You can easily imagine that our ancient ancestors did not have the same kind of sleeping materials available to them. Michael Tetley, a physiotherapist, grew up with, and spent time studying, various native people. In his article "Instinctive Sleeping and Resting Postures: An Anthropological and Zoological Approach to Treatment of Low Back and Joint Pain" for the *British Medical Journal,* he wrote: "I have organised over 14 expeditions all over the world to meet native peoples and study their sleeping and resting postures. They all adopted similar postures and exhibited few musculoskeletal problems. I must emphasise that this is not a comparison of genes or races but of lifestyles…Largely anecdotal evidence has been collected by 'old timers' for over 50 years from non-Western societies that low back pain and joint stiffness is markedly reduced by adopting natural sleeping and resting postures."[19]

Tetley found that the vertebrae would reset when resting against the hard ground and that various resting postures could correct different joints.

One other point was that pillows are not necessary, nor even helpful. I know that pillow thing is going to bother people. For whatever reason, people don't want to give up their pillows. Personally, I have been sleeping without one for over six years now. What I've found is I never wake up with a kink in my neck, like many people find happens from time to time, as I did before making this change.

But if you're used to pillows it may be too much to just ditch it straight, and this is because your body structure is used to it. Still, if you'd like to do this, you can progressively work your way there by using thinner and thinner pillows.

Why am I talking about your sleeping position in a chapter about movement? Because your body adapts to movement as well as the positions it stays in for short or prolonged periods of time. If you want to move well and be healthy, you must look at your resting positions too. Realize that everything you do affects your body, and if you want your body to work well, that means naturally working your body.

Moving in Nature

What has been described here is not groundbreaking information. It is not new, and it is not unique to me. While most of these ideas aren't taught in the conventional fitness gyms, you'll hear them echoed in many places.

Recently, programs such as MovNat have forged "old" ground in helping people get back to natural movement. But they're not the only ones.

One of the seemingly lost aspects of natural movement is to actually move in nature. In many cases, different facets of the types of movements discussed here are taught and recommended but are often done in the flat-floored, fluorescent-lighted, stale air of a gym. It's better than not doing them, but not as good as it can be.

We keep coming back to the principle of stacking the benefits of nature. So why not do your natural movements in nature? Then you will not only practice moving better, but get fresh air, sunlight, grounding, and increased sensory stimulus—including the proprioceptive feedback of feet on ground that isn't completely flat and balanced.

Some early research shows that people feel better exercising outdoors than indoors, and that it supports cognitive function.[20] I find it funny that to properly control the settings in some of these studies the control group rides a stationary bicycle while staring at a wall, while the experimental group watches a video of a forest.[21] And they called that green exercise—as if the visual stimulus is the main, or only, thing they want to know about. I understand the need to try to isolate variables in science, but this is somewhat ridiculous. Still, they found that the video of the forest lowered the blood pressure more effectively.

Another study found that people walking outdoors got all the same physical benefits but had greater emotional benefits in self-esteem and mood.[22]

Even if a person has exposure to a little nature time and some exercise, otherwise living civilized indoor lives most of the time, this supplement can go pretty far in restoring health and supporting performance.

Furthermore, a forest or just a few natural elements can provide a rich playground for movement. Moving your body to this location will likely take walking or running. Then you can hang from and climb the trees. You can probably find something nearby to lift. You can always squat, jump, roll, and crawl across the ground. And it's all free compared to a gym membership or hiring a personal trainer. I would take playing around outside like this to running on a treadmill like a caged hamster any day of the week. I hope you would too.

9
Sun

"The Sun can be your greatest gloom, or your greatest comforter, depending on how you view its shine."
– Anthony Liccione

"Ô, Sunlight! The most precious gold to be found on Earth."
– Roman Payne

We take the sun for granted. Recognize for a moment that without its light and heat all life on Earth could not exist. Yet, I bring up the sun for good reason. Nowhere else is it more apparent how far removed we've become from something natural, even distorting the idea into something evil, putting effort into doing unnatural things to avoid it.

In recent years, we've come to realize that the sun does bring some benefits. But we've pigeon-holed that into one thing, vitamin D, which we instead obtain via pills, thinking that the sun causes cancer.

Everyone reading this does not remember a time when electricity didn't exist. I sure don't. I was born and raised in a time when we had access to light anywhere and anytime we wanted. But this is far from being the case historically. Even now, our lives are still largely ruled by daytime and nighttime, but it use to be much more so.

The average person gets up sometime around sunrise and goes to bed sometime after nightfall. This is a daily cycle that governs the circadian rhythm of the human body. This powerful cycle is at play in many health-related factors, including learning, mood, sleep and much more.[1]

Your health suffers if you don't follow the natural rhythm. There are many studies showing the detrimental effects on people that stay up late, for instance, night-shift workers. This is linked to lower-quality sleep, increased diabetes risk, weight gain, breast cancer, heart attack risk, depression, and more.[2]

As a side note, my mother, who died of breast cancer, worked the night shift for many years as a nurse. I can remember the first time seeing a report of that link, and wondering if anyone so employed was told of such?

We're taught to fear the sun but cast your mind back in time for a moment. Ancients, all around the world, use to praise the sun as one of many gods, and sometimes goddesses too. I think this is important, even logical, that this occurred. From Ra to Apollo, Sol to Tonatiuh, it was common to see this giver of light and life as something holy and transcendent.

Echoing this, Napoleon Bonaparte said, "If I had to choose a religion, the sun as the universal giver of life would be my god."

With our science, we know the sun is almost 93 million miles away, made up of 72 percent hydrogen, and is about 27 million degrees Fahrenheit at the core. But does any of that help you in your daily life?

What if, instead, you worshipped the sun? I'm not saying bowing down and praying to it or thinking of it as some magical being that will grant you miracles or smite you based on its whims. Instead simply by spending time with it, developing a friendly relationship, and giving it the proper recognition as the ultimate life-giver.

It is interesting to note that in many stories and myths, when people were before god they would bow their heads and couldn't look directly at god's brilliance. Just try looking at sun during high noon, and you may find where this idea first came from.

No life would exist without our sun. That's worthy of some devotion, if you ask me.

The ancients' days were ruled by the sun. What you did during the day and during the night were very different by necessity. And based on the amount of sunlight, depending on where you lived, we see one of the most self-evident adaptions in humankind, the color of the skin.

We know that plant life requires the sun. They produce energy based on photosynthesis. Chlorophyll, which is why plants are green, uses the sun's energy to turn carbon dioxide into sugar. They turn light into food.

Humans do their own kind of photosynthesis. It's not the same, and it doesn't necessarily produce energy or ATP directly, but sunlight does produce certain chemicals in the human body. Further, as we showed in the discussion of water, the energy of the sun likely drives the charging of internal water.

And recent research found that true photosynthesis might occur in mammals with a chlorophyll-rich diet. The chlorophyll can modulate mitochondrial ATP.[3]

Since we see that sunlight doesn't just hit the skin but penetrates the blood and cells, perhaps we haven't found or don't understand everything it produces or changes. As you'll come to see, we already know it does a lot more than just make vitamin D. But first, let's look at why we fear the sun.

The Dangerous Sun

Despite its life-giving properties, in recent years, we've come to see the sun as the enemy. We have blamed the sun for cancer and aging. Certainly, it plays some role in those, but how much is the sun to blame?

Were humans suffering from skin cancer to the tune of one out of every five people, hundreds or thousands of years ago? That's the current rate of skin cancer in the United States. No, they were not, as cancer of any type was very uncommon, though not unknown. And remember this was before electricity. This was before people spent all day working indoors. This meant that people spent more time in the sun.

But if skin cancer rates are going up, and time in the sun is decreasing, how did the blame get put on the sun? It doesn't make logical sense.

The standard research links UV light exposure, which includes light from the sun, to increased risk of cancer.[4] More specifically, UVA can penetrate the skin, contributing to skin cancer via the generation of free radicals which damage DNA. UVB causes sunburns when too much occurs and can also damage DNA. All UV exposure is linked to photo-aging of the skin by damaging collagen and destroying vitamin A.

You've heard all these things before, right? Perhaps not the details, but, as I said, this is the standard knowledge that is passed onto people, albeit in a more simplified form of "sun equals dangerous."

Yet, the whole sun-cancer link may not be based on good research either. Dr. Albert Bernard Ackerman, of the Ackerman Academy of Dermatopathology in New York, stated that the link between melanoma and sun exposure was not proven, that "the field is just replete with nonsense."[5]

Here's what you may not know. While higher exposure to sunlight may mean more skin cancer (the link to squamous cell carcinoma is well established, but this cancer is not as serious as most others), having higher vitamin D levels makes those cancers, and all cancer, less deadly.[6]

A twenty-year study, following 29,518 Swedish women, found that those avoiding the sun were more likely to die from all causes by a significant factor. The researchers noted, "Nonsmokers who avoided sun exposure had a life expectancy similar to smokers in the highest sun exposure group, indicating that avoidance of sun exposure is a risk factor for death of a similar magnitude as smoking."[7]

Let me reiterate that. Avoiding the sun is as bad as regularly smoking. So, you can stand naked in the sun, and light up, and be as well off as a nonsmoker who spends all their time indoors, and lathers sunscreen on themselves anytime they're outside.

Further, they found that those who were sunburned more often, died less. That makes you think, doesn't it?

Besides rickets, a specific deficiency in vitamin D, we seem to have forgotten the importance of sunlight. But even in America, one hundred years ago, sun bathing was also used to successfully treat things like tuberculosis and various skin disorders.

Perhaps skin cancer and aging it is not the sun's fault, but something else. You know what else has risen in usage right along with cancer rates? Sunscreen use—the very thing we're told to put on skin to protect from the sun.

What is sunscreen made of? It's a very good question, the answer you probably don't know, because it uses all kinds of chemicals that the average person can't pronounce derived mostly from petroleum. Oxybenzones, PABA, and other chemicals are not heavily tested to verify they're safe. In fact, some research shows they disrupt hormones.[8] And with your hormone levels altered, you're much more likely to get something like breast or prostate cancer. The rates of both of these have risen sharply over the years.

That chemical glop isn't just waiting on the skin but is getting absorbed into your body. Would you eat your sunscreen? If not, then you really shouldn't be putting it on your skin. In either case, it's getting into your body.

Ever since sunscreen use has been widely adopted, and people have been cautioned to avoid the sun, you would think that skin cancer rates would go down. That would make logical sense if the sun was bad and sunscreen was good. But that's not what we see. Skin cancer rates keep going up.

And it's not because people haven't been following the advice. Whenever I go out with a group of people in the sun I always see them slathering on the sunscreen even before they get outside. It's put on babies and children too. Overall, people have heard this message loud and clear and they comply.

People are now cautioned to put sunscreen on every day. Even if they're scarcely in the sun at all. It's recommended as part of the daily skincare routine.

Plenty of other things have also changed in the same time, including increased intake of rancid oils and sugar. Perhaps the sun isn't so much the problem; it's that with our lack of quality nutrition our body can't handle the same exposure we once had.

Because of the importance of looking young in our culture many people may be more worried about sagging skin than cancer. However, if your diet properly supports collagen synthesis, which the average industrialized nation diet does not, then you don't need to worry about this. Normal sun exposure won't cause undue stress here if other aspects are in alignment.

Specifically, your sunscreen should be built in. It is internal in the form of the nutrition you receive. Beta carotene, other carotenoids, vitamin E, vitamin C, flavonoids, and omega-3 fatty acids protect from collagen damage and sunburns.[9]

Early on when I was studying nutrition, I heard stories that people who ate exclusively raw food couldn't get sunburned. This sounded like a super power to me. What was causing it? By having many more antioxidants and phyto-chemicals as well as avoiding the rancid, cooked oils, their bodies were better able to handle the stresses of sun exposure. But you don't need to be a raw foodist to get these benefits, if you still follow the same trends.

Chances are the microbiome of the skin is equally important too. Research has only scratched the surface of looking at the effects of UV light on the bacteria, fungi, viruses and more that live on our skin. These all play a role in our immune system. The effects of sun exposure on your skin's microbiome is likely to have far more research coverage in the future.[10]

In my mind, this sunscreen thing is largely propaganda, further fueled by those that sell sunscreen. Sure, people that recommend it may be well-meaning, but that doesn't make it right.

The sun is a stressor. As such it can be too much and too intense. In many parts of the world the intensity can be felt on a hot day. But this is combatted easily, not by using sunscreen, but by going to the shade or wearing clothing. Common knowledge is not so common anymore.

Yet, as a stressor, it also can be a good thing, done in the right dose. Plus, we don't need to wait generations for adaptation. The skin tans with sun exposure, thus protecting you the more you get.

The fact is that getting sunburned only occurs in people that avoid the sun, those that live in industrial societies. Otherwise, people get tanned which modulates over the seasons with the sun's exposure. This naturally occurs if you aren't unnaturally hiding from the sun all the time.

Personally, I would rather get burned to a slight degree than put my body through the shock of sunscreen. And I would rather get burned than avoid the sun altogether. Remember, according to that Swedish study, exposure and burn will make you live longer.

Like anything, sun exposure can be overdone, but that happens less and less these days. And those things that are meant to protect you actually stop the benefits and come with side effects. So, let's dig deeper into the benefits from sunlight.

Vitamin D

Vitamin D has come hot on the scene in the past decade or so as many people's number-one supplement. For a long time, it was known only for assisting with calcium absorption and thus bone health.[11]

Now, D has been shown to do many more things. It is a major player in the endocrine and immune systems. Normal and optimal levels of vitamin D reduce the risk of heart attack, cancer, autoimmunity, diabetes, infections, depression, and more.[12] It basically has an impact on every disease.

Vitamin D is not so much a vitamin as it is a prohormone. When it was discovered it was misnamed. Its best description may be as a neuroregulatory steroidal hormone that influences almost 3000 genes. In short, vitamin D basically affects everything, either directly or indirectly.

Hormones work as chemical messengers. They send and receive messages. The signal of sunlight sends messages to many different parts of the body. Specifically, the UVB spectrum triggers vitamin D to form in the skin, but, as we'll see, sunlight signals other chemicals too. Overall, that message is healthy functioning. That's how important vitamin D is, and hence how important sunlight is.

But since people fear the sun, and these days simply don't have time to spend in the sun, we take vitamin D pills instead.

I do recommend this for the average person because having normal to optimal vitamin D levels is critical for your health. It is estimated that more than 70 percent of Americans are deficient. If you can't get the sun, or enough of it, then supplement for sure.

But remember that it is a supplement, and, as I'll show you, sunlight does not only equal vitamin D. There is much more at play. For these reasons, I feel supplemental vitamin D is only a fallback position and, while useful, scarcely holds a candle to getting the real thing via sunlight.

Vitamin D doesn't just come in one form. One of the distinctions is between D2, known as ergocalciferol, and D3, known as cholecalciferol. Most D2 is synthetically made by irradiating fungus and plant matter. This is the kind that is prescribed by doctors and given by injection, under the drug names of Viosterol or Drisdol. A meta-analysis was done that looked at 94000 people and the differences between those taking D2 and those taking D3. Those taking D3 saw a drop in mortality, death from all causes, of 6 percent. Those taking D2 saw a slight increase in mortality.[13]

If we looked at this naturally, it makes sense. We're meant to get D3, primarily from the sun, as that is the form created. We're not meant to get huge injections of D2. The body must do a lot of work to transform D2 into the active form of D3.

But D3 from sunlight is still not the same as D3 from a pill. All supplemental forms, and what you get dietarily, is fat-soluble vitamin D. But when vitamin D forms on the skin, it is water soluble. The version that forms on the skin is vitamin D3 sulfate, which can freely travel in your blood. Interestingly enough, it is also the form found inside human breast milk.

Also, if you do not have sufficient amounts of sulfur in your diet, then perhaps your body isn't able to handle the message of the sun as well. There are lots of possible factors at play that can change the sun from being helpful to harmful.

In the liver, vitamin D3 is transformed by hydroxylation into the form of 25(OH)D3. This is the kind that is tested in your standard blood test, as it's easily measured compared to the active form.

From the liver, it goes to the kidneys and other areas including the breast, prostate, lung, skin, colon, pancreas, and brain, where it is made into the active form of 1,25-hydroxyvitamin D3, also known as calcitriol. This is the form that truly acts as a hormone in the human body and is structurally very similar to those.

Almost every cell in the body has been found to have vitamin D receptors (VDR), which are involved in transcription of genes. More VDR binding sites occur in genes associated with cancer and autoimmune diseases.[14] This shows one possible reason why D is so important to these diseases.

While the sun is the primary source, vitamin D can be gotten dietarily too, not just in pills, in 'fortified grains' or milk. It is naturally found in many fat rich sources in nature, including fatty fish, liver, and egg yolks, because these animals create and store vitamin D too. Weston A. Price found that all diets of the natural humans he looked at received some vitamin D from their diets as well.

Overall, food and supplements aren't the mainstay for vitamin D. The sun is. Getting extra D via your diet should be seen as a bonus, or something to aim for more in winter months, but not as the main method.

Research that looks only at D3 levels with no difference in how it is obtained can't be truly accurate for this reason, because the sun provides much more than just vitamin D. Only minimal research has been conducted on these differences so far.

Other Benefits of the Sun

We know that sunlight signals lots of things in the body including genes which interface with your hormonal and immune systems. It is not just vitamin D that is active. Other byproducts of human photosynthesis are:

Cholesterol sulfate - The molecules of vitamin D and cholesterol are very close in structure. One of the issues around high levels of LDL and atherosclerosis may be because of an insufficiency of cholesterol sulfate which is produced on the skin in sunlight. Dr. Stephanie Seneff, senior research scientist at MIT, thinks that most of the benefits from sun exposure come not from vitamin D, but from this molecule.[15] What if that is the case? You're certainly not getting this from your vitamin D pill.

Proopiomelanocortin – This molecule is generated from UV exposure.[16] It is a big molecule that may then be altered to create the following three molecules:

1. Beta endorphins - Got pain? UV exposure has been shown to increase beta endorphins, our endogenous opiate that increases pain tolerance and helps us relax. The melanocytes in skin contain an endorphin receptor system.[16]
2. Alpha melanocyte-stimulating hormone – This hormone limits oxidative DNA damage, increases gene repair, and supports the immune system, in addition to starting the tanning process by producing melanin. This hormone specifically reduces melanoma risk.[17]

3. Adrenocorticotropic hormone – Helps control cortisol release by the adrenals, as well as triggering melanocytes to produce melanin.[17]

Melanin - Melanin is created to suppress the UV skin damage. The body has in-built mechanisms to protect it when you have too much exposure. Sunburns only really occur for people in industrial civilizations because the body tans in response to sun exposure along with the season due to melanin. This is how our body responds so that DNA damage doesn't occur.[18]

Substance P – This neuropeptide regulates the immune system and promotes blood flow.[19]

Calcitonin gene-related peptide – CGRP is a neuropeptide that modulates cytokines and is one of the methods by which sunlight can treat skin disorders. This may be the action through which sunlight helps treat psoriasis.[20]

Nitric oxide – This important cellular signaling molecule dilates blood vessels, reducing blood pressure. Many performance-related supplements for the gym and for the bedroom promise to increase nitric oxide, which is important to those functions. But sunlight, specifically UVA, which is often considered the harmful ultraviolet ray, has been shown to mobilize NO in the body, both in the keratinocytes in the skin and in red blood cells. While this is inflammatory sunlight may also be a performance booster.[21]

Sunlight also helps regulate the immune system through the action of T regulatory cells, specifically in cases of autoimmunity.[22] Vitamin D also induces cathelicidins that fight both bacterial and viral infections.[23]

You can see that several of these interact with the immune system. Years ago, sunbathing was recommended as one of the best curative treatments for many types of diseases like tuberculosis.[4] And there was much success in doing this.

And on and on the list could go. These many molecules in turn interact with many others, producing far-reaching effects in the body, that we have only scratched the surface in understanding what they do. Remember that it was only a couple of decades ago when we thought that vitamin D was responsible for bone health and not much else. Now we understand it is active across many hormones and genes. What else will be revealed by future research, including in all these other pathways?

Virtually none of these are formed from your vitamin D pill. Hence, the name "sunshine in a pill" is not accurate. While reductionist scientists would love sunshine to create one thing, which in turn does one thing in the body, this is far from reality.

Full Light Spectrum

UVA, which is touted for all of its negative effects in cancer and photoaging, is the wavelength responsible for releasing nitric oxide. UVB is often considered the more beneficial of the wavelengths, because it causes vitamin D production. However, as we saw with some of the other components, both A and B are important for different things

Sunlight comprises somewhere around 1500 wavelengths. The ozone removes anything with a wavelength shorter than 290 nanometers. The ultraviolet exists in the 290 to 380 nm range. The visible spectrum in the 380 to 770 nm range. Infrared is in the 770 plus range. For the most part, this is a continuous spectrum of light, besides a few wavelengths being absorbed by particles in the atmosphere.

There are several factors that block the UVB, the vitamin D–producing wavelength. Being indoors on a sunny day is not helpful unless the doors and windows are open, as glass blocks UVB, while still allowing the UVA in.

Clouds also block UVB. Even the angle of the sun matters. UVB rays only comes through the Earth's atmosphere when the sun is above 50-degrees on the horizon. Many people are told to avoid the sun when it's at its peak, but that is actually the best time to get UVB. Lower than this angle and the ozone layer reflects the UVB while still allowing the UVA in.

Unfortunately, this means that in many parts of the world, the sun does not allow you to get UVB light, during certain parts of the year, as the sun is always lower on the horizon. This shows the importance of getting the sunlight when its available, even if this is only in short windows throughout the year.

Sunscreens are designed to block UV, including both UVA and UVB. An SPF 15 sunscreen causes a 99 percent reduction in D3 synthesis on the skin.[24] It likely stops the production of all these other chemicals too. By blocking the light, your body isn't able to absorb and utilize it for the many functions it has.

We think of the sun as just hitting the skin. We don't often realize that it penetrates the layers of the skin. In fact, visible light penetrates all tissues to a certain depth.

Yet the focus is all on the UVB because it produces vitamin D. Perhaps the full light spectrum from the sun is equally important. This is hard to measure outside of the effect of light on the eyes, and of course, we do get the visible spectrum from other light sources too.

And that's not all. Think about lying under the sun on a hot day. Is it only the surface of your body that feels warmth, or does it penetrate into your core? That's largely the infrared heat.

The sun has the full spectrum of infrared rays—far, middle, and near—though some of these may get absorbed by the atmosphere. Still, over 50 percent of the energy that reaches the Earth at the sun's peak is in the near infrared spectrum.

One of the best devices for supporting your health, becoming very popular today, is an infrared sauna. I personally have one and use it regularly. These provide many benefits, and research is looking at their benefits to blood pressure, pain, detoxification, skin health, relaxation, weight loss, and more. [25]

If the benefits are coming from the infrared heat, it's important to realize that the sun provides these same wavelengths too. This seems to be a completely unresearched sun benefit. We can get heat from other sources, but that means you can also get these benefits sitting outside on a hot day, soaking up the rays.

Dr. Mercola writes, "The near infrared wavelengths, especially 800 to 850 nanometers, are what cytochrome c oxidase, the fourth protein in the electron transport chain in your mitochondria, resonates with. This is important if you hope to optimize your ATP and cellular energy production."

The various photoproducts of sunlight cause photochemical reactions throughout the body. This affects more than the skin. It affects the blood, the intracellular fluid and the cells themselves. Because nothing in the human body works in isolation, sunlight exposure or lack of exposure affects either directly or indirectly every organ and system in the body. Contemplate that for a moment.

"The Effects of Light on the Human Body," by Richard J. Wurtmann, raises many important points, including: "The observation that ordinary sunlight or artificial light sources can drastically alter the plasma level of even one body compound (in this case bilirubin) opens a Pandora's box for the student of human biology. It presents the strong possibility that the plasma or tissue levels of many additional compounds are similarly affected by light." [26]

To sum up, it is important that you get sun exposure. Done withing reason, you won't get an excess amount of vitamin D, nor of any of the other chemicals, by doing so. Instead you'll get the amounts you need. This supports vitamin D, nitric oxide, melanin, several hormones, many immune functions, and more.

And it is best done through full-spectrum, natural sunlight. There may be some technologies to mimic some of the processes, but isn't getting some sun easier to do, especially when you realize we're always missing some critical pieces in our replications of natural things?

How Much Do You Need?

There are two very important factors regulating how much sun you need: your skin color and where you live.

People with lighter skin are adapted to places where less sun is available. White people, descending from Europe, are used to places where clouds predominately cover the sky during a large portion of the year. The sun may come out just a few days of the year. The sun also may not be high enough in the sky to provide its full UVB benefits. Thus, their skin is lighter so that they can more easily absorb its rays. And in these cases, things like dietary vitamin D become more important, as they have been historically in those regions.

Contrast this to black people, descended from Africa, where the sun is shining most of the time. The skin is darker to protect from too much exposure. They're adapted to this environment, and thus need to be exposed to the sun a lot more to get the same benefits. For those with the darkest skin color, being in the sun almost all the time may be necessary to maximize benefits.

A pale white person spending thirty minutes in the summer sun can generate 50000 IU's of vitamin D which are released into circulation within the next 24 hours. A dark-skinned person will generate about 10000 IU's in the same sun. And a tanned skin individual gets somewhere in the middle with about 20000-30000 IU's. Not surprisingly, research suggests that non-whites tend to have lower vitamin D levels than whites, and this is true even at their ancestral latitudes.[27]

Remember that this vitamin D is water soluble. That means it can be washed off if you use soap on your skin within that 24-hour period. It is not immediately all absorbed.[28]

But vitamin D is stored in the body in fat-soluble form. Thus, if you can soak up as much as you need in the summer months, it can help keep you optimal throughout the winter months.

So how much do you need? There is debate as to the most optimal amount of vitamin D. It is measured in the blood as 25(OH)D. The Vitamin D Council recommends a range of 40 to 80 ng/mL. The U.S. laboratory reference range tends to be a little lower, at 30 to 74 ng/mL. More recently in 2011, after reviewing over 1000 studies, the Institute of Medicine recommended a slightly lower range of 20 to 50 ng/mL.

Looking back to indigenous peoples, the Masai and Hadzabe tribes of Africa were found to have blood levels of 44-48 ng/mL.[29] This is through being outdoors, not from supplementation.

You'll notice that there seems to be a common range around 40-50 ng/mL, so that is likely a good ideal to shoot for.

Still, this is the level we measure because we found it easy to measure. While it is correlated to many different health factors, this doesn't mean it is actually the most important number in the body. It's just what we can look at with current technology.

Besides race there are many other factors. One study looking at Hawaiian surfers who spent fifteen or more hours outdoors each week over a three-month period of time, saw differing levels from 11 to 71 ng/mL.[30] Sunscreen and other factors were likely at play.

Don't forget that this is just vitamin D. As far as I know no blood test is looking at the levels of all those other compounds mentioned earlier.

So how much sun should you get? The skin responds. Generally, for people of lighter skin once it starts to turn slightly pink, that's an indication you've got enough for the day. If you're getting too much sun exposure find shade or wear layers of clothing. Certain topical oils like coconut can also provide some protection. It can't be SPF rated, because that term is only allowed for sunscreens, but coconut oil would have an equivalent of roughly 4-7 SPF.

In our global community, where we're no longer connected to where we came from, it may be difficult to get the right amount for ourselves. A black person living in Seattle may not be physically able to derive the maximum benefits from the sun. They should still seek it out when it's available, but in cases like this supplementation goes from optional to necessary.

Where to Get Sunlight

There's another piece of the 'where' puzzle I'd like to address. Not where you're at and the amount of sun that is available, but where you expose your body to the sun, and by that, I mean what parts.

To maximize the benefits, it is ideal to get sun where "the sun don't shine," i.e. the private areas. Think about when was the last time that your genitals even saw sunlight? For many people, it's not since they were a toddler, with the parents allowing them to run around naked outside.

But if we think of sunlight primarily as a hormonal signaling system, and knowing the vitamin D is a hormone, not a vitamin, it makes sense for this to occur on the endocrine-intensive tissues of the body. For men, this involves the testicles. For women, getting sunlight on the breasts is going to be important. Just think of the hormonal and immune system benefits sunlight provides; meanwhile breast cancer is one of the biggest killers in industrialized areas. What if there is a connection?

Although the following study hasn't been replicated and it's from awhile back, I thought the idea was fascinating. Measurements of testosterone increases were greater in men who got sun exposure to the genitals compared to those who only received sun exposure on the back and chest. [31]

Perhaps it was just from having more surface area exposed. But I think the testicles crave the sun. Forgive me if you feel this is slightly graphic. After learning about this research, I had to try it for myself. What I found actually spooked me out at first. The testicles and scrotum seemed to move of their own accord under sunlight. And I wasn't the only one either. Several other people have reported the same thing, and if you're a man I suggest you get outside and give it a try yourself. Others have reported that their balls get bigger too! (I hope it goes with saying that naked sunbathing should be done in a private place, or a place where society deems it appropriate to avoid any troubles.)

Not only does sun exposure matter but so does how you do it. Future research is likely to prove this out.

Making It Routine

I pride myself on being healthy. After all, I make it my business to be so. And nothing is worse than a hypocrite. Yet, one day I found myself sitting outside and I was looking at my skin. It was so pale that I could see many of the veins beneath the skin.

It looked sickly, like the skin of a diseased person. Think about what we often see when someone is sick. Pale skin. Now think of someone who is the epitome of health. Chances are they look like they have some sun exposure. A nice, healthy tan.

Bodybuilders use tanning machines, or spray tans, before they take the stage. Why? Because it makes the muscles look better. You'll never see a pale bodybuilder ever win. It just doesn't look as good. This isn't to say that bodybuilders are healthy, especially when on stage most of them are far from it, but just to showcase this point. All you have to do is observe and you'll see the truth to some sun exposure being healthy. I know the China doll white skin is fashionable, but fads like those come and go. And I would not look at the fashion industry to tell us what is healthy and not.

After I was struck by this realization, I made my number-one health goal for the year to get tan. Yes, I actually had it as a goal, which I wrote down. I made it a priority. I found it necessary to do this to get it done. And thus, at the age of 31 I got a tan for the first time in my life.

At that time, the place that I lived at had a little yard area. Depending on the season, the sun only shone there for a few hours of each day in winter, and quite a few more hours in summer. The sun got blocked off by trees earlier in the day, and the house itself later on. So, this was my window of opportunity. Of course, I could go elsewhere to get sun, and sometimes I did. But at home, since I worked from there, it would have to be my first and foremost option.

Previously, I always worked through this time. I'd take a break sometime around noon to do my movement practice, and I'd get some sun then, but I needed to do more to achieve my goal. This meant laying out there. I had to cease working and use this as a break. I started eating lunch while sitting outside, and spent some time reading as well.

In addition to the sun, I want to point out that I was getting grounded, fresh air, some of the other benefits of nature, all the while relaxing. We'll be covering this in more detail later but getting sun while electrically grounded may be important as something that helps amplify the benefits while protecting from possible drawbacks.

That became part of my routine. Of course, it was dependent on the weather. I stopped taking vitamin D supplements as I started getting real sun. It's been a challenge to get enough that my blood tests have come back in that ideal range, but I'm still working at it and getting better.

Then I was in the market to buy a home. One requirement was a good spot where I could sunbathe nude. It's important to my health, so I made sure the house I bought had that option.

One thing I like to think about is the solar rechargeable battery metaphor. You know the battery indicator on your phone? Think of having this for yourself and for the sun. In a sense, the sun truly is recharging your battery of vitamin D and other components. The question is, are you fully charged?

We're still not done with the sun. In the next chapter we look at it, along with light and darkness, the moon and all their effects on health.

10
Light and the Moon

"[The moon] was alive to me this night. I could feel her presence. She seemed very close, and there was an energy emanating from her – not the physical energy we feel from the warmth of her consort, Inti, the sun, but a spiritual energy, one of mystery, inner discovery, hope and redemption."
– John Perkins

The benefits of getting sunlight are evident to most people. Even if they believe the sun causes skin cancer, they at least have some idea that we need vitamin D. And even if they don't spend any time outdoors, the daily cycle of the sun still impacts their lives in some ways. Plus, the other side of the daily cycle is the night phase.

What about the moon? This other heavenly body found in the sky also plays a role in our functioning. The moon has its own cycle with its own effects. In this chapter, both of these areas are explored.

Light and Dark, Serotonin and Melatonin

Light and dark are critically important for regulating serotonin and melatonin, two hormones and neurotransmitters that are needed to keep us happy and allow good sleep. An easy way to keep this in mind is "S" for sun and serotonin, and "M" for moon and melatonin. (Of course, the moon is not out just at night, but we generally think of these as being correlated so we can use this mnemonic.)

While we touched upon the effects of visible light of the sun in the last chapter, I've largely saved that for here, so we can talk about it in relation to darkness, as well as other light sources.

The circadian rhythm is our daily cycle that governs wakefulness and sleep. One of the issues of modern living is dysregulation of these cycles which causes sleep issues that then impact everything. Sleep deprivation of a couple nights can lead to impaired glucose and insulin sensitivity, leading to obesity and diabetes.[1]

Did you know that one of the best things you can do to support your sleep is something you do first thing in the morning, not when you're going to bed? Getting sunlight in your eyes early in the morning means you'll produce more serotonin during the day. This not only supports your mood, and many other functions, but it is transformed into melatonin when night comes, which means better sleep.[2]

Studies with hamsters showed that it is not some internal circadian clock, but the environmental cues from light and the lack of it, that regulate serotonin levels.[3]

Our lights are not nearly as powerful as the sun. Melatonin researcher Russel J. Reiter of the University of Texas Health Science Center said, "The light we get from being outside on a summer day can be a thousand times brighter than we're ever likely to experience indoors. For this reason, it's important that people who work indoors get outside periodically."

Furthermore, it's been shown that brighter and longer duration sunlight lead to more serotonin in the brain.[4]

When people are exposed to morning sunlight, their nocturnal melatonin production occurs sooner, and they enter into sleep more easily at night. Melatonin does more than just help us sleep deeply too. It's the body's most powerful antioxidant and plays a big role in the immune system and cleaning up cancer.[5]

Melatonin production also shows a seasonal variation relative to the availability of light, with the hormone produced for a longer period in the winter than in the summer.

While these effects can be replicated with full-spectrum artificial lights, it is important to recognize that science often misses some details in technologies like these, that aren't revealed until years later.

If you live in a place with little sun, by all means get one of these, but if you live in a sunny place, the best option is to utilize the sun's brilliant light.

There is an ancient yogic method called sun gazing. When the sun is on or near the horizon you can safely look at it with the naked eye. This is considered a way of directly absorbing the sun's energy. (I hope it goes without saying that normally you should not look directly at the sun, aside from when it's on the horizon, as it can blind you.)

Only recently has our science come to find that, through production of serotonin, this does have a real impact. I'm willing to bet that there are other hormones and neurotransmitters affected by such, that later science will show. Research on rats has shown that light entering the eyes affected ovarian growth and function.[6] Who knows what else is happening?

Whether or not you can sun gaze, or get sun in your eyes indirectly, the light spectrum signals the hypothalamus. This, in turn, controls the pituitary, which controls most of the hormones in your body.

The pineal gland, called the third eye, also has light-sensing cells. It is where melatonin is primarily produced. Light passes through your eyes, along a pathway called the retinohypothalamic tract to the hypothalamus, and across further nerve pathways to the pineal gland.

Light and darkness are the main cues to a successful circadian rhythm. Without the proper cues, your rhythm will be off, and all of the issues that come with that begin. Dr. John Ott, the inventor of full-spectrum lighting, coined the term "malillumination" to describe our lack of quality light in similar ways to malnutrition.

Seeing sunlight in the morning is one of the key determinants of this cycle. When we stay indoors, or wear sunglasses any time that we are outside, we don't register the bright light of the sun, and thus, dysregulation begins.

Like sun on the skin, we've gone overboard with protecting the eyes from sunlight too. Many mainstream doctors and opticians will tell you to wear sunglasses all the time to protect your eyes. Like sun exposure to the skin, there can be problems. Overexposure to sunlight in the eyes is associated with cataracts and macular degeneration, but even if it's causal, it is one factor of many.[7]

As with skin, I believe you should get a good amount of sun exposure to the eyes, but don't overdo it. Let's reestablish common sense and not be so fearful of nature.

Dr. Alexander Wunsch, a photobiologist, has stated, "Sunlight induces coordinated endocrine adaptation effects…Our system, via the eyes and via the skin, detects the colors of the light in the environment in order to adapt the hormonal system to the specific needs of the time and place." In short, we need the signals from the sun to be healthy.

No research that I have found has looked at this, but perhaps getting some moonlight at night also helps. Unlike the sun, you can safely stare at the moon at any time. While we know that darkness affects our melatonin levels, perhaps moonlight specifically has some of its own interactions. Perhaps actually seeing the moonlight may have a regulatory effect on these same chemical messengers or other ones.

Recently, I have noticed a number of successful people mentioning "star therapy" as a great way to relax and unwind, that is gazing up at the stars in the night sky. Unfortunately, your ability to do this in most cities is becoming harder and harder. Jack Troeger, a former astronomy teacher, calls the light pollution of urban centers "stealing starlight." While the lack of starlight and the abundance of artificial light is not the only factor, Israeli researchers found that communities with more artificial light at night had a 73 percent increase in breast cancer.[8] Did I mention that melatonin is a strong cancer fighter?[9]

Malillumination and The Blue Light Spectrum

Just like air, just like water, there is certain quality lighting we need to get to be healthy. There also is certain quality lighting we need to avoid or minimize to be healthy.

Electricity has been one of the greatest technological advances that has altered our lives. But this comes with a cost. Albert Einstein once wrote in a letter, "Our entire much-praised technological progress, and civilization generally, could be compared to an axe in the hand of a pathological criminal." While he was talking about the atrocities of war, and the technology used in them, this same sentiment applies in other more insidious ways that we often don't recognize until it's too late.

Recent research has found how the blue-light spectrum, emitted strongly from our various screens and light bulbs, is especially disruptive to melatonin. This hormone helps us sleep, and lack of it is implicated in other issues like decreasing insulin sensitivity.[10]

Why is this? Blue light is normally only in large supply during the day. The sun supplies ample amounts of it. Besides the sun there aren't natural sources of blue spectrum light.

Unfortunately, it's not just our sleep-wake cycles that may be affected by our modern lifestyles. More recent research indicates that these flickering blue lights from our digital devices and florescent lights may be far worse for our eyes than sunlight.[11] These blue-light frequencies may cause photoreceptor death at rates far higher than other spectrums of light.[12]

In one review found in the journal *Molecular Vision*, the authors wrote, "The use of blue light is becoming increasingly prominent in our society, and a large segment of the world population is now subjected to daily exposure (from a few minutes to several hours) of artificial light at an unusual time of the day (night)...Although we are convinced that exposure to blue light from LEDs in the range 470–480 nm for a short to medium period (days to a few weeks) should not significantly increase the risk of development of ocular pathologies, this conclusion cannot be generalized to a long-term exposure (months to years)."[13]

With the amount of time that many people spend working and playing on computers, smart phones, and tablets this could mean very bad things for the future of our eyesight. The trends are already moving in the direction of macular degeneration occurring at an epidemic level. People are getting diagnosed at younger and younger ages.

As one review put it, "Age-related macular degeneration is a complex multifactorial disease that has an uneven manifestation around the world but with one common denominator, it is increasing and spreading."[14] What else is increasing and spreading? The amount of time we spend staring at our devices.

Not just our eyes suffer either. The action on the skin cells can be just as detrimental. One study concluded "that visible light can cause cell dysfunction through the action of reactive oxygen species on DNA and that this may contribute to cellular aging, age-related pathologies, and tumorigenesis."[15]

Furthermore, this may cause epigenetic changes that are passed to the next generation. A study on hamsters found that exposure to certain lighting disrupted both the endocrine and immune systems. The bad news is that these impaired systems were also passed down to their offspring.[16]

Jayson Bawden-Smith, in his book *In The Dark*, wrote, "I am convinced I had what I have begun calling 'blue light disease' – a pre-diabetic state caused by excessing exposure to artificial blue light and harmful EMFs."

Blue light disease. While I'm not a big fan of labelling things as such, because they're not actual things but instead processes, I find this very interesting as it calls out the importance of the negative effects of blue light. Nor is this an isolated case. A study on humans and blue light found that it did alter glucose metabolism.[17]

While different people may have their hormones disrupted more or less, this is a disease that will often only have subtle effects that may take a decade to show up. How many different effects across the body does this truly have?

Before the advent of electricity, we had to live more in phase with sunlight and moonlight. Depending on the weather conditions, night can be pitch black or quite clearly illuminated. Many city dwellers that have never been outside the neon lights are sometimes surprised to see just how bright it can be at midnight in a rural area, depending on the phase of the moon.

Since the moon simply reflects sunlight, wouldn't it have the same spectrum of colors? The fact is that moonlight happens to have much less blue and a lot more red. In rats, pineal function was suppressed only at light levels slightly greater than the light shed by the full moon on a clear night. That means that moonlight, even at its brightest, isn't detrimental to melatonin to the degree that our modern lights are.

Our natural light supply, fire, is also much redder and includes the benefits of infrared energy that was written about earlier, with a minimum of blue.

Ancient humans existed at night by the light of the moon and stars, as well as fire. And here we see that our sleep-wake cycles, even our whole physiology, seem to be uniquely adapted to these light sources. What we are not adapted to is the 24/7 light sources of today's modern age.

To support your sleep, it is best to avoid staring at a screen right before bed. Many people make sure to leave an hour gap between when they're on a computer or their phone or watching TV and when they head off to sleep. I think one of the worst ideas for sleep is to have a TV in your bedroom.

But even with this there is the disruptive blue-light spectrum coming from our light bulbs. And the energy-efficient LED lights, as well as fluorescent lights, are worse than the older incandescent lightbulbs. Why is it that so many technological advances appear to be worse for us?

The good news is there are a couple of technological advances that can help you fight back. On computers, there are apps like Flux that allow you to dim the screens color emissions when the sun falls. This is even built into the iPhone with the latest version at the time of writing, if you head to your settings.

You can also go into your TV settings and reduce the blue light as well as dim the screen. You can also install dimmer switches on your house lights. Even if it's still not the best light, at least there will be less of it, especially before bed.

In addition, you can also get a pair of orange-colored glasses that block the blue spectrum of light. Wear these for an hour before bed and your melatonin will begin to produce, allowing for better sleep. I've never really had problems sleeping, but still I got a pair of these to test out. I noticed they helped me increase the quality of sleep.

Black-out curtains are recommended to shut out the ambient light that comes in through windows. If you live with any artificial lights around you, which means in any urban or suburban area this is highly recommended. But I wonder if it comes at a cost without having the natural moonlight available? That this may in fact be helpful to us, whereas the artificial lights are not.

Understanding that not all light is created equal is important for regulating our cycles and health. To sum up, get sunlight shortly after waking up and throughout your day. Then, avoid any blue light, especially before going to bed. These two things are going to be the most impactful for being healthy.

The Moon Cycle

Earlier we talked about different cycles that occur in nature. That daily cycle is the most obvious and most prevalent. One of the other cycles is shown in the phases of the moon, which is how the moon looks from our place on the earth.

The new moon is when the moon turns invisible because the Earth is between it and the sun. The moon begins to wax, appearing bigger, until finally it reaches the full moon, where the entire disc is present. From here it wanes until it disappears, and the cycle begins again.

This cycle of the moon takes an average of 29.5 days. You'll note that this is close to a month. And in fact, the word month comes from the moon. Think of "moon-th" and you'll see this.

One effect of the moon is on the tidal force. The gravity of the moon pulls on the oceans. Those that are closer to the moon are under more force, while those on the opposite side of the Earth are under less of a pull. This causes a change in the tides.

The human body is made up of 70 percent water. The moon's gravity does pull more and less on us in the same way. Might this have some effect? Most of the research that has investigated things finds nothing, but not all of it. Some effects are shown in human reproduction, and possible links with some forms of epilepsy and hospital admittance.[18]

The lunar cycle appears to be especially important for women. In the majority of traditions, the sun is masculine while the moon is feminine. And we see that the lunar cycle has an impact on reproduction, including fertility, menstruation and birth rate.

While I was in Guatemala, the Mayan shaman Julio explained that the moon rules over the water. This is easily seen in its power over the tides. But it just as easily affects the water of the human body. The element of water is also reflected in each person in their emotions.

Julio described how a waxing moon would increase a person's creativity. New ideas would pop into a person's head. These may be good or bad ideas, either way, just a lot more of them. And this creativity would decrease as the moon wanes. Here was the time to act on the ideas you had from the previous cycle.

I'm also reminded of a conversation I had with Brooks Kubik, author of *Dinosaur Training*. He was an early mentor of mine in the world of strength training and was always careful in keeping a detailed training log of all his workouts. As he worked out in his garage at night with the door open, he observed that he had better workouts during the full moon.

The effects of the moon are subtler than those of the sun. That is the nature of the feminine, plus the longer moon-thly cycle. It is only by paying attention to it that you can begin to sync yourself to it and notice those effects.

The words lunacy and lunatic come from Luna, the moon. Many people have noted that people may act weirder or more dangerously during a full moon. While most research says this is not true, the belief persists.[19]

Perhaps the latest research shows the moon has no effect on us, because we no longer recognize the effect the moon has on us. You go back just a few decades and the effects of lunacy, crime and suicide rates, is shown in studies. Is this because we have more accurate data today, or has how people interacted with the world actually changed? Perhaps its effects would be stronger if our modern people were in sync with the moon cycle, witnessing the light, or lack of it, in our everyday lives, rather than in an abundance of artificial light.

Within our cities, with the pollution and ambient lighting, many times you can't even see the stars. And yet most of the time we're indoors and not even looking for them.

Go out into nature when the skies are clear and look with awe at the night sky. Future research may show that doing so helps us in myriad ways.

Seasonal Cycles

We have the longer cycle of the seasons too. Depending on where you live on the Earth these seasonal changes can be mild or extreme. When we spend the majority of our time indoors we become less attached to these cycles, but that doesn't mean they don't affect us.

Here in Santa Cruz, in the heart of winter, it has been raining a lot. This is great as over the past couple years California has been in a drought.

And I am noticing how it has affected me. Without the sun shining I am less likely to go outside. My routine of sunbathing has been squashed. And I find that I am leaving the house less during these times. But on those days when the sun comes out, I emerge from my hovel and soak up what I can of the sun's rays. Not having it whenever I want, helps me appreciate it more when the sun appears.

The seasonal cycle affects us in many ways. It's a longer cycle so it may not be so apparent to all, once again depending on where you live. But this will have its effects on your physiology and psychology.

Seasonal affective disorder (SAD) is the name for the depression and low energy that come with the winter months. If you're in tune with the natural cycles, the moon and the seasons, your body will better be adapted to them. Our physical and visual disconnection is likely exacerbating issues. That being said, it is part of the natural cycle to pull back in activity at these times. With less light, shorter days, it is quite natural to have lower energy. While humans don't hibernate like bears do, there is some drop in activity that occurs.[20]

But SAD isn't just for fall and winter months either. Some people get some different symptoms during summer months too. The good news is that this can be corrected, ideally with real sun exposure, but also with properly designed light boxes.[21]

SSRI's, selective serotonin reuptake inhibitors, are being prescribed for depression for many people. These could possibly just be done away with if people got the right kind of light, and if they followed the other natural steps that support serotonin and other important neurotransmitters.

Through the light, or lack of it, we have our connection to the heavenly bodies. These have many effects on us, both known and unknown. We are connected to them through our skin and our eyes. Eyes to the heavens and feet firmly on the ground. With that, next we turn to our physical connection to the Earth itself...

11
Earthing

"He who wishes to explore Nature must tread her books with his feet."
– Paracelsus

"When we walk upon Mother Earth, we always plant our feet carefully because we know the faces of our future generations are looking up at us from beneath the ground. We never forget them."
– Oren Lyons

Think about the term "mother earth" for a moment. In a sense, we are born out of the earth as every element that we're made of comes from the earth and various things that grow on the earth. (Of course, everything the earth is made of came from the stars, but, in this way, those are our more ancient ancestors.) Still it's not just the elements and chemicals that create us.

As much as we are chemical beings we are also electromagnetic beings. I hope that became clear in how light signals our skin and eyes in all kinds of bodily processes. And one of the recent discoveries is how a connection to the earth has various health benefits. Recent to science, that is. This was another thing that was well recognized in most, if not all, indigenous communities. This is known as earthing or grounding, and I'll be using those terms interchangeably throughout.

Just as it is critical to have a physical connection, and physical touch, with your mother when you're an infant, leading to physical and emotional well-being[1], we now know that having that same touch with "mother earth" may be equally crucial. That physical connection, which is an electrical connection, allows much to happen.

As one study put it, "Until a few generations ago, most humans walked and slept in direct contact with the surface of the earth. Our modern life style involves wearing insulating shoes and sleeping in buildings that electrically isolate the body from the ground plane. While some people intuitively sense that they feel better when they walk or even sleep directly on the earth (as on a camping trip), most of the population is more or less permanently isolated from the earth's electrical influences."[2]

In a nutshell, the earth is a nearly limitless supply of free electrons. This is because of electric charge of the solar and ionospheric winds, which transfer a negative charge to the ground through lightning. Thus, the upper atmosphere is positive, while the earth is negative.

When we have skin contact to the earth or something that is conductive attached to the earth, these electrons can begin to flow. As we dive into the research, you'll see this lowers inflammation, pain, and muscle soreness, while helping regulate stress, cortisol, and sleep.

And it is possibly more than just the electrons. Who knows what else may be "transferred" in this way?

Think about this process of earthing naturally. Virtually every creature is living connected to the earth close to 100 percent of the time. Exceptions would include birds and insects that are flying through the air. Also, some natural materials may not by conductive. Still, in nature everything is grounded either fully or most the time.

Contrast this to humans and some of our domesticated animals, like a house cat that lives completely indoors. Most modern humans are very seldom earthed. We're indoors most of the time. Dried wood, carpeting, linoleum and most flooring materials are not conductive. And when we go outdoors, the shoes are almost always on, the rubber soles completely blocking any conduction.

But we evolved in connection to the earth. Is it any wonder that we've become disconnected from nature, when we have literally disconnected, in an electrical sense, ourselves from nature? Therefore, one of the first steps in reestablishing that connection is to literally get connected.

Inflammation, Pain, Circulation and Muscle Soreness

These free electrons act as antioxidants in the body. An antioxidant is something that quells oxidative damage occurring through many bodily processes. While many people tout the antioxidant properties in foods such

144

as berries, coffee, and chocolate, and these can be very helpful, the earth itself may be the best antioxidant source.

These electrons help quell reactive oxygen species and lower inflammation.[3] As inflammation is at the root of every chronic disease, this is very important. Thus, by lowering inflammation, earthing will help with pretty much every chronic disease.

Changes in concentrations of white blood cells, cytokines, and various other molecules have been measured when a person is earthed, showing an impact on the immune system.[4]

One of the areas that originally got my attention, because of its applications for strength training, was how earthing affects DOMS, or delayed onset muscle soreness. This specific type of inflammatory response of the body, in response to a training stimulus, has been historically hard to reduce with just about anything. But earthing has been shown to reduce the pain related to DOMS, while changing certain blood parameters, when compared to placebo groups.[5]

Plus, grounding works quite well for chronic pain. If you have chronic pain anywhere this is a very easy experiment you can do for yourself. Note your pain level on a scale of 0 to 10, with zero being none at all and ten being the worst pain you've ever felt. Then get grounded (specifically touch the painful area to the ground if possible, but it's okay if your shoulder hurts and you only touch your feet to the ground). After half an hour grounded, rate your pain on a scale of 0 to 10 once again and note the difference. Most people will find some sort of reduction occurs.

As pain is subjective, measuring it on a scale like this is the best way we have to determine it. For many people in pain, earthing helps lessen it. In one small study, it helped ten out of the twelve subjects.[6]

Part of the reason that these benefits occur is because of the electron flow, which improves circulation. If circulation is better, than more nutrients can be delivered to all tissues, and waste products removed.

How does earthing help with circulation? Zeta-potential is the degree of electrostatic repulsion between similarly charged particles. This can be measured in red blood cells. In effect it shows blood viscosity, or how much the blood cells clump together versus staying separate. And indeed, research has shown that blood viscosity lowers when grounded.[7] That electrical connection allows your blood to be better electrified in ways it needs to be to function ideally. This is important because this may have a significant impact on cardiovascular disease.[8]

Cortisol, Stress and Sleep

But that's not all that happens. Having this electrical connection to the earth helps synchronize your body to the earth. We've already talked at length about the circadian rhythm. Here we find that it's not just the light we see or don't see, but earthing may also affect it. We see that through earthing our circadian rhythm becomes more synchronized.

This is why it is one of the best things you can do to eliminate jet lag. After flying go spend a half hour earthed. While it may not get rid of the jet lag completely, it will certainly help.

One of the daily cycles is that of cortisol, which is known as the stress hormone. Far from being a "bad" hormone, this is critically important for our health. Issues occur when cortisol is chronically elevated. And the fact is the cortisol is anti-inflammatory. It is working hard to quell the damage going on, which is why it's high in many people.

Cortisol naturally rises in the mornings. This is one of the things that helps us get out of bed and begin the activity for the day. After it peaks during the morning, it steadily declines throughout the day, reaching a low point at night. That's a normal cortisol cycle.

Earthing has been shown to synchronize this cortisol rhythm toward a more natural mean. This is true especially in women.[6]

Perhaps most important to many people is that these benefits mean better sleep because of less pain and normalized cortisol.[6] Once again, the effects were even more pronounced in the female subjects.

Some of my predictions for the future include more research coming to light that shows the benefits of earthing on a wide range of physiological functions.

A more recent study found changes in thyroid hormone levels, showing an impact on metabolism as well.[9] Considering the rates of thyroid dysfunction, this is another important benefit.

EMFs

Electromagnetism is a force that exhibits both electric and magnetic fields. They're simply different manifestations of the same force. In addition to the electrical connection to the earth, there is a magnetic one.

EMFs or electromagnetic frequencies are a huge group of many things. Visible light, infrared, radio and cosmic rays and many more all fit into this category. There are both natural EMFs and man-made ones. When the term is used, it is often about these man-made ones that come from our phones, WiFi, and every electrical device we make.

For years industry has been saying that man-made EMFs don't have negative consequences on human health, except by thermal effects (heating). (Just like the tobacco companies swore that the research wasn't in. Unfortunately, it's a common tactic.)

But more and more research is coming to light about what these EMFs are doing to us. It is very clear that mobile phones being carried in pockets negatively affect sperm quality in men.[10] There is a link between exposure to extremely low frequency fields and breast cancer.[11] It's clear that some of these fields are causing damage to DNA.[12]

The "NIH National Toxicology Program Cell Phone Radiofrequency Radiation Study," was large, well-designed, and well-controlled study. It found that "Exposures to 'weak' levels of radio-frequency radiation can have a significant impact. If wireless frequencies were 'safe' and had 'no impact on the body', one would not see such results." One of the lead scientists involved in this study, Ronald Melnick, said, "This study should put an end to those who doubt the capacity of non-thermal levels of wireless radiation to cause biological effects including cancer. The study results clearly show that cell phone radiation can cause adverse health effects. The counter argument has no validity."[13]

The industry has claimed that EMFs can't be harmful because there is no mechanism of action by which we understand how it works. As if that makes it true, just because we can't explain how something works. But Dr. Michael L. Pall has proposed that these EMF effects are occurring through the voltage-gated calcium channels that cause oxidative stress in cells, leading to such things as DNA damage.[14]

While it isn't foolproof, by being grounded, you are effectively shielded from these harmful EMFs to some degree.

In a typical home office setting the grounded test group saw voltages in their body decrease by a factor of 58 on average.[15] Whether it is because the electrical connection allows you to discharge these frequencies or that the earth's own frequency overrides or blocks the EMFs, we can't say for sure. But this effect is yet another benefit that earthing can bring.

Effects on Mood and Neurology

In a study with 27 participants, grounding helped improve heartrate variability (HRV).[16] HRV is a measure of the beat-to-beat alterations in the heart rate and is an important measure of nervous system and cardiovascular function. In this study, they found that HRV kept improving the longer the duration, up to the end of the allotted forty-minute period, showing greater benefit with more time. Along with this were reported reductions in anxiety, stress, fear, and panic.

A double-blind study, where participants were measured with the Brief Mood Introspection Scale, found that those grounded improved mood more than the placebo group, showing greater benefits than relaxation alone.[17]

In measurements with EEG, the tool that measures electrical activity in the brain, earthing has been shown to have neuromodulating properties too.[18]

In essence, earthing affects just about everything. We see benefits to many foundational systems like inflammation, cortisol, and circulation. We see that it is not just physical but affects our psychology too.

Remember the EZ, or liquid-crystalline phase of water, discussed a few chapters back. This structuring of water takes energy to do so. And I'd be willing to bet that earthing is one method that gives your body the energy it needs to drive this reaction. Being that we're made up of water, that is in use in every function, then it makes sense that the effects on the body would be systemic and alter everything.

The question to ask yourself is when was the last time you were grounded?

How to Ground Yourself

Now let's cover the actionable steps you can take to get these benefits. First and foremost, spend time outdoors while barefoot. If you have a yard you can do this easily at your home. If you don't have a yard, there's undoubtedly some parks around at the very least. Take a moment to think of the earth. We've generally only impacted the surface of it by laying concrete and asphalt. Even in a huge city the earth surrounds us. So, you just need to find those spots where it is available.

The more surface area you have contacting the earth the more the electrical flow can take place. Lying on the earth is going to allow for more flow than just the bottoms of your feet. Still, any contact is much better than none at all.

What is the ultimate way to get earthed? It's not actually with the ground, but instead with natural bodies of water. The water is conductive, and you get full body contact if you are fully submerged.

In fact, the one and only time many people get grounded in their daily lives is when they take a shower. If you're close to the water stream and it is steadily supplied, this conducts to the metal pipes, which ultimately are connected to the ground. Perhaps this is why many people look forward to showering, and also why many people have insights while in there. Those benefits on the physical and mental side of things allow more ideas to come forth.

How much time do you need to spend earthing? Because of the electrical connection involved there is some benefit for getting grounded for even just the briefest amount of time. As anyone who has worked with electronics can tell you, this can serve to discharge collected static electricity.

So, if you are walking around town in your rubber soled shoes, you can reach out and touch a tree, or a plant growing up out of the sidewalk, or a bare patch of earth when you see it.

But for the deeper benefits, the more time you spend grounded the better. As a good baseline, spend at least half an hour per day grounded. This shouldn't be asking too much, especially when you realize that for the best benefits it should be closer to 24/7.

This is one of the benefits I like to get while doing my workouts outside. By being barefooted not only do I get the proprioceptive benefits of bare feet on the ground but the extensive benefits of earthing too. It's being proactive in reducing muscle soreness.

If quality sleep is something you're seeking to get more of, then spend the time looking at the morning sun after you rise and do it while getting grounded outside. Take a few deep breaths, and you've stacked the benefits once again. Your circadian rhythm will thank you.

Another great option is gardening. Anyone that gardens knows that health benefits come from the process. By having your fingers in your dirt, you're getting earthed, and that's responsible for some of them.

And if you have children who are playing outside, play with them after kicking off your shoes.

Grounding Technology

While the best option is to actually get outside to get earthed, because this comes with the other benefits of getting some nature time, the fact is that most of us spend a lot of time indoors whether at work, at home, or in recreation.

What about all that time we spend indoors? As you may have gathered from the studies mentioned, there are ways to keep yourself grounded, even as you sleep in your own bed. These grounding products either use a grounding rod that is stuck into the earth or make use of the grounding plug available in almost all homes and buildings.

In fact, I'm grounded right now as I'm writing this to you. I have a connected and conductive pad under my feet, so I can be grounded, and receive all the tremendous benefits, even while I'm working in my office.

There are several different products available to ground you in the comfort of your own home. You can find these at: www.legendarystrength.com/go/earthing

If you think about this as an investment it can be well worth the money because you can reap the benefits long term.

However, this does come with a caveat. Not every house appears to be properly grounded. Due to how it is wired, in some cases you may be plugging yourself into something you don't want to. With the small wrist straps I have felt "zapped" by electricity. If this is occurring, you're probably adding free radicals to your body, not the reverse!

For these reasons, if possible, instead of relying on the grounded outlet, run a wire from your grounded bed sheet, or other device, to a metal rod outside.

Also, it is possible that some areas of the earth may, in a sense, not be properly grounded. If lots of dirty electricity is running through them, you may not receive all the benefits. The good news is that this only appears to be the case in some areas.

Thus, touching the real earth, especially deep in nature, is the best way to do it, but if you do have outlets that are properly grounded you can put them to good use. Because the benefits are big, and we spend lots of time indoors, it is worth experimenting with these devices. With your own experience, you may be able to note changes to pain, your mood, sleep, soreness and more.

Grounded Shoes

Shoes with rubber soles insulate you from the healthful effects of the earth. Rubber is used because it is an easy-to-use material, flexible, resists damage, and ultimately is great at protecting your feet.

(Most shoes also act as a cast, putting your feet into unnatural positions, and thus cause atrophy in the musculature of the feet, as discussed in the Movement chapter.)

Before rubber was used commercially, more natural materials like leather were often used. After leather is worn in and your skin oils are leeched into it, this material is conductive. You can still find traditionally made moccasins in a few places.

Also, since this research has come to light a number of companies that make grounded shoes and sandals have been discovered. While still using rubber soles because of the protective benefits, they use some sort of conductive material that connects your foot to the earth electrically. This way you can have your feet protected so that you're not fully barefoot, but you'll still get the earthing benefits.

I'm currently a big fan of Earth Runners as they are minimalist sandals in addition to being grounded. No one else, at the time of this writing, covers both of these benefits. You can find out more details at: www.legendarystrength.com/go/earthrunners

Also, concrete is still grounded, while asphalt is not. So, depending on where you walk, even in big cities, you may still be able to get the benefits.

Mentally and Spiritually Grounded

This entire chapter has been devoted to the physical and electrical connection to the earth. However, that's not the only thing to be discussed.

Research has been conducted on the consequences of living in high-rise building, on different floors, as well as compared to detached homes. While there are many confounding factors, from air quality, emergency response times, social effects, and more, much of the research shows the negative impacts in living higher.[19]

One part that is not often discussed is the possibility that being further away from the earth may have subtle health effects as well. We know that in space the human body rapidly degrades without the effects of gravity. Of course, gravity is still in effect on the 20th floor, but perhaps something else is going on.

To wrap up this chapter I'd like to go back to one of the concepts mentioned near the beginning of it. In being disconnected from nature, in this case physically by touch, we've further disconnected from nature. Physical and electrical ungroundedness likely leads to mental and spiritual ungroundedness too.

Think about the rise of depression, anxiety, and other psychological disorders. Contrast that to how many people report a feeling of calm while being in nature. The earlier research we looked at showed positive effects on mood. Thus, it is clear that earthing extends beyond just the physical health benefits.

And in the end, a physical connection to the earth may just be the foundation needed for any kind of real, grounded spirituality.

12
Food

"Let nothing which can be treated by diet be treated by other means."
– Maimonides

P ut two nutritionists in a room and you'll get three ideas about diet. Part of me didn't even want to address the topic of food in this book. While food is certainly important, it does not trump the importance of all the other steps found in these pages. Yet, in the West, we have a collective obsession with food and diets.

Trust me, I know, as I have experience in obsessing over food. Orthorexia is the term used to describe an obsession with eating foods that one considers healthy. This is considered a medical condition. Although I was never diagnosed, as I don't need to be boxed into a definition of something that is really just a process, I know I exhibited the characteristics of the condition from time to time.

When I first got into food, realizing it was important for health and performance, I quite naturally sought out the best diet. At the time, this seemed to be the raw food vegan diet. It just made sense. Humans are the only ones that cook their food which destroys all the living enzymes inside. If you want death and disease, then eat dead food. If you want to live, eat live food. Simple as that, or so it seemed.

But raw food proved to be a tough diet to follow. The most I ever did was a month at a time.

While there are still proponents, most of the advocates of the diet in the early 2000s have turned back to cooked food. A lot of them have left veganism too. I personally know a few of them.

Still, for many years, I knew this was how I "should" eat. And if I wasn't eating that way I often felt bad about it. Unfortunately, this kind of self-judgement led to binging behavior. There are times, plural, when I ate an entire half gallon of ice cream in one sitting.

These days I still focus on food, but no longer hold raw food as some ideal. What I see as the best food ever has shifted and I'm happy to say that's what I eat most of the time. However, even when I don't, I'm much more relaxed about it. I largely avoid certain things that I don't even see as food anymore (such as McDonald's) not out of willpower, but from having truly shifted my desires.

I share my story here to reveal the dark side of obsession with food. I don't deny that what you eat is important. But my main point here, one that I hope you take to heart, is that food is relatively unimportant next to all the other aspects of your health covered in this book.

To properly demonstrate this, let me ask a question. Whom do you think would be healthier; the person that ate the best diet ever, but neglected their breathing, sun exposure, their sleep, their water supply, was exposed to toxins in a wide variety of places other than food, and so on, or the person that ate crappy food, but took good care of everything else in their life?

I am sure you would agree that it would be the latter. Of course, what you eat and don't eat must be viewed as a single factor, albeit a significant one, in the complete picture of health. But it needs to be knocked down a peg or two in the place it holds collectively. It's important, but not that important.

If you have struggled with food all your life, I would encourage you not to even worry about it for the next couple months as you instead focus on the other aspects of natural health instead.

That is also why you won't find any recipes in this book about health. Instead we're just going to look at some of the big principles around food, so that we can avoid getting roped into eating fads, as I was with the raw food.

It seems these principles have been lost in the shuffle from diet to diet. In the end, it comes down to eating the most natural food possible, processed in natural ways. This may be tougher than it seems though, because of how our food supply has changed over the years, so that what is natural is far from clear.

154

"You are what you eat"

This is a common saying. It may even be cliché. But I think it is important to look at it closely for a minute. It is literally true in that the cells of your body are made up of the cells of whatever you consume and absorb. Nutrients get broken down and altered, but your food is the starting material.

Thus, if you want to be healthy, you need good starting material. For example, every cell membrane is made up of fats. If these are high quality, natural fats, then the cells are likely to function well. If these are partially hydrogenated, rancid or trans fats, coming from overly processed foods, then your cells will not function as well. Specifically, it looks like the ratio of omega 3 to omega 6 fatty acids is important.[1]

Without the right starting material, your cells cannot function properly. It's as simple as that. Is it any wonder we see "resistance" in cellular receptors like with insulin, as seen in diabetes, if what composes the receptors is poor-quality material?

"You are what you eat eats"

"The whole of nature, as has been said, is a conjugation of the verb to eat, in the active and in the passive," said William Ralph Inge. If you are what you eat, this is similarly true for every other living thing. If a cow eats its natural diet of grass, rather than being fed moldy grain, its cells will similarly be healthier, thus making it healthier to eat. This line of reasoning doesn't apply just to animals.

Plant life "eats" as well. It's not through a mouth, nor digesting in the same way, but they still absorb nutrition. What they eat is largely the soil, as well as the sun and water. If the proper minerals are not present in the soil, the plant will not be as nutritious as it can be. It certainly won't have those minerals present. If this is grass that the cow then eats, up the chain it goes. The cow's cells get made up of the grass which is made up of the soil. If it is lettuce that you then eat, its health depends on the soil. Up the chain it goes. This is true for every living thing.

Masonobu Fukuoka developed "natural farming" in Japan. Another

155

name for his methods is do-nothing farming, because few interventions are done, not even composting or pruning of trees. Instead it is working with the ecology to naturally produce food. He wrote, "Far from being dead and inanimate, the soil is teeming with life." Elsewhere he continued this thought, "Is it really possible to restore the balance of nature by spraying an array of bactericides and fungicides like this into a soil populated with such a large variety of microbes?"

The soil is not just about minerals but about the life it contains. These organisms, about which we know little, are not thought of in the majority of farming operations. Instead we bring in "help" from the outside.

Regarding this, Sir Albert Howard, a botanist and early pioneer of organic farming, said, "When we feed the soil with artificials, it creates artificial plants, which make artificial animals, which make artificial people who can only be kept alive with artificials."

Quality food must come from quality food all up the food chain. Unfortunately, this is becoming tougher and tougher to do in our polluted and depleted world. But it can be done.

"You are how you eat"

How you eat can be looked at in a couple of different ways. How the food is prepared is a big part of this. Is the food raw? Is it cooked? How is it cooked? What is it combined with? While the best methods vary from food to food, how the food is eaten is almost as important as the starting quality.

Certain methods of preparation can turn the best food, let's say an omega 3 fatty acid, into the worst food, rancid oil that will wreak havoc in your body.[2] While this is an extreme example, it underlies the importance of how food is prepared. Cooking will often destroy certain nutrients, or cause certain changes in structure, but there are also times when it enhances nutrition.

Another part of how you eat is in how you consume it. Are you gobbling down food as fast as possible, or eating at a normal or pleasant pace? This blends into the next piece.

"You are what you absorb"

Just because you swallow something doesn't actually mean that it will become a part of your body. Your digestive process determines what is absorbed and what is not.

Because of damage to our microbiome and use of various things that cause intestinal permeability (like gluten, whether you're intolerant of it or not[3]) or lowered stomach acid, many people aren't absorbing most of the nutrients from the food they eat.

And then there is the fact that we absorb more than through just our digestive tract. Our skin is absorbing material, good and bad, as well. In essence, you are also "eating" whatever your put on your body.

"You are what you don't eliminate"

On the flip side of absorption is elimination. Unfortunately, the body is absorbing many things that you don't necessarily want. And that means that these things are a part of you, at least until they are eliminated. The body has multiple pathways of elimination including urination, defecation, sweating, and the breath, and different things may be eliminated with each.

This is added in here because what you eat, and how you eat it, also play roles in what gets eliminated.

"You are who you eat with"

We are social creatures. It's not just the food, but factors like who you eat with that play a role too. Perhaps it is because they influence you in all these other aspects.

Or perhaps it's because you actually end up sharing bacteria with them, as discussed in a later chapter.

A 2009 study showed that that if your friends or family are obese then you are 10 to 45 percent more likely to be obese, depending on how close to these people you were.[4]

157

"You are when and where you eat"

Some dieticians seem to think there is a magic window of 24 hours. All the calories you eat only matters in that time frame. Whether it is morning or noon has no difference.

But the fact is that when you eat can have a very real impact, simply for the reason that your hormones are different at different times of day.[5] Some say that breakfast is the most important meal of the day. Others avoid breakfast completely and stick to dinner as the main meal. And still others tout lunch as the best time to eat the most. I don't claim to have the answer here, besides, it is surely different for different people. I bring it up to say that when you eat is also a factor.

The location of your meals is going to affect many of these things as well. Imagine that you enjoy a meal while sitting outside in the fresh air and the sun, feet on the earth, while relaxed. Compare this to trying to eat quickly because you're on the road and have somewhere to be. Do you think this could change absorption of your food and how it is utilized inside your body?

Obviously, we need to look at many different factors, not just in the food, but our environment too. For now, let's dig deeper into the aspect of food quality, as this is critical.

Food Quality

When we are talking about food quality it comes down to a few things. Sean Croxton, a well-known podcaster, put it succinctly, "just eat real food." This is known as JERF for short. It's a simple idea, but one that will take you 80 percent of the way to a healthier food goal.

So, what is real food? It is food that is natural. It is food you can identify. Most often, it does not come in a package and doesn't have a label.

Weston A. Price was a dentist that traveled the world and looked at the teeth of native populations that maintained their traditional diets as compared to those that started eating "white man foods." His research lays the best groundwork for what humans naturally eat, better than any double-blind study because of its breadth and depth, and the fact that it follows the principles of natural living. These were humans well adapted to their environments.

In the prologue of his book, *Nutrition and Physical Degeneration*, he sums up the research. "The diets of the healthy primitives Price studied were diverse. Some were based on sea foods, some on domesticated animals, some on game, and some on dairy products. Some contained almost no plant foods while others contained a variety of fruits, vegetables, grains and legumes. In some mostly cooked foods were eaten, while in others many foods—including animal foods—were eaten raw. However, these diets shared several underlying characteristics. None contained any refined or devitalized foods such as white sugar or flour, canned foods, pasteurized or skimmed milk, and refined and hydrogenated vegetable oils. All the diets contained animal products of some sort and all included some salt. Preservation methods among primitive groups included drying, salting, and fermenting, all of which preserve and even increase nutrients in our food."

It is obvious humans can adapt to very different diets. But in looking at common ground you can find similarities across the globe in traditional diets. Before we dive further into these, it is important to look at what is not natural.

Slightly Poisoned Food

That there is even debate as to whether organic food is better than conventional food, sprayed with pesticides, herbicides, larvicides, fungicides, and insecticides is laughable. These poisons kill off life. That is their job. To think that they only affect certain types of life and not your own is arrogant, especially since when use of these began, science tended to look only at the effects on human cells, not all of the bacteria and everything else that makes up us.

As one review of the research put it, "There is a body of evidence suggesting that gut microbiota are a major, yet underestimated element that must be considered to fully evaluate the toxicity of environmental contaminants."[6]

Let me reiterate that. When modern agriculture with its various chemicals came on the scene, we did not realize the importance of the gut bacteria. At that time, we were under the impression that all bacteria were bad. As you'll come to see in the chapter on Symbiosis, this is far from the case. And these chemicals have not been heavily investigated to see what they do to our microbiome that makes up a good portion of us.

Let's look at corn, to see how far down the unnatural hole we can go. Corn was one of the main crops for Native Americans. They revered it as one of their staple foods. The original wild grass (yes, corn is a grass, not a vegetable) was a plant called teosinte. Its kernels were 30 percent protein and only 2 percent sugar.

As the natives farmed the corn, rather than just wild harvesting it, it began to change. Up until about a century ago we had sweet corn that was now only 4 percent protein and 10 percent sugar. But it didn't end there.

Modern sweet corn was genetically modified by a nuclear bomb. This sounds impossible, but it is true. Back in 1947, corn seeds, along with other foods, were experimented on by nuclear blast on the Bikini Atoll of the Marshall Islands. This is written up in a government document titled *"Effects of an Atomic Bomb Explosion on Corn Seeds"*, which was declassified in 1997.[7] The irradiated corn was found to be super sweet, so a geneticist working with the radiated corn, John Laughnan, began selling it.

That's a scary enough idea...that very few people know about. But that wasn't all. Further genetic changes were made to corn.

Glyphosate, popularly known as Roundup, keeps pests away by chelating some minerals from the food. In fact, it was first patented by Stauffer Chemical as a chemical chelator. It has been shown to deplete manganese in the plants, as well as in animals that fed on those plants.[8]

Furthermore, the shikimate pathway that is at use in plants, through which glyphosate kills weeds, is also present in bacteria, though not in animals.[9] Some of the most pervasive genetic modifications were not to try to make a plant healthier or more nutritious, but instead to be Roundup Ready, that is able to absorb more of this herbicide.

The latest GMO corn creates Bt toxin itself, or *Bacillus thuringiensis*, as it was mixed with bacteria genes. Since it comes from bacteria, and bacteria swap DNA readily in a process called horizontal gene transfer, these same poison-producing genes may be taken on by the bacteria living in your stomach.[10] Eaten tortilla chips at home or a restaurant lately? Sadly, this poison may now be produced from inside you.

But don't we need these things to grow crops? The real issue with pests and molds is in monocropping products. Nature sees this as unsustainable, because it is, and aims to take it out. Healthy plants will fight off insects to some degree themselves. That old teosinte grew wildly and defended itself just fine without human hands. That's what healthy plants do.

While the promise was better living through chemistry, and later genetics, this hasn't proven to increase yields in the long run.[11]

Plus, we really don't know how far changes in DNA may spread. It's a possibility that in genetically modified wheat, those modifications may silence part of human DNA.[12]

Dr. Steve Klayman says, "Man, in his attempt to improve on nature, is creating a disaster. This disaster, now, is banned in many countries around the world, because they recognize what it is. Unfortunately, in America, the politicians are paid off so that they won't ban it."

Remember that you are what you eat eats. The soils where these crops are grown tend to be far more polluted than those that are grown organically. If the soil doesn't have the proper minerals, or microbes present, the plant itself can't be healthy. Then if you eat it, it can't produce health in you.

In general, eating organic is a step in the right direction. This eliminates GMO's by law, at least for now. It means that poisons aren't directly sprayed, though they're still everywhere in the environment, so neither are these completely clean.

And it is important to note that all organic food is not equal. There are still large monocrop farming operations that have gotten on the organic bandwagon due to customer demand. Generally, from soil quality alone, but also the length and time of shipping, these foods will not be as high quality as something grown more locally by smaller operation farms.

These same concepts hold true of animal foods. Unfortunately, we've polluted virtually all of our oceans, seas, and rivers. So, finding unpolluted seafood is becoming much harder. However, there is research showing that the selenium, also present in seafood, can protect against mercury.[13] Mercury causes damage to the nervous system, yet selenium binds to mercury and detoxifies it. Still, the amounts of mercury, not to mention other contaminants, in bigger fish, such as tuna, should probably be avoided or at least minimized by everyone.

Cows and chickens are "monocropped" in much the same way as fruits and vegetables. They're pumped full of poisons to artificially keep them alive and help them gain weight faster. In animal husbandry, there is something called feed efficiency. Animals gain weight faster when they are on antibiotics.[14] They can be fed the same amount of food, but those on antibiotics turn it into more body mass. Similarly, cows also have increased feed efficiency when estrogen was implanted in them.[15]

This fact alone shows that calories are not the be all, end all answer as some claim. Do you think the same effect doesn't occur in humans?

These animals are fed unnatural diets. Thus, they are not healthy and thus cannot produce health in those that eat them, whether it is eggs, milk products or meat. Fortunately, in all these cases there are better, non-poisoned options available. One of my favorite books about food is Michael Pollan's *The Omnivore's Dilemma*. This gives you an inside look into the different methods of creating food, comparing the industrial to the organic to the beyond organic to the wild.

For example, pastured chicken eggs are much healthier than conventional or even organic eggs. When on pasture land the chicken can eat a varied diet including insects and not just grain that they are fed. A study found pastured eggs, compared to eggs from caged birds, to have twice as much vitamin E, two and a half times the Omega-3 fatty acids, and a 38-percent-higher concentration of vitamin A.[16]

Many people ditch animal foods because they believe them to be unhealthy. And yes, if the animals themselves are unhealthy, then they, or the food products they create, are unhealthy as food. Yet, this same holds true of any food you eat. It's just with animals; being made up of more different food, the effects of bioaccumulation increase the problems of toxicity.

Whatever the food is, the problem is minimized when we strive for the cleanest foods we can find, where poisons are not sprayed, and genetics aren't tampered with, and the highest quality natural diets are in use.

Properly Processed

Although I harped on raw food as an exclusive diet, many foods like fruits and vegetables, nuts and seeds can be best for you in their raw state.

Cooking is just one grouping of processes. You can steam, boil, bake, fry and many more options. Sometimes this is beneficial. For example, tomatoes release far more lycopene when they are cooked.

Despite the assertions of raw foodists, the evidence suggests that cooking is in fact what helped separate us from other animals and made us human. For details on this, read *Catching Fire: How Cooking Made Us Human*, by Richard Wrangham.

Each food seems to have an ideal way to be processed. For example, garlic must be crushed or cut, and allowed to sit for ten minutes or so, for an enzymatic reaction to occur which creates allicin. At that point, the garlic can be used for cooking. Or you can enjoy garlic raw, but most people don't like that intensity. I picked up the above trick from Jo Robinson's, *Eating on the Wild Side*. Throughout that book, you'll learn all kinds of tips and tricks to maximize the nutrition you can get from many fruits and vegetables. It also provides suggestions for which varieties to get.

Nuts, seeds, grains, and legumes should be soaked before use. This deactivates phytates, which are enzyme inhibitors inside of them. This allows more of their nutrients to be absorbed and also stops the phytates from robbing you of iron, zinc, manganese, and calcium. However, phytates aren't completely bad either. There is evidence that some can offer protection against cancer and other diseases.[17]

The term "processed foods" is often used synonymously with bad food, but it really depends on the type of processing. In general, heavily processed foods are bad. When you can't tell what is in the food item from looking at it, chances are it is not be the best choice.

And in general, we want to avoid processing that takes high levels of technology to perform. While there are certainly exceptions, chances are if you couldn't do it at home, it often shouldn't be done.

But processing is not good or bad by itself. It depends on the food and it depends on the process. In general, we want to use processes that minimize any anti-nutrients, while maximizing absorbable nutrition. This may involve soaking, sprouting, cooking, fermenting, combining, and any number of other options.

Local Food and Freshness

While it is amazing that any meal we eat can have foods that come from disparate parts of the world, this too comes at a cost.

What is better? A head of lettuce from the supermarket, or the head of lettuce from the farmer's market? Even if they're of the same variety and both organic, it will almost always be the lettuce from the farmer's market. This is because it has likely just been picked that morning, rather than days or even weeks earlier. By being fresher, more of the nutrition is present.

Even better than that would be lettuce from a garden you pick yourself, or wild greens you forage that day.

Foods that comes from your local environment are going to capture something else from the environment as well.

In a testament to how freshness matters, Price wrote, "I asked an old Indian whom I saw grinding corn between two stones why he did not use larger stones and grind a lot at a time. His reply to all of my questions was 'no good'. When I reduced the time down for the flour to be used in three days he still said 'no.' When I asked him why, he said 'something gone'. His magnificent physical condition at a very advanced age strongly testified to the wisdom of his program."

This principle states that the more local and fresher your food is, the better it will be for you. While certain foods can be processed and packaged in ways that can maximize nutrition, this is a rule of thumb you'll want to follow predominately.

Macronutrients

The average person looks at calories. Some people still claim that calories are the only thing that matter. Even though we saw that with the use of antibiotics increasing feed efficiency, this is disproven as the only factor that matters.

Considering that a calorie doesn't even exist, it seems odd to me that it is considered by some as the only thing of importance. A food calorie is a unit of energy needed to raise the temperature of 1 kilogram of water by 1 degree Celsius. Of course, your body is doing more than heating water with the food you consume. While looking at calories can be useful in certain times, it is not the answer to health.

Other people will then look one step down on the food label and see the macronutrients, fat, protein and carbohydrates. The majority of diets out there involve minimizing or trying to get rid of one or more of these, while maximizing the others. Sometimes they are all seen as important, but the ratio between them becomes paramount.

There's been low fat, no fat, high fat, high protein, low protein, low carb, very low carb, high carb, etc. Every iteration has been tried.

These macronutrients are very important. And changing them can and will have dramatic impacts on health and performance. But it is important to note that a fat is not a fat, a carb is not a carb, and a protein is not a protein. To put it another way, partially hydrogenated GMO canola oil is not fish oil. Fat from a grass-fed cow is not the same as fat from a grain-fed cow. These are all fats, but they are not equal.

High fructose corn syrup, is not the same as table sugar, is not the same as broccoli, is not the same as a sweet potato. All are carbs, but they are not the same thing. Protein from a cow is not the same as protein from rice. Both are proteins, but they are not the same.

These are just generalizations or categories of things. To imagine that they are all equal is ludicrous. Equally crazy is to base our health upon such generalizations.

The Importance of Fat

Our society is carb heavy. While I'm not going to say that you need to cut out carbs or go low carb, I am going to tout the benefits of fat. I think the demonization of fat, as described in depth by Nina Teicholz in *The Big Fat Surprise*, better than anything else explains how we can get far off track based on our science, running blind down the wrong road.

Many in the health field have caught onto this and are sharing it with clients and others, but the message still hasn't quite reached the masses.

Ancel Keys, the main scientist behind the diet-heart hypothesis, actually conducted a study to look at animal fat versus non-animal fat— except he didn't use animal fat. He used margarine, a hydrogenated vegetable oil containing as much as 48 percent trans-fat. Labelling this as saturated fat, he then jumped to the conclusion that animal fats were unhealthy.[18] That is quite a leap, one that is far from scientific.

It has taken many years to correct this idea that spread far and wide. Things like heart disease weren't caused by animal fat. Cholesterol is not the problem. In fact, cholesterol is largely a good thing. And how much cholesterol you eat doesn't really affect your cholesterol levels; instead, most is made in your liver.[19]

And in the latest and best-quality studies done on the topic, there is no relation between saturated fat intake and heart disease.[20] In fact, a higher intake of saturated fats was associated with less risk of stroke.[21]

Not only is fat the best fuel source, but different types of fat are used for many structures, like cell membranes, and functions in the body, like mediating inflammation. Fats coat all your nervous system cells. Fats are used by your heart, your lungs, even your bones.

Of course, as previously mentioned, not all fats are created equal. Far from it. Even if we go a step down in categories. Not all saturated fats are equal. Not all polyunsaturated fats are equal. Not all monounsaturated fats are equal.

Keys and others have largely misled us. Labels state that canola oil is heart healthy, based on flawed science, but that is a lie. Mary Enig, of the Weston A. Price foundation said, "Like all modern vegetable oils, canola oil goes through the process of refining, bleaching and degumming — all of which involve high temperatures or chemicals of questionable safety. And because canola oil is high in omega-3 fatty acids, which easily become rancid and foul-smelling when subjected to oxygen and high temperatures, it must be deodorized. The standard deodorization process removes a large portion of the omega-3 fatty acids by turning them into trans fatty acids. Although the Canadian government lists the trans content of canola at a minimal 0.2 percent, research at the University of Florida at Gainesville, found trans levels as high as 4.6 percent in commercial liquid oil. The consumer has no clue about the presence of trans fatty acids in canola oil because they are not listed on the label."

Japanese research, done for the National Institutes of Health, stated that high omega-6 vegetable oils, "are inappropriate for human use as foods."[22]

Recall my discussion of processing foods. Could you squeeze enough rapeseeds (the origin of canola) or soy beans to make oil at your home? Would you then refine, bleach, and degum it yourself?

Here's how I look at fat, from the foundation of principles rather than hype. Ask yourself, is this fat easily obtained from nature and does it come from a healthy source?

Rich fat sources like avocados, olives and coconuts are all touted for their benefits. If olives are picked at the right time, it only takes a minimum of processes to make oil from it. Sadly, many olive oils are cut with other oil like canola. If you want really good olive oil look for unfiltered varieties. These are much richer in polyphenols and other components from the olives.

Some say fat in red meat will kill you. But that doesn't make the critical distinction between a healthy and an unhealthy cow.

Animal fat is good for you, if it comes from healthy sources. Seafood can be some of the best fat sources there are, depending on what the fish eats.[23] Price wrote, "I have been impressed with the superior quality of the human stock developed by Nature wherever a liberal source of sea foods existed."

Here's what to look for. Wild caught fish from more pristine areas like Alaskan salmon. Farmed fish has been fed grain and have much higher levels of toxic heavy metals and other pollutants. (The good news is that there is news of fish-farming operations that are done right, so this generalization may not always continue to be true.) In general, to minimize toxic exposure eat lower on the food chain. Eat sardines instead of shark.

But it's not just fish. Cows, pigs, chickens, ducks—all of their saturated animal fat can be good for you, if it comes from healthy animals. Some of the best fats, docosahexaenoic acid (DHA) and arachidonic acid

(AA), are found in healthy animal fats. These fats are crucial for brain function as they structurally make up much of the brain.[24] When a cow eats its natural diet of grass, rather than grain, it significantly changes the fatty acid profile of the cow, and therefore of the milk and meat that is taken from it.[25]

Nora Gedgaudas, in *Primal Fat Burner*, points out that human beings thrived, and actually had even bigger brains, before the last ice age. At this time, we hunted mega-fauna, like wooly mammoths and land sloths, that could be up to 50 percent fat.

Micronutrients

When it comes to health, more attention needs to be paid to the micronutrients instead of macronutrients. Most notable of these are vitamins and minerals, though this also includes things like antioxidants and phytonutrients.

You need all of the vitamins, A, B-complex, C, D, E, and K in abundant supply to be healthy and perform at an optimal level. The RDI numbers put out by the government are notoriously low. While these amounts may prevent you from deficiency diseases like rickets for D and scurvy for C, it by no means discusses an optimal amount. Nor does this consider individual differences. Nor that different types of the vitamins may be absorbed or utilized differently. After all, these are generalizations too. It doesn't take into account that when you're fighting an acute or chronic disease your need for one or more vitamins can increase dramatically.

These same facts hold true for minerals. There are the major minerals that many people know about like calcium and magnesium, though that doesn't necessarily mean people don't need more of them. Many estimates are that over three-quarters of the population is deficient in magnesium, which plays a role in over 300 enzymatic functions in the human body.[26] A whopping 3,571 magnesium binding sites have been detected on human proteins.[27] So being depleted of magnesium is going to be a root issue for all kinds of problems.

Then there are the typical trace minerals. Copper plays a big role in our metabolism, as its used in functioning of many critical enzymes, among much else. Zinc plays a role in proliferation, differentiation, and metabolic function of our cells, is critical for sex hormones, among much else. Chromium plays an important role in blood sugar levels, among much else. Cobalt makes up part of vitamin B12, among much else. Selenium fights cancer, among much else.[8]

Every day new research is uncovering more and more about how much these do for human health. Boron wasn't on the radar until recent years. Now it's been shown to be linked to stopping arthritis and osteoporosis and aiding in sex hormone production.[29]

All these described are the major minerals and the "main" trace minerals. But we can go further. The issue here is we don't know much about what many of these do. What do we know about lutetium, ruthenium, scandium, gadolinium, yttrium? Chances are you probably haven't even heard of some or all of those since your high school chemistry class.

Maybe a hafnium deficiency leads to your eyes wearing out. Or an osmium one that stops your hormone production. Or maybe it's a combination issue brought about by lack of dysprosium, erbium, and tellurium that affects your joint pain. I'm making things up here, as I do not know if those elements are linked to any of those things specifically, but I hope you get my point. What if just one part per million makes a difference?

This speaks to the importance of getting trace minerals. The easiest way to do this is with sea salt, which contains many trace minerals, whereas normal table salt does not.

And you'll also find lots more minerals in your food when you eat a diverse, high-quality diet. Price found that native diets typically had ten or more times the fat-soluble vitamins, and somewhere between one-and-a-half times to fifty times the mineral concentrations than the typical US diet. That was during his time. The average American's diet is even worse today.

Furthermore, he wrote, "We human beings of modern civilization are at a great disadvantage in the selections of foods in that we seem to have lost a sixth sense by which we would recognize a specific need for special food. Many of the primitive races and most animals retain the capacity to satisfy the body needs by choosing the foods that will provide minerals and vitamins."

You Must Eat Life to Live

It is important to realize that you must eat life to survive. There is no way to get around this.

I spent six months as a vegetarian because I thought this was the healthy way to go. Many people have been swayed to this line of thinking.

While I recognize that animals should not be harmed needlessly, life takes life. That is natural and there is no way around it. Animals are not the only thing living. As you'll come to see in a later chapter plants have awareness too. Just because they don't have a face, doesn't mean they're not alive.

We are disconnected from the web of life and death because, for most of us, we're brought up completely removed from it. When all your food comes from the market, rather than the field, the river or the forest, you're physically disconnected from the nature of it.

I know I am. Only in recent years have I begun to forage a very small amount of my food. Recently, I went fishing for the first time in my life and have done so a couple times since. I am working to increase the amount of active involvement I have in my food.

Here I'd like to make the case for omnivory. First, just looking at the structure of our mouth and digestion you can see that they are far more similar to carnivores, and nothing like ruminants, those that eat grass.

We have canine teeth for tearing flesh. But we have smaller mouths and teeth and weaker jaws than strict carnivores. We also have flat molars for grinding up food. We only have one stomach, as oppose to a cow's four. Our intestines are far shorter than herbivores. But we also contain enzymes like amylase which allow us to break down carbohydrates, which many carnivores lack, though we can't break down cellulose. Meanwhile food doesn't stay in our stomachs for the length of time it does in carnivores.

Looking at this, it's obvious we're neither pure carnivore or herbivore.

So, what are we like? Katherine Milton found that there were two primates whose guts were very similar to ours. "Capuchin monkey (*Cebus* species) which has a high-quality diet of sweet fruits, oily seeds, and (40–50% by feeding time) animal foods—invertebrates (insects) and small vertebrates. The savanna baboon (*Papio papio*) is a selective feeder who searches for high-quality, nutritious foods."[30]

The term *high-quality* here is used to designate higher-calorie food sources, whether plant or animal origin, as opposed to leaves and most vegetation. The "expensive tissue hypothesis" explains that compared to other animals, our brains use up proportionally more energy than the gut, thus we need richer food sources that take less digestion.[31]

Many people have been swayed to vegetarianism or veganism by work such as T. Colin Campbell's *The China Study*, or a series of recent documentaries like *What the Health*. One problem is that in many of these, the diets are compared with the Standard American Diet. Of course, a vegan diet, when a person starts actually eating fruits and vegetables, is superior to fast food and high sugar intake. But even then, it may only be for a time.

The China Study wasn't even a study so much as some epidemiological evidence where statistics seemed to be used to support the aimed-for argument. One example is the county of Tuoli in China. This was not mentioned, yet these people ate 45 percent of their diet as fat, with an average of 134 grams of animal protein each day. They rarely ate any plant food. The result was very little cancer and heart disease. In fact, they were healthier than the people in areas that were nearly vegan.

Some other direct studies have found things in opposition to Campbell's conclusion. One found that greater fish consumption led to higher cholesterol, and these people were much healthier overall.[32] This is fascinating because one of the people on this study was Campbell himself.

Quotes from that study include, "Our finding that the highest blood cholesterol levels in the Chinese were associated with DHA and fish consumption but with the lowest risk [of heart disease], is also a contradiction of what might be expected…It is the largely vegetarian, inland communities who have the greatest all risk mortalities and morbidities and who have the lowest LDL cholesterols. It could well be that there is a minimum level of LDL cholesterol below which cell membranes are adversely affected."

A study by the Humane Research Council found that 86 percent of vegetarians and 70 percent of vegans go back to eating some meat.[33] Some of this occurs because of health reasons, including loss of vitamin B12, vitamin A, iron, protein, zinc and other deficiencies as well as the symptoms that occur from these.

It is important to realize that veganism is a very new way of eating, made possible only by our modern agricultural and transportation systems. There are very few long-term vegans, and there are no vegans who have existed as such exclusively for generations.

Contrast this to vegetarianism, where dairy or eggs are eaten. This is doable. Many in India have existed and even thrived in doing this for a long time. But it is important to note that they make ghee, or clarified butter, a rich source of saturated fat and vitamin A, one of their most sacred foods.

Once again, I refer back to Price's work. He wrote, "I have not found a single group of primitive racial stock which was building and maintaining excellent bodies by living entirely on plant foods. I have found in many parts of the world most devout representatives of modern ethical systems advocating the restriction of foods to the vegetable products. In every instance where the groups involved had been long under this teaching, I found evidence of degeneration."

Still, the health reasons are only one reason that people change their diet. Others choose vegetarianism for morality—not just to avoid killing animals but in recognition of the environmental impact. Unfortunately, this typically looks at the impact of industrialized feedlots, not animals that are naturally raised. Indeed, in the latter situation, raising animals for food actually can improve the environment. Common arguments include that cows use up much more water, but when different types of water are looked at, grains and vegetables often take just as much per pound as beef does.[34]

Then there are the greenhouse gases that are blamed on cows farting. When cows are on pasture lands, properly done, their excrement improves the soil carbon through carbon sequestration and nitrogen fixing. This, in turn, reduces greenhouse gases.[35] Meanwhile, conventional farming practice further destroys the soil and causes more emissions. Nor does this idea consider that huge herds of buffalo, estimated at 60 million, used to roam the Great Plains for far longer time frames, and this same problem didn't appear to exist then.

Conventional practices are unsustainable, not eating animal products, which humans have done since a long before we were even *Homo sapiens*. For more details on the problems of veganism and vegetarianism I recommend reading *The Vegetarian Myth* by ex-vegan Lierre Keith.

Wild Food

Earlier I mentioned Jo Robinson's book *Eating on the Wild Side*. The title speaks to the idea that wild food—that is, natural food, that hasn't been altered by human hands—tends to have far more micro- and phytonutrients in it than non-wild food. She writes, "To date, four hundred generations of farmers and tens of thousands of plant breeders have played a role in redesigning native plants. The combined changes are so monumental that our present-day fruits and vegetables seem like modern creations."

Eating on the wild side is eating more food that is closer to wild species than domesticated species. Unfortunately, there are very few wild foods that make up our diets anymore. In both plants and animals, we've cultivated and domesticated them to make them easier to handle and eat, but this has come at a cost. And this was before geneticists got involved! The mighty auroch no longer lives, but we have today's modern cows instead.

I enjoyed Robinson's book but felt that it missed the big idea of actually going for getting wild foods in your diet, not just selecting certain cultivars that are closer to the wild versions.

There are also some foods that you can regularly buy that are wild. Brazil nuts are touted for their high selenium content. What most people don't realize is that this is because these come from massive trees that have resisted all efforts of domestication. And by the way, it is best to buy them in the shell, to prevent mold growth and ensure the oils are not made rancid by air exposure.

Seaweeds are another wild food. You'll want to make sure these come exclusively from clean waters, which unfortunately is becoming harder. You'll find tons of minerals in these, and a high supply of iodine in many like bladderwrack, kelp, Irish moss, and dulse.

Of course, many fish and other seafoods are also wild, except those that are farmed, which is becoming more and more common.

If you want to go deeper into food, then one thing you might want to take up is wildcrafting. This means going out into the wild and foraging for edibles. To do this takes knowledge of the area and is best learned with a mentor. Not only can you find foods but also many medicinal herbs. One of the great things about herbs is that they still possess the medicinal qualities of wild food, even if they're cultivated. I'll provide more on that in an upcoming chapter.

In the beginning, this may just be nibbling on a few things here and there. But with practice in identification of the right plants and locations where they grow in abundance, you can start collecting amounts that can make up a significant part of your diet. Collecting food in nature is one of the best ways to get connected to nature, because what you eat literally becomes a part of you. This way you establish a real connection to your food.

Since taking a class with Kevin Feinstein, and reading his book *The Bay Area Forager*, co-authored by Mia Andler, I've started doing much more of this. I have foraged for and consumed acorns, blackberries, thimbleberries, black nightshade, nasturtiums, common mallow, wild radish and more. More recently, I wild harvested seaweed, finding abundant amounts of kombu, nori and bladderwrack. And I'm just getting started.

Buhner writes, "The !Kung bushman of the Kalahari Desert, as an example, regularly eat more than seventy-five different plants in their diet in one of the harshest ecosystems on Earth; cancer is virtually unknown. (They additionally work less hours than we do, have a high caloric intake by American standards, and spend most of their time in what we call 'leisure pursuits.')"

In foraging, you'll gain many of the other benefits of nature, while accomplishing the gathering of some of your food supply. Be patient with this process if you undertake it. But it doesn't have to be too difficult. You can begin by collecting dandelion leaves or roots from your yard, as long as no one has sprayed them with poison.

Unless you begin to engage in this process, it is important to realize that 100 percent of your food comes from domesticated foods. These are foods that have been bred and hybridized, even if not genetically modified by radiation or actual gene-splicing techniques, typically to be more fit to grow and store, and not for nutrition purposes.

As Yuval Noah Harari, author of *Sapiens*, described it, "We did not domesticate wheat. It domesticated us. The word 'domesticate comes from the Latin domus, which means 'house'. Who's the one living in the house? Not the wheat. It's the Sapiens." He goes on further to state, "This is the essence of the Agricultural Revolution: the ability to keep more people alive under worse conditions."

This, in turn, takes us farther away from nature. Wheat is now grown on 215 billion acres across the world, making it one of the most successful plant species on the planet, if spreading is looked at as an evaluation of success.

Again, this has come at a cost. From the very beginning the domestication of wheat caused problems. And as the pace of society accelerates in the modern era, it seems we have accelerated those issues too.

Lost Food Groups

Besides wild foods, there are certain food groups that were always a part of the natural human diet, that we have largely gotten away from. Many of these, assuming they come from healthy life, are going to be healthy for you to consume.

The first up is organ meats. Although veggies like kale are touted for all the nutrients they pack, these pale in comparison to something like liver. In many different organs, you can find abundances of B vitamins, vitamin A, K, D and E, choline, coenzyme Q10, omega 3 fatty acids, trace minerals and much more.

These fell out of favor from our parents and grandparents because of their taste. The average American today probably has never tasted organ meats. But taste is malleable. And if they're prepared properly they can be very tasty as well as nutritious.

My favorite way to prepare liver so far has been lightly fried along with bacon and onions. Liver is the best source of vitamin A and B12 there is, as well as being rich in folate and choline. The good news is that it's cheaper than muscle meats despite being far healthier. (That is if you can find liver, since most stores do not carry it.)

One story from Price regarding liver is as follows. "Some of the tribes are very tall, particularly the Neurs. The women are often six feet or over, and the men seven feet, some of them reaching seven and a half feet in height. I was particularly interested in their food habits both because of their high immunity to dental caries which approximated one hundred per cent, and because of their physical development. I learned that they have a belief which to them is their religion, namely, that every man and woman has a soul which resides in the liver and that a man's character and physical growth depend upon how well he feeds that soul by eating the livers of animals. The liver is so sacred that it may not be touched by human hands. It is accordingly always handled with their spear or saber, or with specially prepared forked sticks. It is eaten both raw and cooked."

While all of the natural peoples Price looked at were healthier than moderns, there were key differences. Those that relied on more animal foods, and less plant foods, overall seems to be even healthier, like the tribe mentioned above.

Heart is hands down the best source of coenzyme Q10 which all your cells need to produce energy. I like to grind heart up along with other ground meat and make things like burgers or shepherd's pie.

Something that has caught on, because it tastes good in addition to the nutrition, is bone broth. This can be made with beef bones, a chicken carcass, chicken feet, fish or other options if you have the bones. Very highly mineralizing, this also gives you gelatin, collagen, glycosaminoglycans (GAGs), chondroitin sulfate, hyaluronic acid, keratin sulfate, glycine, and proline which are all good for the joints and skin, and digestive tract.

For a long-time chicken stock was recommended to the sick as something that would help speed recovery. In one of very few studies actually looking at this, chicken soup was shown to reduce inflammation and support neutrophils.[36]

Another food group that makes people more squeamish than organ meats is insects. Yet these are catching on in high-end restaurants and certain other places, because not only do they provide a lot of nutrition, but they are easier, cheaper, and less resource-intensive to prepare than larger animals. An easy way to get started is something like cricket powder or meal worm powder where you can't tell it came from insects.

Fermented foods are not a staple in the diets of many people, yet they ought to be. These provide bacteria that is so critical to our digestion, immune system and so much more. More details are in the Symbiosis chapter.

Sprouts are also packed full of nutrition. When a seed is spouting it is a fury of enzymatic nutrition. Broccoli sprouts have significantly more sulforaphane, a potent anti-cancerous compound, than broccoli itself.[37] A rat study also found that a related compound, glucoraphanin, could help obesity by turning white fat into brown, which burns more energy, and improve gut bacteria.[38]

Herbs are another lost food group that will be detailed in an upcoming chapter.

Remember how this chapter started off talking about my reluctance to even get into food? I'm sure that there are people that will otherwise like this book but disagree with what is brought up here. And because diet is often treated religiously, they'll throw out the baby with the bathwater.

The fact is that humans can have a varied diet. That is clear looking at people all over the world. Yes, for the average person, our nutrition has improved since hundreds of years ago. But it has degraded since the time of thousands of years ago before the advent of agriculture.

Modern and scientific agriculture has got us to where we are today. More of the same is not the solution. While we can't go back to eating as our ancestors did long ago, as the human population is too big to do so, and much of that food no longer exists; we can, however, make steps toward that. We can get back to having an actual relationship with our food. Doing so, we will get closer to nature and best support our health and performance.

When I say eat healthy food and you will be healthy, I am talking about the health of the animals, plants, fungi and bacteria, involved in whatever food you're eating. If whomever they ate down the chain, were healthy, then you will be too.

Lierre Keith sums up her book and what is best to eat by having yourself ask the following questions: "Does this food build or destroy topsoil? Does it use only ambient sun and rainfall, or does it require fossil soil, fossil fuel, fossil water, and drained wetlands, damaged rivers? Could you walk to where it grows, or does it come to you on a path slick with petroleum?" Most of us could not even accurately answer these questions. Thus, we all have a long way to go. As with everything else, be patient with yourself over this lifelong process.

A final piece of wisdom comes from Dr. Claudia Welch who wrote, "The more complicated your physical, emotional or spiritual life, the simpler your diet should be." In this way, you may also be what you don't eat. This is every bit as important and we move into doing that in a conscious way next...

13
Fast and Feast

"Fasting is the greatest remedy--the physician within."
– Paracelsus

"Fasting is not so much a treatment for illness but a treatment for wellness."
– Dr. Jason Fung

We certainly haven't lost the feasting part in our modern world. For many people feasting is a day to day regimen. Unfortunately, the balancing factor to that, fasting, has largely been forgotten. This is despite having big proponents throughout the years from Hippocrates, Plato, Galen, Benjamin Franklin, Paul Bragg, Jack Lalanne, and today a whole slew of new proponents with various forms of intermittent fasting.

Herbert Shelton, a physician who supervised over 40,000 people doing fasts, stated, "Fasting must be recognized as a fundamental and radical process that is older than any other mode of caring for the sick organism, for it is employed on the plane of instinct."

Even Mark Twain said, "A little starvation can really do more for the average sick man than can the best medicines and the best doctors."

I've decided to title this chapter fast and feast, rather than the words feast and famine. The definition of famine is an extreme scarcity of food. This is an idea I want to get away from, because, by and large, people fear going without food. Sure, it's a natural fear, in that lack of food eventually would lead to wasting and even death. However, to think this will happen if you skip a meal or two, or even fifteen, is ridiculous.

Right now, as I write this, I am heading into the third day of a nutritional fast. At this time, this is the longest I've ever done so. My energy and clarity of thinking has varied a little bit over the past couple days, but overall it hasn't been bad. In my schedule was plans to write a different chapter, but upon meditating I was called strongly to do this one.

My introduction to nutrition was with *The Warrior Diet*, written by Ori Hofmekler. It came about a decade before the more recent intermittent fasting buzz, and in that sense, was a little before it's time. But that led me back to read a book called *The Power of Fasting* by Paul Bragg.

Fasting has come hot upon the scene in recent years. Specifically, different types of intermittent fasting as recommended by people like Brad Pilon who wrote *Eat, Stop, Eat*, and Dave Asprey with his bulletproof intermittent fasting, through the use of the fat-fueled Bulletproof coffee.

Right now, it seems like it is touching the mainstream. But after a few more years it will likely fade in popularity once again, only to be re-discovered again. And so, the cycle continues.

Speaking of cycles, it is of prime importance that you realize that fast and feast are to come in cycles. While most people have this conception that food was always hard to come by in the past, they just don't realize how abundant nature can be when you know what you're doing. The average hunters and gatherers spent less time getting food than we do in our average work days. The rest of their time was spent in leisure.

Of course, there were times of food scarcity too. The human being evolved with this cycle in mind, and thus, actually benefits from it happening. Think about that for a second. Not having food, because it is a natural thing that happens from time to time, actually benefits human health, not detracts from it.

For the average industrialized person, the idea of starving is just that, an idea. They've never even come close. Yet the fear of it may still stop them from engaging in this time-tested strategy.

To allay your fears, did you know that a man has been recorded doing a 382 day fast? That's over a year! A 27-year-old Scottish man, starting at a weight of 456 pounds and ending at 180, took only noncaloric fluids, a daily multivitamin, and other supplements under supervision.[1]

With that in mind, does a 24-hour fast sound so bad, now?

As we continue there are three main aspects we'll be covering. First are the physical health benefits that are involved in fasting. The second is different types of fasting and how to get started. The last part is about going beyond the physical benefits of fasting.

Physiology of Fasting

Isn't it fascinating to know that the human body basically possesses a back-up metabolism? Under certain conditions, how the human body produces and uses energy changes radically.

Most people are not aware of this, because it is not taught in our schools. If you study physiology deeply, as in college, you might learn about it, but it is often labeled as something to be avoided.

This alternate form of metabolism is known as ketosis, where the human body uses ketones, produced from fat, for energy, rather than carbohydrates. While there does seem to be a switch, this shouldn't be thought of as black and white. The body is still using some glucose, even while in ketosis.

Some of the benefits from fasting are because of being in ketosis. Ketosis can be gotten into and maintained not just through fasting, but through a high fat, low carbohydrate diet. (Even protein must be kept low, as protein is also converted into glucose, the typical metabolic energy, through a process called gluconeogenesis.)

It's been known that a ketogenic diet is great for helping control seizures for a long time.[2] More recently, a lot more investigation has gone into the other health benefits that come from this, including for weight loss, cancer, diabetes, PCOS, acne, neurological disorders, respiratory and cardiovascular risk factors.[3]

However, knowing more about these benefits has been stymied by how many thought of this as a disease, confusing it with the harmful ketoacidosis, which sometimes occurs in diabetics.

Thinking back ancestrally it might be quite difficult to maintain ketosis while eating, because people wouldn't have as ready access to refined forms of fat typically used in today's low-carb diets, completely devoid of protein or carbohydrates. Exceptions might include those peoples that hunted large mammals, before the last ice age, and the Inuit, or others on a similar diet.

Thus, ketosis was historically created most exclusively through

181

fasting. I think that is important to recognize. While some advocates are promoting everyone get and stay in ketosis permanently, we're likely to find that this comes with its own set of health issues over time. Going into ketosis sometimes, like our ancestors did, is probably the best way to do it.

The research points to us having developed ketosis as a means to preserve our energy-hungry brains. Compared to other animals our brains use up a much larger percentage of our total energy intake. Contrary to common opinion, and what science told us for a long time, the brain doesn't run only on glucose, but can also use ketones known as beta-hydroxybutyrate and acetoacetate as fuel.[4]

A metaphor helps illustrate and explain these energy sources, one that I originally heard from Nora Gedgaudas, author of *Primal Fat Burner*. Carbohydrates are thought of as kindling in a fire. They light quickly but then burn out quickly. You have to keep throwing sticks on the fire to keep it going, which is what people are doing by eating up to six times per day. A carbohydrate meal with fiber may be slightly bigger twigs and branches. Something like high fructose corn syrup is more like newspaper in the fire.

If your blood sugar crashes and you're hungry a few hours after a meal, this is what you are doing. In a sense, your body forgets how to use fat as a fuel, through habitual disuse, and must rely on consistent supplies of glucose. The more often you do, the harder time your body has making the switch. And here we see why so many people struggle to lose fat. It's because their bodies have forgotten how to utilize it for fuel.

Fat as a fuel is more like a big log. It may take some time to get started, but when it is burning, it will continue to do so for hours. If you have a big supply of logs you can keep the fire going for days and weeks with ease.

The human body stores a limited supply of glucose in the muscles and liver. It stores much bigger supplies of energy as body fat. Remember also that carbohydrates have four calories of energy per gram, whereas fat has nine. While I'm not a big proponent of looking at calories, this is helpful to see that fat is over twice as useful for energy purposes.

We know that humans can burn carbohydrates and fat for energy. And we know a fair amount about the metabolic pathways of doing do. What is not well researched is how one person, regularly fasting, will have more metabolic flexibility than a person that never does so. This isn't an easy thing to study. And then, how this impacts all sorts of other health factors is only beginning to be explored. In addition to switching fuel sources, there are other changes that happen.

In fasting, with no food to digest, digestion stops happening. With a constant supply of food, the digestion is always at work, and is a very energy-intensive process for the human body. The average person spends 10 percent of their energy each day just digesting food. It's higher or lower depending on the type of food and can vary by a large amount. In an odd study, a "whole food" cheese sandwich took almost 50 percent more energy to digest than a processed cheese sandwich.[5]

When food stops coming, the digestion finishes up what is still inside the human gut, and then goes quiet. This frees up energy for other functions.

A number of different hormonal effects occur. Most notably, insulin goes down. While carbohydrates are mostly known for their insulin-signaling effects, the fact is that all foods trigger insulin to some degree. As such, stopping eating is the best way to lower insulin and begin to reestablish its sensitivity, which is important for anyone the with type 2 diabetes or metabolic syndrome.

Another thing we see is that, in the beginning, the hormone ghrelin increases. This hormone is named because it is growth hormone release inducing.[6] While most of the ghrelin is found in the stomach it is also present in the hypothalamus, the master endocrine organ.

In one study, just 24 hours of fasting brought about a 2000-percent increase in growth hormone in men, and a 1300-percent increase in women.[7] And in another study of healthy men, five days of fasting brought about further increases in growth hormone, with more frequent releasing as well.[8]

As I wrote in my book *Upgrade Your Growth Hormone*, "growth hormone" is a slightly unfortunate label. It was first identified in relation to puberty and children hitting growth spurts. That is where the name came from. But, as is always the case in the human body, things are more complex then we initially see. Growth hormone is responsible for a lot more than a growth spurt. I find it is more helpful to think of it as the repair and recovery hormone.

The time that it naturally peaks throughout the day is during sleep, where it rapidly increases after falling asleep.[9] This occurs to help the body physically repair. It also happens to be the one time of day when people are not eating. The term breakfast is because it is the meal when you *break* your overnight *fast*.

The big spikes of growth hormone seen with fasting trigger the body to repair damaged tissues and basically reboot the system. Without a constant influx of food, the body can amp up its detoxification efforts. The liver and kidneys are always at work helping the body rid itself of both endogenous and exogenous toxins, those that are produced inside the body, and those we get from our food, air, absorbed through the skin and other places. Limited research has shown that a 36-hour fast increased drug clearance via cytochrome P450 metabolism.[10] While looking at an isolated function, this, taken together with all the other changes, shows a likely uptick in systemic detoxification throughout the body. I hope more research on this is done soon.

A process called autophagy begins. Autophagy, derived from the Greek *auto*, meaning self, and *phagein*, meaning to eat, means "self-eating." Autophagy occurs best under fasted conditions and can be completely stopped by consuming any carbohydrate or protein sources.

Specifically, this process doesn't go for healthy tissue, unless you're in starvation, but instead eats up the junk. Old worn out cell parts, dead and diseased cells that should be killed with apoptosis, and more get recycled. This further removes toxins from your body.

It may be the combination of autophagy and the elevated growth hormone that brings many of the benefits of fasting. Out with the old cells and in with the new. Fasting induces the body to make the cells more resilient to stress. Inflammation is reduced, and DNA is better protected.[11]

Autophagy appears to occur all over the body. Contrary to earlier opinion, this study found autophagy occurring in the brain and neurons, showing its importance for a cognitive tune-up and prevention of Alzheimer's and other neurodegenerative diseases.[12] Fasting also helps regenerate myelin, the coating of nerve cells.[13]

Autophagy has also been shown to be active inside muscle stem cells.[14] Furthermore, prolonged fasting may be able to activate dormant immune stem cells, effectively giving your body an immune system reboot too.[15] The question is, and more future research will likely bear this out, what other stem cells get activated? Is it all kinds?

Dominic D'Agostino, an associate professor in the Department of Molecular Pharmacology and Physiology at the University of South Florida Morsani College of Medicine, has heavily researched fasting and ketosis. He stated that, "If you don't have cancer and you do a therapeutic fast one to three times per year, you could purge any precancerous cells that may be living in your body." What if he is right and that is all it takes?

One review of the literature on autophagy showed that it inhibits aging through multiple pathways. The authors Petrovski et al., write, "There is overwhelming evidence that cellular mechanisms and signaling pathways regulating aging are related to autophagy. An increase in autophagy extends life span via [calorie restriction] and insulin signaling."[16]

One of the leading fields of study in aging is that of mTOR, or the mammalian or mechanistic target of rapamycin pathway. This pathway regulates many cellular processes, including autophagy. While mTOR is not bad, as it is responsible for growth, too much signaling is implicated in cancer, obesity, diabetes, and neurodegeneration.[17] Fasting is one of the best ways to suppress mTOR.

Once the body stops receiving carbohydrates from food, the liver increases production of a hormone called glucagon. Glucagon in turn activates the lipase enzyme, which breaks down fat cells to be used for fuel, also releasing toxins that are stored inside them.[18] This then allows the stored fat to be turned into ketones for use as fuel.

It is not just the subcutaneous fat that you can see that is used. Visceral fat that surrounds your organs also gets used up in this fashion. This is important because visceral fat is linked to diabetes, obesity, and other inflammatory issues. Fasting may be one of the best ways for your body to eat these fat stores.

Despite all of this information, overall, the studies on fasting in humans are sparse. Probably because there is no money to be made in people not consuming anything. Not only is fasting available to everyone, it is better than free. You save money because you're not paying for food!

You can even save time because you're not spending that time preparing and eating food.

The few specific studies on humans show improvements in weight, coronary artery disease, and diabetes.[19]

Gandhi, a big proponent of fasting, who even used it politically for hunger strikes, said "Fasting is a fiery weapon. It has its own science. No one, as far as I am aware, has perfect knowledge of it." While the science we just went over shows many benefits, this isn't the complete picture. Future research will show even more. But I hope you don't wait until then to start receiving what fasting can deliver.

Durations of Fasts

There are almost as many different types of fasting as there are eating. Here I will break fasts down into a few different categories. This helps identify where to get started and where to progress to. Overall, I aim to clear up confusion.

As with everything, there are some changes that come with different types. Each fast has some advantages and disadvantages.

Intermittent fasting is any type of fasting that done intermittently— that is, with frequent periods of starting and stopping. The typical intermittent fasting involves eating dinner one night, sleeping through the night, skipping breakfast, then eating lunch as your first meal.

Others shorten this window even more. Some will do a twenty-hour fast each day, eating only in a window of four hours. Going from dinner to dinner the next day.

Either of these can be done day after day for long periods of time. Or it can be done occasionally, with a return to more typical eating patterns afterword.

I personally think of intermittent fasting as anything 36 hours and under. If you go from dinner one night to dinner the next night, this is a pretty short fast. During that time, you're not going to get into full blown ketosis, nor induce the full autophagic process. But you will give your digestion a break. And you will get a spike in growth hormone.

Contrasted to intermittent fasts are extended fasts. I think of this as 36 hours and beyond. Of course, 36 hours is quite a bit different from 30 days.

Typically, the second or third day of an extended fast is going to be the most difficult as the body is still trying to burn sugar for fuel. But somewhere in this time frame the body begins to go into ketosis. Note that this is variable. If you are practiced at fasting your body will enter much easier, versus if you've never done it before and not entered into ketosis ever. (Actually, most people have as an infant. If fed exclusively breast milk, which is mostly fat, a baby is in a state of ketosis.)

Many people who have never experienced fasting are surprised to find that you don't get hungrier and hungrier the more time passes. After two or three days, hunger diminishes and may even go away completely. It's like the body understands what is happening and thus catches up to the idea. When digestion ceases, the signals of hunger can also cease.

About five days or a week into the fast you'll likely have entered into ketosis fully and the process of autophagy should be working full-time. And you just might be surprised how much energy you have and how clear your thinking is.

Types of Fasts

The terms intermittent and extended speak to the duration of the fast. The other categorization is in what you are and are not ingesting during the fast. A fast is typically free from "food" but as we can see this definition is fuzzy.

There is the dry fast. In a dry fast you not only completely fast from food, but from water as well. As most people are already chronically dehydrated, and just a little dehydration can impair body functions, this is generally not recommended.

That being said, there is likely a time and a place for it. One thing I have heard is that by alternating dry and water fasting the body can detox certain radioactive elements that it doesn't seem to be able to let go of otherwise. This has been investigated in Russia, but not at all in the West. (Except some Native Americans who engage in this type of fasting regularly.) It being a more difficult fast would also extend the mental benefits further. While I plan to try this in the future, this absolutely should not be your first attempt at fasting.

Then there is the water fast. In this fast you abstain from all food, and in fact everything else, besides pure water. During a water fast, you drink a lot of water. This helps in hydrating your body and supporting detoxification.

Those are quite simple. Then you have all the various forms of nutritional fasting. A nutritional fast is where you are getting some sort of nutrition in addition to water. Here are just a few types.

A micronutrient fast involves the supplementing of some kind of vitamins and minerals. This may be full spectrum or focused on certain ones. Although the human body can thrive off of just body fat stores from some time, it is still using certain vitamins and minerals throughout that time. By adding this in you can help support various body processes, without any caloric intake.

Various teas are also used often in fasting. Whether green or herbal teas, these provide nutrients, via phytochemistry, that can aid in various processes during fasting. Often detoxing or laxative teas are used to assist in those areas more so. Coffee is sometimes used as well. Unless any fuel source is added to these they are calorie free and thus won't change some of the other details of the fast.

Juice fasting involves drinking large amounts of fruit and/or vegetable juice. These can help aid the body in detoxifying and act as a vitamin and mineral supplement. However, there will be some sugar, and if there is too much sugar it could slow or even stop the transition into ketosis and may impact autophagy as well.

Broth fasting is another method that acts similar to juice fasting. Again, this supplies many micronutrients. Broth doesn't have any carbohydrates, but it does have some protein. Remember, it is the lack of ingesting protein that really gets autophagy going. Thus, too much broth could slow or stop that from happening.

Fat fasting is a newer method which involves taking some isolated fat source. Specifically, MCT oil, typically derived from coconut or palm, is rapidly transformed into ketones in the human body. Thus, MCT oil or other forms of exogenous ketones, can be used as a method to help ease the transition into a fasted state. Without any carbohydrates or protein, you won't stop ketosis or autophagy. Taking some fat can be done throughout a fast, or just in the beginning of an extended fast in order to ease the transition into it.

These various forms can be mixed and matched. There are specific protocols that are used for different purposes, but these cover the broader types of fasting that involves more than just water.

Lastly, there are food fasts. These involve some type of food. This may involve something you eat, like a watermelon fast, where you eat just one food, a mono-diet, and nothing else. Another example is a spirulina fast. Spirulina has all kinds of micronutrients and is also a complete protein. You can live off the stuff, and I know someone who went over a hundred days living just off of spirulina.

There are liquid fasts that involve things like soups and stews. Basically, you can eat any food, it just must be in liquid form. In these, because you are getting some calories and a mix of macronutrients, it will alter what occurs in the fast, though will still bring some of benefits.

If you are doing an extended fast you can also do different stages. For instance, you may enter and/or end the fast with some sort of nutritional fast but do a day or a few of strict water fasting in the middle. In my next extended fast I plan to do one day of a dry fast in it as well to see what I experience.

How to Get Started Fasting

Start small and start easy. If you have never fasted before you'll want to begin with a small intermittent fast. Eat dinner one night, go to bed, skip breakfast, and then eat again around noon.

Those that say breakfast is the most important meal of the day, don't understand the power of fasting. And you can enjoy your breakfast meal at lunch time just the same.

With any fasting, there is some overcompensation in eating, but it's small. If we're looking at calories after a 24-hour fast there is typically an increase of about 20 percent in the amount of food eaten. That may sound like a lot but if you see that you just ate 100 percent less the day before, it balances out to a deficit.

If skipping breakfast was easy, the next time you plan to fast, make it a 24-hour fast. The easiest for most people is to go from dinner to dinner.

With intermittent fasting I don't see a lot of reason to do many of the types of fasting recommended. You won't run low on micronutrients in one day. You can drink teas, but I would skip anything with a caloric load. Give your digestion the break it deserves.

Though, as mentioned, those fat sources can help you get some ketones going faster, thus that can be something to look at doing. Dave Asprey recommends his bulletproof intermittent fasting, which involves coffee and sources of fat from butter and MCT oil, but no other food. Because this does provide some fuel, while not having the effects of carbs or protein, this may work well for some people.

Paul Bragg, as well as others, have recommended a 24-hour fast done once a week. For a couple years that was something I regularly did. At times, I got away from it, then got back to it like I have now. For health purposes, I think it is hard to beat in its simplicity and effectiveness. Figure out the day of the week that works best for you, then just do it routinely.

And when I mention these numbers, it doesn't have to be exact. If you eat dinner at seven at night and then start dinner at five the next night that is okay. You have just done a 22-hour fast. Close enough is close enough.

Nowadays, I often do intermittent fasting while traveling. Skip the airport and airline food, which tend to be low-quality food anyway, and fast instead. For me this appears to help with time adjustments and any jet lag as well.

Get used to 24-hour fasts and then you can begin to go longer. The next step is a 36-hour fast. Eat dinner one night, completely avoid food the next day and night, then break your fast at breakfast the next morning. This is a bigger step in that it'll be your first entire day without food.

I believe to get all the benefits of fasting you need to do extended fasts. Intermittent fasting is good, and can help you become used to fasting, but many of the best benefits come later in the process. Intermittent fasting is like the regular tune-up, but in longer fasts you get the "reset" effect.

After you have done a 36-hour fast choose when you're going to go longer. As I am doing right now, during the writing of this chapter, select a time to go for a five day or one-week fast. At this stage, you may want to do some type of nutritional fast. I've heard multiple people say, and it is my experience as well, that these are easier than a strict water fast.

After you have done a week, the decision is up to you if you'd like to do a longer fast. A good protocol is to do a weekly fast at least once a year. Some people do them once a quarter, especially during the change of seasons.

Experiment with different lengths of time. Experiment with different types of fasts. At some point, I would recommend doing a strict water fast, but find what works for you.

One other important point is that how you break a fast is worth paying attention to. With intermittent fasting you can eat a full meal as soon as you choose. But in an extended fast your digestion shuts down, so to have a huge meal as soon as you refeed can be problematic. A study with rats showed that eating a high-protein meal after fasting for 48 hours brought about liver damage.[20]

It is best to ease back into eating with some easy nutrients. Some people recommend juices. Some recommend broth. Then add some solid foods that are easy to digest like fruit, a salad, or plain rice. Eat small amounts and feel how your body responds. Only go for heavier meals after having done this. In general, the longer the fast you've done, the longer a window of careful refeeding is necessary.

Is there anyone that shouldn't fast? Generally, children should not engage in the practice as they're growing. A short fast once in a while, especially for teenagers, shouldn't be a problem, but extended fasts are not recommended. The same goes for pregnant women.

People with certain diseases may best do fasting under medical supervision. But overall, this is a great thing for all humans. Remember, it is part of our nature to do so.

The Nature of Fasting

Thus far, we have covered only the physical and physiological processes the body goes through, and the steps involved in doing fasts. But that is only part of the picture.

The Complete Guide to Fasting, by Dr. Jason Fung and Jimmy Moore, recently came out, and it is a great book. It is one of the most detailed books on the health benefits of fasting. However, it is incomplete in that it scarcely touches on the mental, emotional, and even spiritual side to fasting.

One trait that fasting of any type helps to strengthen is that of willpower. Willpower isn't the end-all, be-all, like some people claim. It certainly has its limitations. But who wouldn't like to have more willpower? Fasting may be the best way to practice it.

If you'd like to go deeper into other aspects of fasting, then I recommend Stephen Harrod Buhner's *The Transformational Power of Fasting*. As he states there, "Traditionally, fasting concerned itself with the emotions—our psychological selves—and with the soul and our souls' communication with the sacred...Fasting, it was recognized, increased human sensitivity to the nonmaterial world, enhanced personal experience of the sacredness of both self and Universe, and helped the fasting person regain a sense of orientation and purpose."

Cast your mind back once again to our ancestors. Yes, there were periods of time when food was scarce, and fasting was enforced simply by the lack of food. But the fact was that this didn't happen often in many places. The ancients were not so concerned with the physical benefits of fasting but engaged in it consciously more for spiritual purposes.

A vision quest would often involve fasting while isolated from other humans, immersed in nature. Often this quest would not be for a set amount of time but done until some sort of vision occurred. Basically, the person would fast in nature until they were struck with some profound meaning, experience, or vision. We do not engage in this in our culture. Yet some form of it was done by many ancient cultures.

What have we lost in losing this practice? Gandhi said, "What the eyes are for the outer world, fasts are for the inner."

One of the greatest fears of people is to face themselves. When fasting your physical body is going through the process of hunger. This can bring up all kinds of emotions including other fears. This will bring up all the emotional attachments you have to food; most people have plenty.

Furthermore, by spending time away from other humans, and the constant stimulus that is modern life, you'll be left with ample time to think and feel for yourself. Fasting doesn't just have to be about food. You can fast from media. You can fast from cell phones. You can fast from speaking. All of these can be done by themselves, or in combination with food fasting.

By fasting, from food but also from constant distraction, you have fewer demands on your mind. This leads to greater awareness and an increase in your senses. Just try to go out to the forest or the desert one week into fasting and not feel the aliveness of the place.

The nature of fasting is to spend time in nature. Yes, we can get some health benefits by doing a short intermittent fast and going about our routine, daily lives. But the deeper nature of it requires you to dig a little deeper and open the space for it.

Enter into a fasted and meditative state while in the bosom of nature and you'll likely gain insight that may just transform your world. Engage in your own vision quest, not leaving until this occurs, and there's a very good chance it will eventually happen.

"Spiritual fasting, especially in the wilderness, allows the person to step out of a confining life by initiating an intentional encounter with death and suffering and, eventually, rebirth.," writes Buhner. "It reconnects each person to the Universe around them and supplies new direction for life."

By no means will this be easy, but nothing worthwhile ever is.

As of writing this, it is now day five of my fast. I made the couple-hour hike up to the old-growth redwoods in the Santa Cruz mountains. The hike was exhausting but I made it. There I sat in that fatigued and fasted state with my friends, the redwoods. A powerful end to this five-day fast.

Feasting

The name of this chapter is Fast and Feast. As you have just read, the majority of it has to do with fasting. Why? Because that is the missing side of the coin in our modern-day society. It not only is great for physical health, but much more too.

But I would be remiss if we didn't talk about the benefits of feasting as well. You can't fast all the time. There is a time to stop eating food, but there is also a time to eat. Its one of the natural cycles to engage in.

With fasting we see that isolation from other humans can be an aid in doing it. This allows for a deeper connection to the web of life along with nature. In feasting, this is the ideal time to be spent in community. Although many people engage in feasts on the daily, a big feast was always done in celebration of some event and done with the community. Of course, community has been shown to be an influential aspect of our health.[21]

When you feast, enjoy it completely. Enjoy the food. Enjoy the drink. Enjoy the company. Enjoy the celebration, whatever it happens to be.

Just like fasting isn't something you do all the time, neither is feasting. For the most part, you eat regularly and moderately, but in exploring both the extremes you can gain the benefits of both.

And just know, to follow up a feast with a fast, can help rebalance the excesses that may have occurred. This is a good lesson to learn for our big feasting holidays like Thanksgiving, Christmas, and birthdays.

14
Herbalism

"Human beings have used plants for food, clothing, building, and healing as long as we have been. Medicinal herbs have been found in a 60,000-year-old Neanderthal grave, and written records over the past 6,000 years have recorded the regular use of more than 80,000 different plants as medicine. People (like soil, bears, butterflies, and monkeys) have made their medicine by percolating water through plants, eating them whole, soaking them in water for teas, or rubbing them on their skin. They have worked very well for us, and for all life on Earth, for a very long time."
– Stephen Harrod Buhner

"Herbalism is based on relationship – relationship between plant and human, plant and planet, human and planet. Using herbs in the healing process means taking part in an ecological cycle. This offers us the opportunity consciously to be present in the living, vital world of which we are part; to invite wholeness and our world into our lives through awareness of the remedies being used. The herbs can link us into the broader context of planetary wholeness, so that whilst they are doing their physiological/medical job, we can do ours and build an awareness of the links and mutual relationships."
– Wendell Berry

While the Paleo movement has grown by leaps and bounds, and for good reason, they have left out one critical part of the diet. This irks me. The advent of pharmaceutical drugs was not an idea that sprung from nothingness. Ancient peoples needed medicine too. They got this from nature, predominately from herbal plants.

Hippocrates said, "Let food by thy medicine and medicine be thy food." Most people narrow in on the first part of this statement, let food be thy medicine. That means that you should eat food that has medicinal properties, that food should be used both for its preventative and curative powers.

The second part of the statement is medicine be thy food. Hippocrates wasn't just being repetitive. That means that medicine is part of the regular and natural diet of every human being.

Pharmaceutical drugs are an extreme of this idea. They're seen as the best and safest method of medicine out there. In looking at the world this way most people haven't given a thought to herbs, besides a handful of culinary herbs that are used to make food taste better. This older method of herbal medicine has been forgotten in our technologically advanced time. This is unfortunate.

Our daily modern food is on the other extreme. Our food has been genetically modified in many cases, or at the very least hybridized and bred to remove most of the medicinal components from it. One of the reasons for this is that too much medicine is poison. The difference between helping and hurting lies in the dose.

Take the wild lettuce plant, *Lactuca virosa*. This potent plant oozes a latex that is a pain reliever or analgesic. A Polish review of the plant stated, "The action of the substance was weaker than that of opium but free of the side-effects, and medical practice showed that in some cases lactucarium produced better curative effects than opium."[1]

Wild lettuce is far removed from the iceberg or romaine lettuce (*Lactuca sativa* variations*)* you eat in your salad. Here very little "medicine" remains. But you cannot eat a big bowl of wild lettuce.

Essentially, medicine has been removed from our food supply so that it can be added back in, prescribed by doctors at hugely marked up prices.

Why not just get it from food in the first place? And that is where herbs come in.

But it is not just food vs. medicine. Instead these things exist on a spectrum. Here is how I see it:

<Food--Superfoods--Herbs--Full Herbal Extracts--Isolated Herbal Extracts--Drugs>

Regular food really doesn't have much "medicine" in it. But even among supermarket fruits and vegetables there is some, depending on the variety and freshness. Yet, in many of these the stronger phytonutrients have been bred out of them.

As we move up the scale we find superfoods. This label is attached to some common food items like berries or cruciferous vegetables which still have some potent components like anthocyanins, ellagic acid, or indole-3-carbinol. Also in this category are other superfoods like spirulina. Often packed with vitamins and minerals these foods start to have more punch. We can add in the organ meats described in an earlier chapter here too.

Further up the scale we come to herbs. Here there are fewer calories and macronutrients so that it's not really a food item. They won't feed you in that sense. Instead these are used more for their phytonutrients to maintain, optimize, and restore health.

Some herbs are used specifically in the treatment of certain diseases. These were known as inferior herbs. Other herbs, called superior herbs, in the Chinese Taoist tradition, are those that are preventative, yet gentle, and thus can be taken long term. Herbs that can be eaten as or with food, because they are gentle like food, nourishing your body in a different, yet still potent way.

Traditionally, herbs would be eaten raw, used topically, or made into tea or even put into food, like stews. Only with advancing technology have we extended this spectrum further to the right.

A full herbal extract is one in which the whole plant part used is present. (For instance, sometimes you use only the roots, not the stems, flowers, fruits, etc. of a plant.) This may be a strong decoction or tea. It may be a powdered extract or an alcohol-extracted tincture. Often this allows for the medicinal components to come out and work better whether by being concentrated or simply unlocked. Many herbs can't be assimilated in their raw state, just like many foods. But the whole of the plant is present, and thus it still maintains some of its food-like qualities, as far as being balanced.

Many of these, at least those in the superior class of herbs, do not come with a list of side effects. That's one of the components of making it into this class as opposed to inferior herbs. While inferior herbs are useful in acute diseases and injuries, you don't necessarily want to be on them long term, because of such side effects.

Our scale can be taken further by isolating one component of that herb. This is most often the so-called "active constituent" of the herb. I put that in quotes because this idea is a fallacy. A great example of how this can be wrong is in St. John's Wort which has been shown to work in cases of depression. Early on scientists thought that hypericin was the active and extracts were standardized for that. Now many more think it's hyperforin.[2] Except wait—new research is showing that adhyperforin may be the one.[3]

Limited research has shown that whole herbs used against malaria, like *Artemisa annua*, have often been found to work better than isolated nutrients or drugs, the artemisinin extracted from it, because of the synergistic effects available from multiple compounds.[4]

The whole plant is active. Different elements all play a role. While one or more may play the major role in a specific action, this discards the idea of synergy, and also arrogantly puts us in a position of thinking we're smarter than nature. Sure, there may be times where a single molecule may be better in certain cases. But until everything has been adequately tested, in isolation and in combination, and mind you there can be over 300 constituents in a single herb, we won't know for sure.

This plant chemistry can have very complex interactions inside our bodies; we know only a tiny bit about that. To think we can improve upon this level of complexity from an isolated compound approach without fully grasping everything involve is absurd.

At the very least, it's important to recognize an active isolate is something different from the full herb. In these cases, an isolated nutrient from an herb can become very concentrated. Here the effects are likely to become much stronger. However, so too may the side effects.

This is what most drugs are, or at least started as. While estimates vary, around 50 percent of approved drugs during the last 30 years are either directly or indirectly from natural products.[5] Before that time, it was even more.

However, other drugs are synthetically made. It may be a molecule that is close to the one from nature, but with an added or tweaked part. This is often for patenting reasons, so that a pharmaceutical company can protect a cash cow, though it also changes the action of the molecule too. We really want financial and legal reasons to drive our health choices, right?

Again, here the list of side effects grows, as many of these unnatural drugs, have never previously been processed by the human body. They achieve an effect, often at the expense of other systems.

Of course, some drugs are better than others. Some have their rightful place and have helped many people. However, overall, I would say that the industry has done more harm than good. Had we never gotten away from natural medicines, working in a holistic model, I believe we'd be in a better place. Part of this is because people would have never abdicated their responsibility for health to doctors, that seemed to come with this healthcare model.

Buhner writes, "Pharmaceuticals, on very short timescales, produce better outcomes than plant medicines, just as the short-term use of pesticides produces better crop outcomes. When viewed on long scales, however, the superiority of pharmaceuticals and pesticides vanishes."

That is why I am morally against drugs and choose not to partake in any of them, except in the most extreme of situations, which as of yet have not happened.

Let's revisit the scale:

<Food--Superfoods--Herbs--Full Herbal Extracts--Isolated Herbal Extracts--Drugs>

The problem is that most people are existing only on the extremes of this spectrum. Food and drugs. A wild chaotic swinging back and forth. Is it any wonder that the state of health for many people is not good?

Furthermore, the medical complex brings other issues. In a report on Greening Hospitals, the Environmental Working Group, wrote, "'First, do no harm' is the credo of the health care professional. The very nature of their work requires health care professionals to err on the side of safety when it comes to the well-being of the patients they serve. This must include special care to eliminate any environmental health problems that medical care facilities, particularly hospitals, may cause. Ironically, many hospitals pollute the environment with highly toxic substances that actually contribute to public health problems. Of particular concern is the long-standing overuse of incineration for the treatment of medical waste and continued use and improper disposal of hazardous chemicals."[6] By-products of our medical care, further pollute the environment, causing more health problems. This is a vicious cycle.

To bring your health to balance, it is important to restore the natural part of our diet that is superfoods and herbs. Having more of a base in the middle of this chart can make it so that you don't need drugs at all. After all, it is not the lack of drugs that causes problems in the human body. Therefore, introducing them can never fix the root cause, because it doesn't go to the cause.

We do need medicine, we can just choose more natural places to find it. And few things will give you as great a respect of nature as when you find out just how powerful herbal medicine can be.

Want better workouts and recovery? There are herbs for that.

Want better sleep? There are herbs for that.

Want improved cognition? There are herbs for that.

Want to improve your sex life? There are herbs for that.

Want greater energy? There are herbs for that.

Whatever your problem or concern, there are certain herbs that can help you out. I got involved in herbalism to support my health and performance, starting in fitness. After practicing this for years myself I got involved in it as a business. In the beginning, it started simply because my brothers, who are partners in the business, and I just wanted to find the best-quality stuff for ourselves and make it available to others too. Since that time, our company, Lost Empire Herbs, has grown significantly and will continue to do so.

Many of the herbs I will be talking about are ones that we sell. The reason I'm talking about them though is because I am most familiar with them, personally use them, and not just because we sell them.

You're welcome to check our website, www.lostempireherbs.com, to find out more. We pride ourselves on delivering lots of information to help you best guide your choices. Since herbalism is largely a lost art, the average person needs education to even get started.

And even if you choose not to do business with us, I would hope you would still investigate using these and other herbs to help support your health and performance. They are available from countless other places

200

too.

Herbalism is a massive subject that could fill volumes, but just as an introduction let's explore a few of the functions and classes of herbs available and what they can do for you. This is just a glimpse to give you an idea of a few things available that are out there.

Most of the herbs that I mention here would fall into the superior class of herbalism. These are herbs that contain one or more of the three treasures, jing, qi, and shen, according to the Taoist philosophy used in Chinese medicine. The superior herbs help in living a long life, promote radiant health, and work not just on the physical body. Importantly, they have no negative side effects even when taken for long periods of time.

One more important aspect of superior herbs, according to Ron Teeguarden, is "their remarkable ability to *regulate* body functions rather than force physiological activity in just one direction…If an herb does not have double-direction activity, it is a drug—and inferior herb." This shows the ability of certain herbs to intelligently work with your body.

Also, note that I use the term *herbalism* in the holistic sense. Herbs are not just leafy plants but can also include things from the animal, fungal and mineral kingdoms as well, anything natural that can be utilized effectively.

Medicinal Mushrooms

No, not magic mushrooms, though we'll cover those in a bit. Medicinal mushrooms is the name given to a grouping of mushrooms that have some potent effects, most notably on the immune system. The majority of these are tree mushrooms, but there are a number of ground mushrooms too.

Paul Stamets, one of the world's foremost mycologists, wrote in his book *MycoMedicinals*, "Scientists have only recently confirmed what ancient cultures have known for centuries: mushrooms have within them some of the most potent medicines found in nature. Long viewed as tonics, we now know that their cellular constituents can profoundly improve the quality of human health."

I recall seeing Stamets speak at a conference I was attending and talking about how mushrooms helped support the health of his mother who was going through cancer. At the time, my mother had recently passed away. This launched me deeper into using mushrooms. I found that one of the best for cancer, known as turkey tail, grew in the woods near where I lived.

The most popular of these mushrooms is reishi (*Ganoderma lucidum*). Many herbalists have stated, and I agree, that if everyone in the world took reishi mushroom, it would be a far better place. Reishi has been called "the mushroom of immortality" and even the "god herb." Because of its revered status, it is the topic of artwork all throughout the Orient. Reishi is amazing for the immune system, highly regarding for its cancer-fighting properties, also studied for use in HIV, autoimmunity, and more.[7]

Some other top ones, heavily researched for cancer, are the aforementioned turkey tail (*Trametes versicolor*), chaga (*Inonotus obliquus*), and shiitake (*Lentinula edodes*). A scientific review of the evidence stated that, "Medicinal mushrooms represent a growing segment of today's pharmaceutical industry owing to the plethora of useful bioactive compounds. While they have a long history of use across diverse cultures, they are backed up by reasonable scientific investigation now. The mycologists around the world, firmly believe that a greater knowledge of mushroom can ameliorate many forms of cancers at various stages."[8]

Speaking of cancer, if I was ever to be diagnosed with cancer, one of the first things I would do is take massive doses of medicinal mushrooms. This could be done in addition to any other treatment, conventional or alternative. I would similarly recommend this to anyone going through such.

And remember the old maxim, an ounce of prevention is worth a pound of cure. Taking these regularly helps support your health and immune system in a way that is likely to hinder these problems from arising in the first place. (Just like fasting.)

All of the medicinal mushrooms are good for the immune system. They have dual direction activity, meaning that they can help the immune system become stronger when it needs to be, and turn it down in cases where it is overboard, which is anything autoimmune in nature.

In essence, these fungal intelligences help your immune system become smarter. Because of their similarities in how mushrooms look to plants in many ways, and grow out in nature, we often think of them like plants. But in several ways, they're closer to us than plants. Like the fact that some mushrooms will produce vitamin D, like we do, although in a different form. While we use cholesterol as the starting molecule for hormones, and fungi use ergosterol, we both use a component called lanosterol, which is absent in plants. Many of our proteins are similar. And according to research, we share a common ancestor with fungi closer than we do with plants.[9]

Because plants and mycelium (that is the network of the fungal colony) very often work hand in hand, they benefit each other symbiotically. The mycelium does a lot of the immune system work for the plants, in exchange for nutrition. Perhaps they work in our bodies in much the same way.

There're other benefits too. Reishi helps to support your mood, helping people simply be happier and calmer. These "shen" effects, as they're known in Chinese medicine, are less well researched than the immune system benefits, but they're beginning to be, showing how reishi helps with depression and anxiety.[10]

The mushroom that first grabbed my attention and introduced me to the wide world of herbalism in the first place was cordyceps (*Cordyceps sp.*). It's effects in aiding the endurance in my workouts was notable. Along with that, it brings many other benefits to the immune system, endocrine system, and various aspects of anti-aging.[11]

Lion's mane mushroom (*Hericium erinaceus*) is being heavily researched for aiding in Alzheimer's, dementia, and all forms of cognitive decline. This is because it has been found to support nerve-growth factor.[12]

I am not telling you to begin picking random mushrooms from the forest. There are some deadly ones out there. But if you learn about these fungi, they can be powerful allies in your health and beyond.

Adaptogens

The term *adaptogen* is relatively new in the world of herbalism. It was coined by the Russian toxicologist, Nikolai Lazarev in 1947. Adaptogens are those "that increase resistance to a broad spectrum of harmful factors (stressors) of different physical, chemical and biological natures." Basically, they help the body to adapt better to any sort of stressor.

For an herb to be considered an adaptogen it has to meet the following three criteria. These were defined in 1969 by Brekhman and Dardymov.[13]

1. The substance must be nontoxic, suitable for consumption by just about everyone, even at large doses.
2. It must be non-specific, in that it doesn't target just one problem, or one area of the body.
3. It must be normalizing, meaning that it can regulate function, not just increase or decrease.

For these reasons, adaptogens have become very popular recently. They might even be considered trendy.

Some of the most popular adaptogens include ginseng, rhodiola, ashwagandha, eleuthero, schisandra, shilajit, licorice, tulsi and others. Many of the medicinal mushrooms previously covered are also considered adaptogens, including reishi, shiitake, and cordyceps.

In Ayurvedic medicine, the name *rasayana*, meaning a restorative tonic that helps promote health and longevity, is similar in nature.

If you take adaptogens what are they going to do for you? They will help your body better adapt to stress, both mental and physical. This means that your capacity to handle stress will grow larger. Things that previously stressed you may not affect you as much.

What many people notice when they take adaptogens is more energy. Be warned that this can be a double-edged sword though. Just like stimulants, such as coffee, adaptogens can be over-used. If you take them too much, while neglecting to get plenty of quality sleep, good nutrition, time in nature, or any of the other areas covered in this book, just so you can handle a big workload and get by, you may end up digging yourself a deeper hole. Adaptogens are powerful, and as such, they should be used responsibly.

That being said, if you are working on your health in many areas, taking one or more adaptogens can be of great benefit.

Research has looked at the effects of adaptogens on the hypothalamic-pituitary-adrenal (HPA) axis and the sympatho-adrenal-system (SAS). Specifically, the difference in how they compare to stimulants is the difference in recovery periods after forced workloads. With stimulants, you see a high peak, followed by a dip. With adaptogens there is a less-high peak, followed by a smooth elevation. Some of the mechanisms of action investigated include synthesis of proteins and nucleic acids, energy regulation, and release of stress hormones.[14]

Some of the well-known adaptogens, rhodiola, eleuthero, and schisandra were shown to have increases in mental performance and working capacity with even just a single dose.[15] Although this may be the case, most people will want to take them regularly for extended periods of time to maximize the benefits.

Nervines

Nervine herbs are those that act on the nervous system. Generally, this term is used to refer to two different groups, nervine relaxants and nervine hypnotics. For those that want to aid their sleep, you'll want to pay attention here.

For those that want more energy, many are focused on stimulants like coffee and tea, and the adaptogens just covered. But you should also pay attention here. By relaxing and bringing down your nervous energy at times, you will have much more energy at other times.

With the pace of society these days, this category may be one of the most important in herbalism.

Nervine relaxants are those that are gentle in action. This includes lemon balm, gotu kola, ashwagandha, chamomile, catnip, lavender, blue vervain, albizia and others. You can take these in the morning and throughout the day and they'll support your mood and nervous system staying a bit more relaxed. My personal favorite for stress relief is blue vervain.

Chamomile (*Chamomilla recutita*) is thought to have mild tranquilizing and sleep-inducing effects because the flavonoid, apigenin, binds to benzodiazepine receptors in the brain. Meanwhile other similar compounds also bind to these sites and GABA receptors.[16]

Gotu kola (*Centella asiatica*) has mild sedative effects believed to be because of the brahmoside and brahminosides. Meanwhile, the antidepressant effects appear to be from the triterpenes.[17]

The nervine hypnotics are stronger. These are most often used before going to bed, or to literally support falling asleep. Some examples include skullcap, valerian, passionflower, kava, hops and wild lettuce. In addition to helping with sleep, many of these are anodynes or pain relievers.

For instance, passionflower (*Passiflora incarnata*) contains a high amount of GABA and has a direct effect on GABA receptors, needed for sleep and well-being.[18]

Ever get sleepy from drinking beer? Hops (*Humulus lupulus*), which are used to give beer its bitter flavor and preserve it, have long been used in herbalism for their properties. Recent investigation has found their interaction with GABA and NMDA receptors in the brain which may be responsible for their sedative and anxiety-reducing effects.[19]

Other herbs that act on the nervous system can be considered nootropic. Nootropic means a substance that promotes the enhancement of cognition, memory, and learning. Although this term is typically reserved for drugs or isolated supplements, it can be applied to herbs too.

My favorite herb for this is bacopa (*Bacopa monnieri*). The first time I took this herb I could feel my mind immediately focus. This effect occurs every single time I take it. Although I, and many others, can feel it right upon taking it, the research shows that the best effects come from consistent use over time.[20] Some of the adaptogens like schisandra, rhodiola, and ashwagandha also have nootropic effects.

Endocrine Tonics

An area of great interest to me is that of endocrine, or hormonal, support. The adaptogens play a big role in this, with their effects on cortisol, epinephrine and norepinephrine. But what I'm referring to here is the sex hormones like testosterone and estrogen.

Pine pollen is the pollen from pine trees. It is interesting in that in contains several of the same hormones as we do, including testosterone,

DHEA, and androstenedione.[21] The amounts of these are very small, but then again hormones don't take much for signaling. There are other plant hormones too, called gibberellins and brassinosteroids that exert similar actions.

Still, I can't say if it's the hormones or simply the energetic structure of the pine pollen. Whatever is happening, pine pollen seems to work very well for many people that take it. Although it is considered primarily a male herb, it works great for many women too. Ladies shouldn't let the word testosterone scare them off, as they absolutely need this hormone too, just in amounts about one-tenth as much as men. If you're looking for athletic or sexual benefits this is a great herb to try out.

If you live in areas with pine trees you've seen how at a certain time in spring this yellow pollen will be everywhere. Pine pollen is not only active in pollinating pine cones. It is active everywhere. This hormonal signal is acting on all of nature that it touches and indeed may be one of the things that helps Spring spring up like it does in those areas. This clues us in to what it can do for us. For men, especially, this pollen can help with everything related to your pollen—i.e. your sexual function and sperm quality.

Another important functions that pine pollen appears to have is in combating the endocrine disruption that is rampant in our environment, from our own making. Xeno-estrogens and various other endocrine-disrupting chemicals, found in plastics, pesticides, tap water, skincare products, cleaning supplies and more, are part of our daily lives. The phyto-androgens, and other components inside of pine pollen, appear to help combat these, being a much-needed ally in what seems to be a war we're losing.

There is an overall population-level decline of testosterone in men, and this is not because of age or weight gain.[22] Based on my study of the subject, this is mostly because of man-made chemical pollutants. Similarly, a recent study stated, "In this comprehensive meta-analysis, sperm counts…declined significantly among men from North America, Europe and Australia during 1973–2011, with a 50–60 percent decline among men unselected by fertility, with no evidence of a 'leveling off' in recent years. These findings strongly suggest a significant decline in male reproductive health, which has serious implications beyond fertility concerns. Research on causes and implications of this decline is urgently needed."[23]

It is just possible that we could kill off our species by rendering ourselves infertile completely from the chemical pollution we're spreading.

Sadly, very little research has been done at this time on pine pollen, but when it is finally done, we'll likely find it backing up all of what was just said.

Another great hormonal herb is tongkat ali (*Eurycoma longiflolia*). This doesn't work in the same way as pine pollen, but through different mechanisms. The theory is that it helps by triggering the body to increase its own testosterone production and keeps it more freely available by limiting aromatization (the conversion of testosterone into estrogen), and sex hormone–binding globulin, which binds to testosterone.[24]

Since cortisol is inversely correlated with the sex hormones, primarily because it steals precursor material, many of the adaptogens like ashwagandha, ginseng, eleuthero, and others are also known for supporting the hormonal system, especially where stress is a contributing factor.

While certain herbs may be known as male herbs or female herbs, the fact is that all can be used by both sexes for benefit, just dosage and usage will vary. Still, to even it out, let's talk about two of the best "female" herbs.

Shatavari (*Asparagus racemosus*) is considered the primary female tonic in Ayurvedic medicine. There, it is given to both the young and old and is often used throughout the course of a lifetime. Shatavari possesses phytoestrogens, which bring some of the benefits. It has been investigated for helping mothers produce milk, increasing libido, supporting the uterus and every phase of a woman's health. It's also under investigation for adaptogenic properties, helping the immune system, supporting the mood and more.[25]

From Chinese medicine, the top herb for women is dong quai (*Angelica sinensis*). Considered one of the best blood builders, dong quai has a strong anecdotal history of aiding in sexual desire, menopause, PMS symptoms and more, though research backing these claims is conflicting.[26]

Psycho-actives

There's one last category that I would like to address, the so-called psychoactive herbs or drugs as they're commonly referred to. I use the term psychoactive humorously, because when you realize the holistic nature of herbs you'll realize that they are all active on your psychology to one degree or another.

Still, this term is usually referred to those that "heavily alter" your psyche, at least for a time. Other terms include hallucinogens, psychedelics, and entheogens. Many people the world over continue to break laws and use these. Is it pure escapism, or is there a real reason for this?

Back in high school I smoked cannabis and took psilocybin on a few occasions. This was purely for fun. These days, when I partake, it is something quite different. As I got into herbalism, and began to learn about shamanism, I saw that these plants weren't to be misused, but respected. As the shamans will tell you, these are great teacher plants (and fungi).

I started this book talking about Ayuhuasca, but the fact is that I have used psilocybin mushrooms the most, and to greatest effect. These mushrooms have helped me communicate better with nature, building a relationship with Mother Nature, even giving a glimpse into her mind. They have helped with depatterning my mind allowing me to get rid of longstanding bad habits and creating new helpful ones.

These aren't just something random we can take to "trip out". Animals seem to use these regularly too. In an explosion of examples, Lierre Keith writes, "Bighorn sheep will chew their teeth down to the gums to eat psychoactive lichen off of rocks. Cattle will return to eat locoweed until it kills them. Birds get stoned on cannabis seeds, and jaguars eat the bark off the yaje vine to hallucinate. Elephants make wine from palm sap. Birds fill up on fermented berries until they're drunk and disoriented enough to die by flying while intoxicated. Ducks seek out narcotic plants. Monkeys and dogs love opium smoke. Chimps will surmount their fear of fire to smoke cigarettes, and tobacco is addictive to a number of animals, including parrots, baboons, and hamsters. Reindeer will ignore food to pursue hallucinogenic mushrooms if they smell them in use by Lapp shamans. Now consider that the poppy was one of the first domesticated plants – ain't nobody harvesting those tiny little seeds to make a meal."

Instead these form an active part of nature that help to allow nature to do much the same, learning and growing. Buhner writes of these psychoactive chemicals, "The neurochemicals in our bodies were used in every life-form on the planet long before we showed up. They predate the emergence of the human species by hundreds of millions of years. They must have been doing something all that time, you know, besides waiting for us to appear."

With the illegalization, research was suppressed, but now this is beginning to turn. Use of psychedelics has not been negatively associated with mental health issues, despite the press. In fact, those that used them were found to be associated with lowered rates of mental health problems.[27]

A review of individuals' experiences in their use found that, "for psychologically mature individuals, the psychedelics, while not constituting a path to deep awakening by themselves, could facilitate psychological growth when used in the context of an ongoing discipline. Advantages were said to include an opening to new realms of experience and belief, deeper understanding of depth psychologies, religions, and consciousness disciplines, more rapid working through of psychological barriers, and insights that provided guiding visions in subsequent life."[28]

The Multidisciplinary Association for Psychedelic Studies (MAPS) has investigated several specific uses of specific psychedelics. MDMA is being used to treat PTSD. LSD-assisted psychotherapy is being used for anxiety. Iboga, an African medicine, can get people off of heroin without any symptoms of withdrawal.[29]

Psilocybin is being investigated for helping terminally ill cancer patients make the end-of-life transition more peacefully.[30]

The best way to use these are under the guidance of qualified administrators. In some cases, this could be doctors and psychologists. In other cases, it's a legitimate shaman. In my opinion, doing natural drugs in a natural setting is one of the best ways to help restore your connection to nature.

This path may not be suitable for everyone. If you do choose to partake in them, please be careful. Be aware that certain drugs are more dangerous than others. For all their potency, this can lead to good as well as bad. Not everyone benefits.

There are other ways to reach similar states. Just in communicating to the plants you can learn from them. But taking these psychoactive medicines can be like getting hit on the head with a sledgehammer. It's powerful. It's intense. In can have a huge impact. And you must be careful in doing so. This is true of anything that has this kind of potency.

That being said, the use of more regular herbs, not just psychoactive ones, is the path for all human kind. It's a forgotten part of our diet that simply cannot be forgotten if you want to experience radiant health and perform at the highest levels.

Nor are the psychedelics even necessarily the most fascinating of plants. Some have reputations for magical abilities. Agrimony is one of these. Herbalist Matthew Wood says, "It will change the environment around the person using it." You certainly won't find an 'active constituent' inside the plant that has this effect. Is that Semmelweis reflex kicking in for you, yet?

This chapter was meant only to be a brief overview. Herbalism is a complex subject. To understand it properly you need training at least as long and intense as any doctor goes through. In fact, your whole lifetime could go into just knowing a few plants well. I invite you to begin your exploration of the topic.

Experiment

A word on individuality. You may read a study that says this herb works for this function. Or you may hear about how it does so in other people. That's a good clue, a starting point, from which to go off of. But it doesn't guarantee that it will work for you. It might. It might not.

Even if it doesn't work, that doesn't mean that it doesn't work in general. Individually it may not be suited for you. Or the quality of what you're using is not up to par. Sadly, this is a big issue in the industry. There are also things like lack of hydration, lack of micronutrients, and similar things that could be in the way of getting the benefits that you want.

Then there is the whole constitutional component that is at use in every system of herbalism, but not taught in how the West looks at health. This involves matching up the constitution of the plants to your constitution.

Although with some herbs you can feel effects right away, especially if you train your sensitivity to do so, most people will not note any difference for a while. It is best to take most herbs every day for at least a month to really try them out. At that point, you may feel different. Sometimes you won't even note any difference until you stop taking the herbs. It subtly builds up its effects over time, then, when you stop, the contrast is what makes it apparent.

In any case, it is up to you to do the only experiments that really matter, those that work for you. In doing so, in time, you will find those plant allies that are best for you.

Did one or more of the herbs mentioned spark your interest as you read through these pages? Did it call out to you? If so, that would be a great place to get started.

15
Symbiosis

"A human being is actually a giant swarm. Or more precisely, it's a swarm of swarms, because each organ - blood, liver, kidneys - is a separate swarm. What we refer to as a body is really the combination of all these organ swarms...The control of our behavior is not located in our brains. It's all over our bodies...'Swarm intelligence' rules human beings...We don't have conscious control over ourselves at all. We just think we do. Just because human beings went around thinking of themselves of 'I' didn't mean it was true."
– Michael Crichton

"This is what medicine looks like when you understand that microbes are not the enemies of animals, but the foundations upon which our kingdom is built. Say goodbye to dated and dangerous war metaphors, in which we are soldiers hell-bent on eradicating germs at whatever cost. Say hello to a gentler and more nuanced gardening metaphor. Yes, we still have to pull out the weeds, but we also seed and feed the species that bind the soil, freshen the air, and please the eye"
– Ed Yong

D o you recall the movie *The Matrix*? In it, Agent Smith, from the technological artificial intelligence, discusses with Morpheus his viewpoint on human kind:

"I'd like to share a revelation that I've had during my time here. It came to me when I tried to classify your species, and I realized that you're not actually mammals. Every mammal on this planet instinctively develops a natural equilibrium with the surrounding environment; but you humans do not. You move to an area and you multiply, and multiply, until every natural resource is consumed and the only way you can survive is to spread to another area. There is another organism on this planet that follows the same pattern. Do you know what it is? A virus. Human beings are a disease, a cancer on this planet, you are a plague, and we...are the cure."

This gets to the heart of how most humans in this day and age generally view ecology. Let me explain.

For many years, after Louis Pasteur's discovery, bacteria were all labeled bad, and man's goal was to destroy them. Pasteurization, named after the man, is defined as the process of heating a liquid or food to kill pathogenic bacteria to make the food safe to eat. This discovery has led to better sanitation, antibiotics, and more that have saved countless human lives.

However, via pasteurization's definition, it doesn't even mention the existence of beneficial bacteria. Nor that this genocide has some friendly fire involved. At the same time, in leading to some advances, this error in philosophy has demonstrated devastating effects to both human health and that of the ecology.

Most people now recognize that most bacteria are not really bad—the majority of the bacteria being either good or neutral. Or the more complex reality that there aren't really good or bad bacteria, but amount and location are critically important.

For example, 1,000 bacteria per mL are normally found in the upper small intestine. SIBO, or small intestine bacterial overgrowth, occurs when there are 100,000 to 1,000,000 bacteria per mL. In addition, the types of these bacteria matter, like the *Klebsiella* species which can produce toxins that damage the mucosa and impair absorption.[1] SIBO then leads to symptoms such as weight loss, nutritional deficiencies, osteoporosis, chronic diarrhea, and more.

So why is Agent Smith off in his assessment? The "all bacteria is bad" kind of thinking has not yet extended to viruses. Most People still think of a virus as an exclusively bad thing. Don't you? You can see this thinking implicitly in the writers of Agent Smith's monologue, how the virus is immediately made equivalent to disease and cancer. However, just like bacteria, this is not the case.

You've undoubtedly heard that the human body is made up of roughly 90 percent bacterial cells, and only 10 percent human cells. While often stated, this happens to be one of those inaccurate scientific myths that spread widely. More accurate and recent analyses point to it being closer to a 50/50 split of human and bacteria cells.[2] (That is at least until the next scientific revision.)

And while the gut microbiome is given the majority of the attention, for its role we'll be exploring more in a bit, it is important to recognize that bacteria are everywhere in your body. Evidence points to the womb not even being the sterile environment it was once thought to be.[3]

And each body part you have contains entirely different ecologies. According to one study, your right hand and your left hand only have about 17 percent of the same species of bacteria.[4] And this, in turn, will vary widely with the next person.

But neither are we just human and bacteria cells. The microbiome is made up of all different types of microbes, including bacteria, fungi, archaea, and viruses. The fungal component of what makes up part of a human is called the mycobiome. Here again we focus on the bad or negative aspects of fungus, whether it is in athlete's foot, toe fungus, or candida, but this mycology has beneficial functions too. Yet we don't even have words to discuss it in the sense of a positive symbiosis—only diseases.

Research on this aspect is far more limited than with bacteria, but some is starting to come to light. Diseases that previously were thought to have no association to fungi, such as inflammatory bowel disease, cystic fibrosis, and hepatitis B, are now all associated with particular mycobiomes. Organs like the lungs, once thought to be sterile environments, are housing many types of fungi.

A review of the sparse literature about the mycobiome states, "Like the mycobiome as a whole, individual members of the mycobiome may also play a beneficial or commensal role in the host. Beneficial fungi have been found to be preventive and therapeutic agents…The limitation of today's immune therapies is that most target only a single fungal species, ignoring the overall mycobiome composition. To date, our knowledge of the mycobiome suggests that interactions among fungi within an environment and between mycobiomes found in different body sites may play an important role in pathogenesis."[5]

Many of the fungi, as well as bacteria, cannot be cultured, and, thus, we know very little about them. Sometimes bacteria and fungi are found together. Other times, when one is in supremacy, it suppresses the others.

Then there is what has been labeled the virome, the viral component of the microbiome. Here the numbers are more staggering. There may up to one hundred times as many viruses as there are human cells. These viruses play active and important roles in our health just like bacteria.

As Herbert Virgin, M.D., Ph. D., put it, "Virome interactions with the host cannot be encompassed by a monotheistic view of viruses as pathogens. Instead, the genetic and transcriptional identity of mammals is defined in part by our co-evolved virome, a concept with profound implications for understanding health and disease."[6]

And this is why Agent Smith is wrong. Not all viruses are bad. It's the same early sentiment we had towards bacteria, and now we're finding just how wrong that is. Hopefully, we can learn from past mistakes.

For technical reasons, these viruses are much harder to identify than even bacteria and fungi. An estimated 1 percent of the virome has been sequenced, and this is likely a high estimate. If understanding everything that makes us up is important to understand health, then we have a long way to go.

Dr. Virgin concludes, "The early findings from studies of the virome, and other aspects of the microbiome, point to the need for a new science of metagenetics, defined as the integrative analysis of the impact of genes of the host in the context of the genes within the microbiome including the virome...The virome is in us and on us, and is likely to be recognized through metagenetic analysis in the future as a friend at times, and, at other times, as a more complex enemy than we supposed."

Even with bacteria, the emerging picture is that we might not really be able to talk about bacterial species, as they swap around DNA and genes too much.[7] As W. Ford Doolittle, Ph.D., said, "There's no single such thing as a microbial species...The species concept is doomed to radical irrelevance because we don't actually need it any more. Metagenomics will come in and shift the paradigm for it...More [novel] organisms are created through [genetic] recombination than through mutation." This horizontal gene transfer allows one microbe to pass on traits, its DNA, to another, such as antibiotic resistance or the ability to digest certain foods.

Antibiotics were supposed to wipe out infectious diseases by the end of the twentieth century according to many people. In arrogance, we did not realize how smart and adaptable bacteria were. Buhner writes, "In an extremely short geologic time period Earth has been saturated with hundreds of millions of tons of nonbiodegradable, often biologically unique pharmaceuticals designed to kill bacteria...It has, as Levy comments, 'stimulated evolutionary changes that are unparalled in recorded biologic history.' In the short run this means the emergence of unique pathogenic bacteria in human, animal, and agricultural crop populations. In the long run experts suggest the possibility of infectious disease epidemics more potent and deadly than *any* in human history."

This is part of the problem of thinking that technological advances will always save us. Antibiotics were absolutely helpful, but in our shortsighted, widespread use of them, they may no longer be. And this could very well setup a worse future than if we hadn't used them in the first place. Only time will tell.

Nor is symbiosis just about tiny, microscopic living things. There are even creatures from the animal kingdom inside of us. While thinking of this might make your skin crawl, that just goes to show how far we've been culturally indoctrinated against what is completely natural and ecological.

In a paper titled *"Equal Rights for Parasites"* Donald Windsor wrote, "Because parasites and hosts co-evolved, the concept of a parasite-free host is an unnatural derivative of our human experience. We strive to raise animals and plants without parasites. In fact, we douse ourselves, our livestock, and our crops with tons of poisonous pesticides to maintain this artificial pest-free status. This very act demonstrates how natural the host-parasite bond really is: like the chemical bond, we have to introduce energy to break it."[8]

We are not just humans, but a complex system, a swarm in Crichton's words, of basically every different kingdom of life. Researchers have called the human skin a "virtual zoo of bacteria," and compared the diversity of the gut to a rainforest.

Ecology. Keep that word in mind as we dive deeper inward, and then

217

expand bigger and outward.

We all live symbiotically. Although that word is typically taken to mean living in harmony, that is not necessarily the case. This is further broken down into different living arrangements.

Mutually beneficial symbiosis is when both, or multiple, unions benefit all of the individuals involved. This does not necessarily mean every cell is benefitted, but the community or the collective is. This is also known as mutualist symbiosis. Then there is also commensal symbiosis, where the organisms benefitted, but the host was not affected for better or ill.

Of course, even this is too simple. As Ed Yong writes, "The world of symbiosis is one in which our allies can disappoint us and our enemies can rally to our side." It's not always the type of the microbe that matters, but also how many of it exists, its relationship to others, and where it is.

Yong continues, "We have evolved ways of selecting which species live with us, restricting where they sit in our bodies, and controlling their behaviour so they are more likely to be mutualistic than pathogenic. Like all the best relationships, these ones take work."

Finally, parasitic symbiosis is how we think about parasites. These are things that live off of the host, hurting the host to better support itself. Mosquitoes and fleas are insect examples we're all aware of externally. Although we'll point to our dog dragging is hindquarters on the ground as having parasites inside, we don't like to look at the fact that so many of us do too. This is not relegated exclusively to un-hygienic people living in the "third world."

In alternative health circles parasite cleanses have often been advocated and used. Get those nasty things like roundworms, tapeworms, and liver flukes out of me! But even here we find that certain parasites, meaning animal life, multi-cellular complex creatures, living within us may be beneficial.[9]

This isn't to say that there are not harmful parasites, bacteria, and viruses that we should do our best to avoid. I don't think I need to belabor that point. But I do question the destructive power of these, if our own immune system and ecology is in check.

Hygiene and Old Friends

Our modern lives of trying to pasteurize away all bacteria and infuse soaps and even objects with anti-bacterial drugs, shows this fear, this flawed paradigm. But the fact is that this attitude is coming with a health cost. The dirtier we are, the healthier we seem to be.

The "hygiene hypothesis" is that, especially in early childhood, lack of exposure to bacteria and other infectious agents, including parasites, may lead to a compromised immune system, as it is not being properly trained. This then leads to issues such as autoimmunity, allergies and other problems throughout life.

This is in stark contrast to the "germ theory of disease" where all germs were labeled as bad and has been the mainstay of medicine for a century, up until recently. In this Darwinian struggle for survival it was either us or them. That's what science thought, though it didn't mean it was true. In 1938, William Bulloch published *The History of Bacteriology*. In this book, our mutualist microbes are not mentioned at all.

Graham Hook is one of the leading researchers of what he calls the "Old Friends Hypothesis." He wrote of this, "This failure of immuno-regulation is partly attributable to a lack of exposure to organisms ("Old Friends") from mankind's evolutionary past that needed to be tolerated and therefore evolved roles in driving immunoregulatory mechanisms. Some Old Friends (such as helminths and infections picked up at birth that established carrier states) are almost eliminated from the urban environment. This increases our dependence on Old Friends derived from our mothers, other people, animals, and the environment. It is suggested that the requirement for microbial input from the environment to drive immunoregulation is a major component of the beneficial effect of green space, and a neglected ecosystem service that is essential for our well-being."[10]

The statement of "cleanliness is next to godliness" may just be false. Unless you mean that by cleaning up, i.e. getting rid of all the "dirty germs," that you'll accelerate your death and then be closer to god.

There are about one million microbes per gram of food you eat. You can't avoid them. No amount of germaphobia and being like Howard

Hughes will save you.

Comparisons between people exposed to more bacteria in infancy, compared to those that weren't, showed less inflammation, as measured by C-reactive protein, later in adult life, in those with more exposure.[11]

Furthermore, it appears that these inflammatory effects even extend to our central nervous system and our well-being.[12] Without some of our old friends, it appears that we just don't feel right.

To study the effects of the microbiome, special mice have been raised that are completely germ free. These have been found to have both higher risks of autoimmunity as well as being more prone to infections and suffer from higher stress, all while eating more but weighing less.[13]

Intercellular Symbiosis

This symbiosis extends further than just one species supporting another. Over history, two or more species have merged, becoming inseparable. In fact, it seems that this is one of the most critical components of evolution. It is not random mutation, but a process called symbiogenesis. Two merged to create something new. Lynn Margulis put forth the idea that some cells evolved through this act of symbiosis or joining up together.[14]

Out in the wild, you can see this in all plant life. Chloroplasts in green plants closely resemble cyanobacteria. And indeed, when the DNA of these were analyzed they were found to be much the same.

In us, it is most apparent with the mitochondria. These are commonly called the powerhouses of our cells, with between one to ten thousand of them in each cell. There are so many that, by body weight, they make up about ten percent of us.

The mitochondria create ATP, the energy we use to do everything we do, to the tune of up to about six hundred molecules per second. Long ago, they were free-wheeling bacteria. But at some point, they joined with cells, that would eventually become all of animal life.

Are these independent bacteria? Or are they human? Or are they both?

When you take an antibiotic to purge a pathogen from your body, might you also be causing destruction to not only your friendly bacteria, but even your own cells too?

"Any organism, if not itself a live bacterium, is then a descendent – one way or another—of a bacterium or, more likely, mergers of several kinds of bacteria," wrote Margulis. "Bacteria initially populated the planet and have never relinquished their hold."

Perhaps more importantly, do they have a mind of their own? Dave Asprey, in his book *Head Strong*, explores this idea that much of our behavior is driven by the quality of our mitochondria. He writes, "I've started to see my own body as a big walking petri dish supporting a quadrillion mitochondria, doing whatever they want."

Birth and Biome

When we are born, we are meant to go through the vaginal canal as nature intended. Being able to do a Cesarean section is great to save the life of the baby or the mother, but there is a hidden downside to it that was only recently discovered.

The baby's digestive tract is inoculated by bacteria in the vaginal canal.[15] Even fecal matter may be important to this process. Once the baby is born, this is meant to be its first contact with the bacterial world. And not getting this contact, the baby may never again take on the bacterial population it was meant to have.

Fortunately, if a C-section is necessary (or god forbid, planned), then a sponge can be inserted into the vagina and then placed on the baby's mouth and nose area, as a roundabout way of accomplishing this.[16]

Next, breast feeding is important to feed not just the baby, but the bacteria too. In fact, human milk ogliosaccharides, a major part of milk, are not digested by humans, but by the bacteria. This prebiotic food is important for setting up the right colony. Research has found that human milk ranges in having over 200 different types of ogliosaccharides, and they seem especially important for setting up the *Bifidobacteria longum biovar infantis*.[17] Think about that for a moment. We've lived with bacteria so long that the human body produces food for the baby and the bacteria too.

Nor is this just good for the baby or the bacteria. Research shows that mothers who breastfeed are less likely to get breast or ovarian cancer, and the longer they do so, the better the results.[18]

Speaking of birth, a symbiosis if there ever is one, I'll provide this short tangent. Alice Dreger Ph.D., a former professor at Feinberg School of Medicine, was quoted in *The Vaccine Friendly Plan*:

"According to the best studies available, when it came time to birth at the end of my low-risk pregnancy, I should not have an induction, nor an episiotomy, nor continuous monitoring of the baby's heartbeat during labor, nor pain medications, and definitely not a C-section. I should give birth in the squatting position, and I should have a doula—a professional labor support person to talk to me throughout the birth. (Studies show that doulas are astonishingly effective at lowering risk, so good that one obstetrician has quipped that if doulas were a drug, it would be illegal not to give one to every pregnant mother.)

"In other words, if the regular low-tech tests kept indicating I was having a medically uninteresting pregnancy, and if I wanted to *scientifically* maximize safety, I should give birth pretty much like my great-grandmothers would have: with the attention of a couple of experienced women mostly waiting it out, while I did the work. (They call it *labor* for a reason.) The only real notable difference was that my midwife would intermittently use a fetal heart monitor —just every now and then—to make sure the baby was doing okay."

This may be surprising to hear for most people. And so might be the following. We think we're technologically advanced, which makes us superior. But, in the United States we have the highest infant mortality rate of any industrialized country, due to our overuse of interventions.[19]

While these ideas are important to know if you, or anyone you know, is giving birth, let's shift focus to what you can do now for your microbiome, whether you were vaginally birthed and breastfed or not.

The Gut Microbiome

Despite being one of the most popular supplements, most probiotics might be close to useless. For one, many of them do not have the count of bacteria that they claim to have. Secondly, even with that count, it is likely not enough to sway your microbiome.

Probiotics first came on the scene in the early 1900s with the research by Nobel laureate Élie Metchnikoff. However, his ideas didn't catch on in a big way until recently. Now, probiotic supplements sell annually over $30 billion across the globe.

To change your microbiome, you're going to have to change the food of the bacteria. By changing the food, the ratio of bacteria is going to change. Different bacteria can setup shop. The many foods for bacteria are different types of carbohydrates, specifically ones that we can't digest but that they can.

One experiment with ten people split those into two groups. One fed primarily on fruits, vegetables, and grains, while the other group ate meat, eggs, and cheese. The microbiomes of these volunteers changed within a single day.[20] Yong wrote of this, "These two kinds of community looked a lot like the gut microbes of herbivorous and carnivorous mammals, respectively. They were recapitulating millions of years of evolution in less than a week."

And if you want to support your microbiome, the best way to do that is with fermented foods. According to some measurements a single serving of sauerkraut may have up to 10 trillion bacteria cells. Yet, the best probiotic pills typically only measure in the billions. Perhaps as important is that these bacteria are multiplied on food for the bacteria. When you eat it, not only are you providing bacteria that can colonize you but also the food supply with which to do so.

Also important may be the role of parabiotics. These are probiotics that have died. While all the attention is on the living cells, the dead bacteria we consume may also be a factor in their health effects.[21]

There are countless fermented foods. Every culture has its own favorites. I recommend you try them all in this multicultural world and find what you like. There's kim chi, beet kvass, miso, natto, pickles, and many more. Kombucha is a popular drink that is not just bacteria but also symbiotic fungus too. While many of the store-bought versions still have too much sugar in them, this can be a great probiotic drink.

Fermented dairy is another option. Yogurt, kefir, and all cheeses are fermented. While most of these found in stores are touted for their probiotic benefit, the majority of them aren't useful for this purpose. You'll want to go to a more natural form, or even make it yourself.

Even alcohol comes from fermentation. Yeast, which is in the fungal kingdom, eats up the sugar coming from grapes, barley, or other sources, to make carbon dioxide and alcohol. Sure, alcohol has its drawbacks, but it is important that we look at the fact that many of the longest-lived people drink alcohol, even in some cases a lot of it, rather than being non-drinkers. Sadly, most of the beer and wine these days is pasteurized to kill off what is living inside of it. But if you look around you can find some that are not pasteurized. The probiotic qualities of certain alcoholic drinks may be an important factor that has been overlooked.

There is also fermented meat. Essentially this is rotting meat. While this may be hard to stomach, it is fascinating to note that this is common in many different ancient cultures around the world. While the taste is likely off-putting, this may only be at first. Once you're colonized your taste buds change, and you may begin to crave this more. Or is it the bacteria that is making you crave it?

In the Amazon rainforest, I got to drink chicha with the Achuar and the people of Sarayuka. This is made from the women chewing up the manioc root and spitting it out, which then ferments. Essentially, it is spit beer. While I can't say it was the best flavor, I know that overtime I could come to enjoy it. For these indigenous people, it makes up the mainstay of their diet, providing the majority of their calories, as well as hydration, since they don't drink water.

Not every fermented food is going to work for every person. There can be difficulties with certain types of bacteria that may not coincide with what is in you, at least currently. This is something that will likely change over time, especially if you're working on becoming healthier.

You want to eat good bacteria and feed them the right food. It is also important to avoid certain things. Many poisons were let out into the market because they're shown not to harm human cells. This largely happened before we knew the importance of the microbiome.

These days we know that glyphosate, the active chemical in the pesticide in Roundup, may well have a negative impact on the microbiome.[22] Artificial sweeteners, such as aspartame, also change the microbiome, inducing glucose intolerance.[23]

Research on the effects of the microbiome are still sparse. Whether one thing causes a change in the microbiome, or the microbiome changes and then causes issues, is still up for debate. Likely both are true to some degree. Still a few studies have shown that certain populations of bacteria may lead to more chance of becoming obese, as well as higher chances of rheumatoid arthritis.[24] Both of these we previously believed not to have anything to do with microbes.

Special germ-free mice have been used and compared to their normal brethren. The germ-free mice have 40 percent less total body fat, even though they consume 29 percent more calories. The microbiome changes how nutrients are absorbed and used. Some research has shown that the *Bacteroidetes:Firmicutes* ratio was linked to obesity at least in mice.[25] But not all of the research confirms this.[26] Working with microbes proves to be tricky.

Polyphenols, which include compounds found in coffee, chocolate, wine, berries, artichokes, and many more fruits, vegetables, and seeds, interact with our gut bacteria. The microbiome is both changed by our ingestion of polyphenols, and responsible for absorbing and metabolizing them so that you can use them.[27]

Fiber of different types is important for feeding the bacteria too. There are certain prebiotic types, such as inulin, resistant starch and oligosaccharides that can be found in bigger or smaller supplies in certain foods. In mice, a low-fiber diet was shown to dramatically crash the biodiversity of the gut. What's worse is that this diversity did not come back when they resumed eating fiber. And this lower diversity would even get passed down through generations.[28]

A review summed up this information, "As carrying out a controlled dietary intervention study in humans is difficult, the complex interaction between diet, age, host environment, and host genetic background in the modulation of gut microbial ecosystems is not fully understood. Nevertheless, a recent report suggests that alteration of the gut microbiota by behavioral changes, including new dietary habits and use of antibiotics, could be the main driver of the obesity pandemic."[29]

Our gut plays a big role in our immune system. Part of it is us, and a part of it is the microbiome. Ed Yong wrote an interesting way to look at the ecology and our immune system. "I think it's more accurate to see the immune system as a team of rangers in charge of a national park – as ecosystem managers. They must carefully control the numbers of resident species and expel problematic invaders. But here's the twist: the creatures of the park hired the rangers in the first place. They taught their guardians which species to care for and which to evict."

Oh, and don't have your appendix removed unless you need to. It is important for your immune system and as a "safe house" for bacteria.[30] And when appendicitis does happen, it is likely because of this ecology being thrown off.

The Microbe Gut Brain

The gut has been called the gut brain (showing how brain-centric the dominant worldview is at this point). It appears that a large part of this is not because of the human gut itself but because of the microbiome. These microbes have been shown to communicate with the central nervous system, through the neural, endocrine, and immune systems. This in turn causes changes to cognition, anxiety, pain, and mood.[31]

One method by which they possibly do this is through their production of the short chain fatty acid, butyrate, which helps retain the integrity of the blood-brain barrier. Butyrate also lowers inflammation, prevents colon cancer, and prevents insulin resistance.[32]

The new term *psychobiotics* has been used to describe live organisms that produce health benefits in people suffering from psychiatric illness. Microbes, such as *Bifidobacterium infantis*, deliver neuroactive substances such as GABA and serotonin which can then help with symptoms of depression and chronic fatigue.[33]

Selective serotonin reuptake inhibitors (SSRI's) are one of the main psychiatric drugs, which work by increasing serotonin levels in the brain. While they do appear to work in some people, they don't in others, and can leave people worse off, even more suicidal. It turns out that 90 percent of your serotonin is produced in the gut, and the microbes play a big role in doing so.[34]

This microbiota-gut-brain axis is an important part of how you think and feel. That means your thoughts and feelings are not just you but based on your ecology as a whole.

Nor is it just that bacteria influence our nervous system. They think for themselves and communicate…linguistically. In a paper titled *"Bacterial Linguistic Communication and Social Intelligence,"* Becker et al. write, "We propose that bacteria use their intracellular flexibility, involving signal transduction networks and genomic plasticity, to collectively maintain linguistic communication: self and shared interpretations of chemical cues, exchange of chemical messages (semantic) and dialogues (pragmatic). Meaning-based communication permits colonial identity, intentional behavior (e.g. pheromone-based courtship for mating), purposeful alteration of colony structure (e.g. formation of fruiting bodies), decision-making (e.g. to sporulate) and the recognition and identification of other colonies—features we might begin to associate with a bacterial social intelligence."[35]

They have language. They are social. They make decisions, and thus, are intelligent. This is a far cry from the old idea of them being pesky invaders which must be destroyed at all costs.

James Shapiro takes it further, "Forty years' experience as a bacterial geneticist has taught me that bacteria possess many cognitive, computational and evolutionary capabilities unimaginable in the first six decades of the twentieth century. Analysis of cellular processes such as metabolism, regulation of protein synthesis, and DNA repair established that bacteria continually monitor their external and internal environments and compute functional outputs based on information provided by their sensory apparatus. Studies of genetic recombination, lysogeny, antibiotic resistance and my own work on transposable elements revealed multiple widespread bacterial systems for mobilizing and engineering DNA molecules. Examination of colony development and organization led me to appreciate how extensive multicellular collaboration is among the majority of bacterial species. Contemporary research in many laboratories on cell-cell signaling, symbiosis and pathogenesis show that bacteria utilise sophisticated mechanisms for intercellular communication and even have the ability to commandeer the basic cell biology of 'higher' plants and animals to meet their own needs. This remarkable series of observations requires us to revise basic ideas about biological information processing and recognise that even the smallest cells are sentient beings."[36]

I know this has a lot of scientific jargon. Still, I include it because when you understand what Becker and Shapiro are saying it changes the paradigm of how you must look at life.

It's not just that "you" have a gut brain, but that everything in your gut thinks too. You are not just you, you are an ecology. We'll be coming back to the intelligence of bacteria, cells, and nature later.

And the gut is not just about microbes either. Many people with Crohn's disease, as well as some other bowel issues, are now experimenting with transplants of pig whipworm eggs (*Trichuris suis*) and finding remarkable results.[37] This is an example of one of those beneficial parasites, that perhaps we're all supposed to have living along with us.

The Skin Microbiome

The skin is the largest organ on our body. Besides the gut, it's also the place with the most ecology, because of its size. And it might surprise you to learn that each part is a bit different than the rest. The bacteria that lives and thrives on your right armpit is different than that of your left. The bacteria that lives on your foot is different from your stomach, is different from your face. Your genitals also possess a unique microbiome.

We even have spiders that live on our faces. *Demodex folliculorum* and *Demodex brevis*, are mites, in the arachnid class, that live within the pores on our facial skin.[38] I know that may make your skin crawl, but perhaps but that's only because there are living things on it that do crawl!

When we use harsh chemical cleansers, what are we doing to this ecology? We're changing it dramatically. We are destroying its ability to self-regulate. We may even be committing genocide, as we wipe out whole genera!

Research in this area is still in its infancy, however we know that these organisms play a role in the modulation of skin health, both in the innate and adaptive immune system, far more than previously anticipated.[39]

There is also the hypothesis that a healthy skin microbiome plays a role in protecting from skin cancer too.

Microcosm Reflects the Macrocosm

All of these things, as much "not us" as "us," exist within and around us. Inside and on top of us, all over our skin, is an entire world's worth of living things. Your body is like a planet to this vast ecology.

And so, we humans are on the body of the earth, also teeming with living things. You are like an insect, a cell, or a bacterium, as compared to Gaia. The earth itself is just a small speck, like a cell, in the Milky Way. The Milky Way, a small part of the Universe.

Mystics and meditators have long recognized this as part of the oneness of nature. It's a fractal pattern, seemingly repeated over and over again.

We can go more microscopic. Down to the atoms themselves that make up cells. Long thought to be indivisible, atoms were discovered to contain protons, neutrons and electrons. Long thought to be indivisible, quarks, were discovered. Long thought to be indivisible, other parts will be discovered.

We can go larger on the scale too. How big is the universe? We don't know. With our more advanced technology we can only see so far. And several theories, like string theories and M-theories, propose multiple or even unlimited universes. This fractal pattern appears to extend ad infinitum. We can perceive only a few of the levels from our human position.

Ecology and life extends both ways up and down the size scale. Being so human-centric is missing out on so much more. To think our level of thinking and comprehension is the only one that matters is pure vanity. And it may be our undoing.

Being a Steward

Since we are not simply human, but a conglomeration of things, this may change how we want to focus our ideas of health. If we are not just us, but a collection of living things that can work harmoniously together, supporting the health of the whole is a matter of supporting health of everyone involved.

You cannot think merely in parts but must instead think of yourself as an ecology and part of ecology.

But there really is no ecological "self" in reality. You are not independent from the bigger picture. This ecological thinking must extend beyond your body too. You are like a cell in the body of the earth. Ecological health is reflected both inside and outside. The border is a thin line if it even exists at all except in our minds.

Plastic, full of BPA, phthalates, and other chemicals, that screws with your human endocrine system, your microbiome, also screws with the greater ecosystem as well.[40] Those same chemicals will disrupt the plant and animal life just as easily.

That pharmaceutical drug you take is created to be persistent so that it is not broken down in the human body to exert its action. But then it is eliminated. Not "poof" out of existence, but through the bathroom—out the pipes and through the water treatment plant, it makes its way back out to the environment where it continues to exert its action. Some persist longer than others. Some have massive half-lives. Out in nature in the bacteria, in the mycelia, in the plants, in the animals, that pharmaceutical is now part of the ecology.

Professor of Biology at New York University, Efrain Azmitia said, "The reality of the situation is 'neurotransmitters' predate the formation of nervous tissue. Serotonin is found in all animals, plants, and most unicellular organisms." Does nature want your SSRIs? Or your chemotherapy drugs? Is it helping or harming? I'd be willing to bet that you hadn't thought of how what you consume has that kind of impact. Until it was revealed to me, I certainly had not.

We must see ourselves as greater parts of the whole. Not because it is some mystical way to enlightenment, but because it is simple natural law.

Until we do this, humans will continue to act like a harmful parasite or virus on this earth. Using up resources at an alarming pace, spreading ourselves far and wide. At some point, we may kill our host, or more likely, the host will get fed up with this action and do something to cleanse it. If you had a massive parasitic infection ravaging your body, wouldn't you do the same?

In 1941, the author of an article in the *Canadian Bee Journal* wrote, "If the bee disappeared off the surface of the globe then man would only have four years of life left. No more bees, no more pollination, no more plants, no more animals, no more man." Colony collapse disorder among bees has seen as much of 50 percent of bees disappear in certain areas.

If we don't realize how our ecology affects all ecology, and do so soon, making some major changes, it is only a matter of time, before we throw something off so bad that there is no return.

The world is experiencing an extinction-level event. We can see the large mammals disappearing. What may be devastating to us is how our microbiomes are disappearing. Rural peoples have more microbiome diversity than those in Western, industrialized societies. And hunter-gatherers have far more than the rural people. [41] When it comes to ecology, more biodiversity generally equals a more healthy, stable, and adaptable ecology.

We may just multiply to the point where there aren't enough resources to sustain us and then there is nothing left to do but die off, at least to a point where sustainability is possible again.

With a mutually beneficial symbiosis there is a give and take. Different organisms evolve to support each other in this way. The earth is here and is abundant in resources. We do need resources to survive and thrive. The question is whether we are taking more than we're giving. Are we mutualistic or parasitic?

Doing this individually is important, but this must be done in a collective way. If one bacteria cell in us goes rogue, whatever that may mean, chances are that nothing changes for the host. But if the whole bacterial colony shifts, those differences will be noticed.

You are a collective to make up you. We are a collective to make up us. As Wendell Berry said, "You cannot save the land apart from the people, or the people apart from the land."

All of the steps in this book are not simply to optimize human health through natural living. It is to help restore ecology, internal and external, individually and collectively.

PART 3

A true connection to the beings in nature

16
Fear of Nature

"It is those who believe only in science who call an insect a pest or a predator and cry out that nature is a violent world of relativity and contradiction in which the strong feed on the weak...These are only distinctions invented by man. Nature maintained a great harmony without such notions, and brought forth the grasses and trees without the 'helping' hand of man."
– Masanobu Fukuoka

It is likely you have heard the phrase "Nature, red in tooth and claw." Used many times, this was originally written in a poem by Alfred Lord Tennyson. It speaks to the violent nature of the natural world.

This is what most of us are brought up to believe.

Much of what stops us from enjoying the benefits of nature is this misguided fear pervading our culture. This is further exacerbated by shows like *Naked and Afraid*. But realize this "non-reality" TV is specifically set up for high drama that will give it ratings. Someone sitting peacefully out in nature, easily getting by wouldn't make for a good show, so they venture to harder places than most.

People that have the know-how can quite easily live in nature, especially when a community is involved. If it was nearly as bad as many people imagine it to be, humans would have never survived as a species. It's just that so few of us "moderns" do have these skills.

When I had signed up for the excursion to the Amazon rainforest it was amazing to see the level of fear that different people would express.

Bugs. This may be the biggest hurdle for many. Indoors we don't really have bugs. Outdoors they are everywhere. Thus, indoors is a better, more comfortable place.

In the Amazon, swarms of mosquitoes will not only eat you alive but give you malaria and Zika virus. Chances are this is one of the first things that pops into the minds of Westerners. Nor is it just the Amazon. For many all of Central America and South America are this way.

And while these things do truly exist, the overblown fear drives disconnection. (Actually, there is doubt to the whole Zika–birth defect link.[1] Other theories involve chemicals that are driving microcephaly.)

As I was preparing to travel to the Amazon I was faced with a whole list of packing supplies and preliminary steps to follow. One warning had to do with contracting malaria. Specifically, they said:

"The rainforest region we will be visiting has a history of malaria, and we recommend that each participant take preventative medicine. Prescription Malarone has proven most effective without strong side effects, and the herbal tincture Artemisia (Wormwood) is a good option."

Seeing as I don't do "drugs" I got some of the herb recommended. But then another update came down the pike:

"Our colleagues in the Ecuadorian rainforest have notified us that there has been an outbreak of malaria (at latest notice 105 confirmed cases) over the past weeks. We want you to know of this increased level of infection by the mosquito population and to strongly encourage you to choose an allopathic preventative to protect yourselves from contracting the disease."

Uh oh! What do I do now? I literally have not so much as taken a Tylenol in many years. So, I looked into it.

First of all, there would be the difficulty in obtaining Malarone seeing as I don't actually have a doctor to prescribe it for me. Secondly, the list of possible side effects is still pretty large even if they aren't super common. Being sensitive to drugs, since I don't use them, this didn't sound fun. Besides, it isn't even 100 percent effective

Ultimately, after meditating on it, the decision came down to this…I practice what I preach, even in a potentially risky matter such as this.

I would place my trust in herbs.

I would place my trust in my own immune system.

This is who I am, and I would affirm that in this decision. So, I loaded up on Artemisinin, an extract of sweet wormwood.[2] (It wasn't until later that I found out that the whole extract was even better.)

I totally forgot about this, but my brother Zane pointed it out to me later. Tongkat ali, one of the popular herbs that we sell at Lost Empire herbs, primarily for hormone support, has been used over the years in traditional medicine to treat malaria.[3] Several studies have been done to back up this historic use, including one that saw a combination of artemisinin and tongkat ali extract suppress 80 percent of infection in mice.[4]

In the end, the mosquitoes weren't even bad at all. I could count the number of mosquitoes that landed on me on my two hands. I got a few bites and no malaria, nor Zika.

The fact is I have seen far worse mosquito swarms not in the Amazon, nor in Guatemala, but in Tahoe, California.

Now, do I recommend you do this if you head to a malaria-infected area? The short answer is no. Every person must make their own choice. I share this just to reveal my personal decision, my reasoning for it, and as a possible alternative to the medical monopoly.

There were other fears too. Don't go in the river. You'll be eaten alive by piranhas! The truth of the matter is that piranhas are there, but they have no interest in you. It was recommended that we not go in the water if we had an open wound, but besides this it was quite safe. And with the hot, muggy Amazon weather, swimming in the river was very enjoyable.

One night we went on a hike. Trekking through the rainforest with flashlights, at one point we were instructed to stop and shut off our lights. Pitch-black darkness surrounded us. But it was far from silent. The cacophony of insects, amphibians, and other creatures buzzing, chirping, and ribbiting is almost deafening.

Here we were deep in the rainforest. My body releasing tension as I fell into the perfectness of that moment. I could feel this culturally held belief in the danger of nature melt away into the black of the night.

This isn't to say that nature doesn't hold any danger. It certainly does. But it is over emphasized. And it is in this fear that our disconnection begins.

Most of us live far from true wilderness. There may be parks or even national forests. But deep wilderness, untouched by man, is unfortunately a rare thing. Yet, wilderness is something to be experienced if you have the opportunity.

Our state parks are very safe in comparison. Most of the large animals that would possibly be dangerous to us are no longer around, as we've killed off most of them. For these reasons, they tend to avoid humans more than hunt them.

Closed off indoors and in our cities, nature takes on this appearance of something out there and scary. But when you actually explore it you'll find it anything but.

Plus, by being without nature it seems that this exacerbates anxieties and fears. Richard Louv, whose work we'll be exploring more in coming sections, writes, "Humans living in landscapes that lack trees or other natural features undergo patterns of social, psychological, and physical breakdown that are strikingly similar to those observed in animals that have been deprived of their natural habitat."

Fear is at the root of our disconnection, but it is not the only thing...

17
Disconnect to Reconnect

"Returning to nature feels like going home, or reconnecting with the source of life. But few people want to return to nature for too long at a time. After all, we are the inheritors of a culture and a way of life that emphasizes our separation. We are the lords of creation, the conquerors of nature. All the ancient fears are still in the background to haunt us: the breakdown of civilization, famine, pestilence, barbarism. Our political and economic systems help to separate us from the destructive powers of nature and human nature, from forces that arouse our most basic fears, from the ever-present threat of chaos. A variety of theories and habitual attitudes reinforces and extends this primary distancing, especially the habits of scientific detachment. And then the greater the sense of separation from nature, the greater the need to return."
– Rupert Sheldrake

"Thousands of tired, nerve-shaken, over-civilized people are beginning to find out that going to the mountains is going home; that wilderness is a necessity; and that mountain parks and reservations are useful not only as fountains of timber and irrigating rivers, but as fountains of life."
– John Muir

The Mayan shaman walks around the sacred fire pit, chanting to the Mayan energies, the *nowals*. Suddenly, the loud sound of a phone ringing cuts into the ceremony. I glance around at the other participants thinking "Who the hell has their phone here?!?"

After the second ring, the shaman reaches into his shoulder bag and pulls out the phone. Not to silence it but to answer the call. After doing so he hands it to the other, younger shaman as the call was for him from our bus driver.

This was pretty funny to all of us in the ceremony. But later that day

John Perkins made a great comment. To the shamans, it was no big deal. It didn't disconnect them from the ceremony. Perhaps they didn't think it ideal, but it was no breach of the sacred that we were all engaged in.

In the West, we tend to think of a phone ringing in such situations as anathema to the process. Earlier that week during a cleansing ceremony, feeling great joy in my heart, a bunch of us started laughing hysterically. One person reflected later that this felt like a violation, that it distracted her from her meditation and she felt bad for the shamans.

But the shamans were laughing too. As John put it, "Don't take it too seriously, it's only the most important thing in your life."

John likened it to the Achuar people coming from the Amazon rainforest to visit San Francisco such as when the Pachamama Alliance puts on big fundraising events. People often wonder how the Achuar feel about such visits. What is the urban jungle like compared to the real jungle? Do they fear muggings on the streets like our people fear swarms of mosquitoes? He stated that all in all, they have a great time. They don't feel disconnected as they're still with Pachamama, the earth, the heavens and everything, at all times.

Can we be like the Achuar? Can we be like the Mayan shamans? Can we be immersed in cities and our technology and still maintain this connection to nature?

The entire week in Guatemala I had been thinking about such issues. And as with most things, I believe the answer is multi-faceted.

First, the Achuar and the Mayans grow up in nature. They're never far removed from the elements and natural processes occurring all the time. It pervades their thinking and spirituality throughout life. They are raised in this way.

Most of us in modern civilization are not raised this way. I know I wasn't. And thus, we may have missed that deep embodiment of nature that builds the unbreakable core connection that is always felt.

Secondly, we spend a lot of time in civilization with our high-tech gadgets. Certainly, a lot more time than we do interacting with the natural elements. How many hours of each day are spent indoors, in vehicles, and staring at screens?

"The cause of the present sickness is our modern technological civilization and its underlying ideologies," writes Rupert Sheldrake. "If we are to enter the new millennium with any hope for the future, we need to recover a new vision of human nature and of our relationship to the living earth." This is important to realize, the foundations of what led us here. How technology and civilization drive this. But this doesn't mean we have to go backwards. Instead, we need a new path with which to move forward.

Richard Louv, in his book *The Nature Principle*, notes that as we go more high-tech, we need to counterbalance this with being high-nature too. Some who only glance at his books or mine, may think they rally people to become luddites and anti-technology. But in neither case is this the message. As he states, "Tech isn't the enemy, but it can certainly be a barrier."

Meanwhile, the nature principle "holds that a reconnection to the natural world is fundamental to human health, well-being, spirit and survival."

I enjoy technology and am excited about new advances coming forward in the future. At the same time, I recognize that many, if not all, of our technologies have hidden costs that we're only beginning to realize and that most people are kept in the dark about. Even if the technology causes no ill effects itself, by its use in disconnecting us, it can. Our removal from nature has other costs, I hope now much revealed, in the same way.

Many of us, myself included, live in the digital landscape of computers and the internet for hours and hours each day. My current role and mission in life requires this to some degree, though I'm working to lighten the digital load.

Take a look at how many people are staring into their smart phones in any public space and you'll see we're not far off from being literally plugged into the data-sphere as long imagined by our science fiction writers. This is only going to increase, not decrease, with the direction the world is going. The logical conclusion for all this is for us to become cyborgs. Wearables are becoming more common and implants are hot on their heels. The dreams of the technocrats would have us leaving all of our natural biology behind. Whether you like it or not, many people and companies are driving towards this future.

Louv's idea is to bring it into a balance. "The more high-tech we become, the more nature we need." High tech and high nature. His idea is to develop a "hybrid mind," especially in children, to get the best of both worlds. A mind that's able to use computers to maximize their computing power and processing of data, as well as using natural environments to support our senses, creativity and learning.

Some people may be more called into the modern technology side of the world and may only feel the need for a little bit of nature. Others will be called to more fully immerse themselves in a naturalist lifestyle, living close to the earth. Neither is necessarily right or wrong, but some nature time does seem to be a necessity for human health and well-being.

A complete immersion into a "modern" lifestyle comes with physical and psychological health issues. This much is clear.

Meanwhile, complete immersion in nature helps creativity. Ruth Ann Atchley, in a study called *Creativity in the Wild: Improving Creative Reasoning through Immersion in Natural Settings*, found, "Four days of immersion in nature, and the corresponding disconnection from multimedia and technology, increases performance on a creativity, problem-solving task by a full 50% in a group of naive hikers. Our results demonstrate that there is a cognitive advantage to be realized if we spend time immersed in a natural setting. We anticipate that this advantage comes from an increase in exposure to natural stimuli that are both emotionally positive and low-arousing and a corresponding decrease in exposure to attention demanding technology."[1]

That shamanic ceremony with the cell phone interruption occurred at the end of my trip to Guatemala. Throughout the journey, I thought about these ideas of disconnecting from the digital landscape, and into the natural one. For me, it was helpful to disconnect to reconnect. In talking to others about some of the ideas from this book I would say the statement, "Being in nature doesn't come naturally to me." Observe that statement for a while and realize the absurdity of it.

Yet, despite the oxymoron, it contains an element of truth. Not being raised with a close connection to nature, it was like learning how to ride a bicycle for the first time. The details seem impossible at first, until you practice and practice and it eventually becomes second nature.

That we need connection with nature to become second nature to us, rather than it simply being first nature, is an endemic issue of our modern society, leading to health issues as well as the destruction of nature.

This is further reinforced by the fear of nature, the desire to conquer and control it, that is constantly pounded into our minds by our society. That I need to write this book at all in order to clear up misconceptions and drive toward the goal of harmony with nature is a reflection of how far we've come down a wrong path.

Yuval Noah Harari writes, "The transition first to agriculture and then to industry has condemned us to living unnatural lives that cannot give full expression to our inherent inclinations and instincts, and therefore cannot satisfy our deepest yearnings. Nothing in the comfortable lives of the urban middle class can approach the wild excitement and sheer joy experienced by a forager band on a successful mammoth hunt. Every new invention just puts another mile between us and the Garden of Eden."

This is echoed in such books as *Ishmael* by Daniel Quinn. There the biblical story of Adam and Eve being cast out of the Garden of Eden is reflective of the shift from a hunter-gatherer lifestyle into agriculture.

Upon arrival in Guatemala, I left my phone off and wouldn't even use it until the return journey home a week later. No phone. No internet. Not a thought of the websites I visit in my everyday life back home. Unlike the shaman, I needed to do this.

This vacuum left a free space to connect with the other people on the journey. It drove a deeper connection with my wife who journeyed there with me. The free space allowed nature to more deeply enter me. And the presence, to actually be present, rather than thinking constantly, planning out the future and reflecting on the past.

While I didn't get the joy of a mammoth hunt, I had experiences that I'll never forget, that are not possible in my everyday plugged-in life.

The question is, why couldn't I simply make the time to unplug back home? Why was it necessary to travel halfway around the world to do so? Because being wrapped up in "real life" simply makes it harder to do. We have routines and habits that drive our constant connection to the digital world. And many of us did not grow up with counterbalancing natural

241

routines because our parents didn't have them either. So, the call to action now is to set conscious routines to make up for the previous lack.

"In relationship with nature, the high-performance human will conserve and *create* natural habitat – and new economic potential – where we live, learn, work, and play," says Louv. It may not be easy in the beginning. It may not feel natural to be in nature. And that is okay. If that is the case for you, just like it has been for me, here are two helpful things I found that can support the journey.

It is helpful to disconnect from technology to connect to nature, if for no other reason that it frees up the time and space to do so.

It is helpful to disconnect from thoughts of the future and past, to become present. This is one of the benefits of meditation. It is also one thing that naturally comes from time in nature.

The technological part was pretty obvious to me. But with my businesses and other aspects of my life that I'm always working to improve toward a greater future, the second part may actually be the bigger block, at least personally. I know there are many times I've felt resistance to going for a walk in the woods because I have stuff I have to do. Sadly, the to-do list will never be done, thus it isn't about that, but about priorities.

Beliefs tend to be built from experience. They're true in the sense that they've been your experience up until that point. Yet, it was in the final day of shamanic ceremonies that I was able to let go of the belief that I wasn't good at being in nature, whatever that meant. In a drum journey, I shed it like a snake skin. As it happens a green snake came into our circle visiting a few people at that time.

Since shedding this idea of my 'unnaturalness,' spending more time in nature and becoming present and connected has been much easier. However, it is still a work in progress.

If it helps you, disconnect to reconnect. And with time, perhaps we may all be able to embody the spiritual connection to the earth that the shamans and indigenous people appear to have at all times, whether a phone rings or not.

18
The Multi-Level Benefits of Time in Nature

"We need the tonic of wildness."
– Henry David Thoreau

"Nature is not a place to visit. It is home."
– Gary Snyder

Even if you are not sunbathing, gathering food or water, earthing, or doing any of the other steps we've covered in detail in part two of this book, you're still going to benefit by simply being in nature.

A Norwegian term, "friluftsliv," roughly translates to free air life. It's an idea that being active in the outdoors supports all aspects of health. Over the course of this book, we've covered many of the specifics, and here we'll go a little broader.

Howard Frumkin, Dean of the School of Public Health at the University of Washington said, "If nature contact were a medication, we would be prescribing it to everybody." But the fact is that no medication can come close to the wide-ranging healthful effects nature brings.

Recent research suggests that simply being in nature lowers cortisol, blood pressure, and pulse rate. In addition, there is greater parasympathetic nerve activity and less sympathetic activity, meaning it reduces stress, turning down fight-or-flight mode.[1]

One study that looked specifically at the immune system found that natural killer cell activity was higher for even 30 days after a trip to the forest, indicating a longer-term boost to immune activity.[2]

And another study, in the *American Journal of Preventative Medicines*, found that greener neighborhoods, not even what we would commonly call nature, equaled lower body mass index in children. They concluded that "Greenness may present a target for environmental approaches to preventing child obesity."[3] There's a good chance that the same is true of adults too.

How is all of this happening? Breathing fresher air is one of them. Plus, many plants give off essential oils or phytoncides which could be at the root of some of these effects, as was discussed in the section on air.

Then we have the bacteria that we've talked about. Even if you're trying to stay clean you'll be interacting with bacteria in the air that enters your lungs and gets on your skin. And if you aren't trying to be clean you'll get much more.

In fact, nature is so potent in its effects, that just having a view of a tree from your hospital bed leads to faster recovery times, better mood, less pain, and less complications, than those who had a view of a wall.[4] A single tree can do this much!

Once again, the effects are not just physical, but are also psychological. In a report titled, *Healthy Parks, Healthy People*, from the Deakin University School of Health and Social Development, Dr. Cecily Maller et al, wrote: "The experience of nature in a neurological sense can help strengthen the activities of the right hemisphere of the brain, and restore harmony to the functions of the brain as a whole. This is perhaps a technical explanation of the process that occurs when people 'clear their head' by going for a walk in a park and emphasises the importance of parks in providing communities with access to nature."[5]

Memory performance and attention span increased 20 percent after just one hour in nature, as reported in *Psychological Science*.[6]

Scientists may not be pleased that nature doesn't boil down to one isolated variable which would make it easy for studying. Yet this is a good thing, because all the benefits aren't coming from any one thing, but more likely it's the combination that gives the far-reaching effects.

One aspect is the sensory component. Simply looking at the fractal patterns of nature appears to do something important. These complex environments, of which nature is far more abundant than anything man-made, have been shown to lead to "enhanced brain structure and function, including increased brain weight, dendritic branching, neurogenesis, gene expression, and improved learning and memory."[7]

Nor is it just sight either, but the sounds of nature too. How many people listen to soundtracks that mimic these because they can be soothing and relaxing? The same level of complexity exists in sounds as with visuals. In fact, it exists across all the senses.

The human species was developed in nature. We can't get away from it. Yet if we try to do so, is it any wonder that we begin to suffer consequences?

In *Homo Deus*, Yuval Noah Harari shows that modern day life is not necessarily so much better than the far past, as it is commonly assumed. He does this by describing two vacation package options you could take.

"*Stone Age package*: On day one we will hike for ten hours in a pristine forest, setting camp for the night in a clearing by a river. On day two we will canoe down the river for ten hours, camping on the shores of a small lake. On day three we will learn from the native people how to fish in the lake and how to find mushrooms in the nearby woods.

"*Modern proletarian package*: On day one we will work for ten hours in a polluted textile factory, passing the night in a cramped apartment block. On day two we will work for ten hours as cashiers in the local department store, going back to sleep in the same apartment block. On day three we will learn from the native people how to open a bank account and fill out mortgage forms.

"Which package would you choose?"

It is clear that one of these would be considered a vacation to the vast majority of people, while the other is simply crappy working and living conditions. But in the past, the first package was simply everyday life, not a once-in-a-year (or lifetime!) getaway. The question is why are we working so hard to simply be moving in the wrong direction?

I know some people would not enjoy the first package nor the latter. But that just shows how far civilization has driven a wedge between some and our natural inheritance. How that civilized fear of nature makes us what to avoid the bugs, dirt, and elements.

Therefore, in this section I wanted to spend some time discussing options for how you can spend time in nature. This might sound elementary, yet, with the average person not spending any time in nature, we have to go back to square one. Collectively, we've forgotten how to interact with nature, and we're suffering for it.

I know I did. As a kid, I didn't give much thought to nature. I played outside a fair amount then. Computers and video games were just beginning to become popular. As I hit my teens there was a shift and I spent a lot less time outdoors. Since devices became even more prevalent in the generation after mine, less and less time is being spent outdoors.

As I became an adult I got busy, as happens to everyone in the Western world. Working, then running my business, while making time to be social, kept me indoors most of the time. And this went on for years. So, is it any wonder that actually making time in nature a daily part of my routine took some effort?

Part of the exploration of what it meant to be an emissary of nature involved spending a lot more time in nature. That's not surprising. I went from going out to the woods maybe once every other week to doing so a couple to a few times a week.

For me the next step was to make it daily. For me that meant putting a hard stop on my work day at six hours, and then spending two hours in nature.

The sad thing is that this would be considered extreme. No one has time for that. I thought so as I set out to do it. Two hours in nature every single day, that's a lot! Yes, for a modern. But not compared to our ancient ancestors, who spent every minute of every day surrounded by nature.

But I figured I could make it work. When you see all the components of nature we've covered in this book it can take some time to do them all. Doing natural movement, sunbathing, gathering food and herbs, all take some time.

The important part was making the decision to do so and then setting up my life and routines to support it. While I was able to keep up with this for some time, at other times it slipped away as I was dragged back into working more. The irony of spending long hours writing a book on nature, so that I didn't have the time to go in nature, is not lost on me. (Fortunately, after printing out some pages, I could at least do some editing outside.)

Of course, my prescription for you is not to spend two hours a day in nature. That is, unless you're at a place where that is the appropriate step for you. Even small amounts are effective. Remember, a view of a tree was far better than a view without a tree.

In a meta-analysis of ten studies, Jo Barton and Jules Pretty found that everyone involved, young, old, male, female, showed benefit from movement in nature, though the young and the mentally ill saw the most benefit.[8] While greater benefits were found with longer durations, being dose-dependent, just small amounts saw marked increases with tapering returns. Barton stated, "A walk a day should help keep the doctors away – and help to save the country money."

Recall that this is not just physical health benefits but mental health benefits too. Patricia Hasbach Ph.D., discusses the new field of ecotherapy or ecopsychology which extends "the traditional scope of treatment to include the human-nature relationship."

E. O. Wilson, a biologist at Harvard University, put forth the biophilia hypothesis, which is "the urge to affiliate with other forms of life." Having been with nature throughout our ancestry, we humans need the direct experience to be whole. It is necessary to our genetic expression. Wilson wrote, "The brain evolved in a biocentric world, not a machine-regulated world."

And while recent research is showing this is true in so many different ways, we still understand little about how it works. As Eleonora Gullone put it, "Given that our modern ways of living, as prescribed by Western industrialised culture, stand in stark contrast to our evolutionary history, it is proposed that we may currently be witnessing the beginnings of significant adverse outcomes for the human psyche."[9]

Aren't we already? If nature indeed is a need, that means that meeting it will lead to satisfaction and healthy outcomes. Meanwhile, not meeting this need, will lead to stress and pathology.

In a review titled *"Psychological Benefits of Nature Experiences: An Outline of Research and Theory,"* John Davis, Ph.D. outlined even further benefits and said, "there is also limited, but suggestive research that these findings are cross-cultural and universal." He continues, "I would hypothesize that a wide range of nature experiences (from gardening to wilderness) will increase a sense of hardiness, healthy and realistic internal locus of control, and self-efficacy…I expect direct encounters with intact, healthy ecosystems (i.e. ecosystems exhibiting a high degree of coherence) leads to a greater sense of psychological coherence...Furthermore, nature is an important element in many transpersonal experiences."[10]

Beyond just the physical and the mental, research shows nature is important for creating "peak experiences" as defined by Maslow and reaching states of "flow" as defined by Csikszentmihalyi.

Wuthnow found that 82 percent of the general population have "experienced the beauty of nature in a deeply moving way." Of these, 49 percent felt this experience had a lasting influence on their lives.[11]

Davis writes, "Wilderness experiences trigger the sense that the world is enchanted, alive, whole and meaningful. By realizing our part in nature, we also come to feel more enchanted, alive, whole and meaningful. Wilderness fosters the sense that we are each unique and individual and, at the same time, part of the larger whole."

A sense of meaning. Doesn't it seem that so many people living today in developed nations are having a crisis of meaning?

When I look at health, or, in fact, just about anything, I look at it holistically. I see that something like an injury is not just physical. There is always a mental, emotional, and even spiritual component to it. And that is why simple physical treatment works only sometimes. If the block is on another level entirely, no amount of physical treatment will fix it. And so it is with nature. It does not work on just one level but pervades them all.

Being deep in nature you won't have EMFs or Wi-Fi which then allows you to get connected to nature. You won't have noise pollution of vehicles on highways or other sounds of civilization either. Generally, the farther away you get, the more natural it becomes. While I think being deep in wilderness may bring the most benefits, just little bits of nature still bring a lot of benefit.

Let's say you are a city-dweller. Let's say that deep nature is going to take you an hour or more of travel to reach. I highly recommend you make the journey, perhaps on your weekends when you can. But this may not be suitable for you on a daily basis.

Fortunately, all city planners recognize the need for some nature, and parks tend to be within walking distance of most places. Some parks certainly are more natural than others, but any park will do. Even a tree on the street, or a dandelion growing out of the cracks in the sidewalk is showing that deep in the city, nature is still present.

Whatever you have available, spend time with it. In the beginning, can you spend just ten minutes a day, three times a week? Start small and grow it from there.

There are days when I am traveling, so I don't have the opportunity to carve out hours of time. What do I do then? I can always make fifteen or twenty minutes. And I'll do exactly what I just said. Perhaps I'm visiting a city, then I'll find a local park.

I used to regularly drive up to Medford, Oregon to train under one of my mentors, who runs a martial arts school there. On the way up from Santa Cruz, California I drove by Mt. Shasta. This is my favorite place to get fresh spring water. It is the best-tasting water I've ever had and flows quite quickly. I'd routinely fill up twenty or more gallons to take back home.

In the past, because I was always in a rush I would simply gather my water and go. But after reflecting on what I've written here I decided to pause to spend a bit of time with the spring, showing my gratitude and appreciation.

I'm far from the only one that goes to that spot. The place becomes crowded at times. On this visit I explored the surrounding area a bit and noticed some wild cherries and horsetail, a well-known herbal medicine that helps support the joints and bones. These were growing in massive abundance.

Up in Medford as I attended a workshop, I didn't have two hours each day. Just an hour drive in any direction could have taken me to some amazing natural spots. Oregon is full of them. But I carved out twenty minutes to walk down to a park that was only a few blocks from where I was staying in the heart of the city there. It was a typical park with play structures and a well-tended field. And there were a variety of trees and rocks around. By spending some time there, I noticed that the trees had littered the ground with their yellow pollen, which was everywhere.

The park was named Hawthorn Park so I looked around for the Hawthorn tree, *Crataegus oxycanthus*. While I knew a little of the medicinal benefits of this plant in promoting the health of the circulatory system, helping in angina, arrhythmias, high blood pressure, and congestive heart failure, I didn't know the tree itself.

I found it there, got to taste the ripe berries, which have a flavor like that of apples, and collected some to make a tincture later. On my drive home, I spotted a bunch more Hawthorn trees. I had begun a new relationship with the tree and my eyes could not un-see what I had now seen.

In a couple chapters, we'll get to how I established a relationship with that tree, as well as so many others. But first, it is important to realize just how alive nature, and everything in it, really is.

19
The Life and Intelligence of Nature

"It was only when science convinced us that nature was dead that it could begin its autopsy in earnest."
– James Hillman

"I went no place the corn did not first tell me to go."
– Barbara McClintock

A fruit-fly has an incredibly short life span of just about one day. Can you picture your entire existence squeezed down into such a condensed period of time? But research shows that the perception of time changes along with life span and metabolic rate.[1]

The seventy years, give or take thirty or so, of a human is incredibly lengthy in comparison. But we're far from the longest-living things on this planet.

Contrast that to a tree's life span. Of course, there is a huge variety among different trees. But some of the longer-lived trees, like a redwood, can live thousands of years. While the time scale is different, so too is how life is lived. Imagine if you couldn't move besides mere millimeters of growth every month. Imagine your life spent in one place.

Pando, also known as the Trembling Giant, is a colony of male quaking aspen trees in Utah. All of these trees are clones, with one massive root system, meaning this is a single living organism. Its weight is estimated at six million kilograms. Its age is estimated at 80,000 years. But others estimate it may be as old as 1 million years.[2] And it's still going. How long will it survive?

Buhner writes, "Judging the actions of these plants, their functions in ecosystems, and their chemistries through the timescale of a human life often misses what can only happen in decades, centuries, or millennia. It is our temporal limitations that prevent most of us from noticing what plants do over such scales of time."

How we humans even categorize life is a subject matter fraught with some difficulty. Life is sometimes defined as the quality that distinguishes a vital and functional being from a non-living or dead body or purely chemical matter. In biology, seven criteria are used to determine whether something is living or not. These can be simplified into the following seven processes:

1. Movement
2. Respiration
3. Sensitivity
4. Growth
5. Reproduction
6. Excretion
7. Nutrition

By this definition viruses are not alive. Although they exhibit six of the seven processes above, they do not reproduce, at least by themselves. Instead, viruses take over cells of other living things and use them to produce more viruses. The livingness of these things is still debated.[3] Of course, that is just because we don't see their form of reproduction, which is different from ours, as being a valid form of reproduction.

As Buckminster Fuller put it, "Virologists have been too busy, for instance, with their DNA-RNA genetic code isolatings, to find time to see the synergistic significance to society of the fact that they have found that no physical threshold does in fact exist between animate and inanimate."

In fact, the materialists would have you believe nothing is really alive, that we're all just machines with complex algorithms that run us. "In the last three centuries, growing numbers of educated people have come to think of nature as lifeless. This has been the central doctrine of orthodox science—the mechanistic theory of nature," writes Rupert Sheldrake.

But ever since this theory—and that is all it is—has been around, it has been fought by others. Vitalism is an old theory, that they will tell you is gone, but still our modern science has not explained life. Just because you can look at constituent parts of a cell, doesn't mean it has no life.

That is the problem with reductionist thinking. Talking about atoms, or protons, neutrons, and elections, or quarks, does not help explain cell or human behavior in the least. And it never will, because the whole is greater than the sum of the parts.

Sheldrake continues, "Mechanistic biology grew up in opposition to vitalism. It defined itself by denying that living organisms are purposive, mind-like principles, but then reinvented them in the guise of genetic programs and selfish genes."

Another aspect that is looked at to determine living or not is the cells themselves. But then this brings up two questions: If the cell is alive, what about parts of it? Does the cell itself have awareness?

There's also the unexplained incident of how life first started. According to evolutionary theory living matter, somehow, at some point long ago, emerged out of dead matter. This is still one of the biggest unexplained gaps in science. The idea that it sprung up from nothingness takes just as much faith as any other idea, because as a theory, it is not testable. The same unexplainable gap problem is true of how human consciousness came to be.

What about the earth itself? James Lovelock proposed the 'Gaia hypothesis' that the earth itself is "a self-regulating entity with the capacity to keep our planet healthy by controlling the chemical and physical environment."[4] Some people like to look at this as a metaphor, while others believe that the Earth truly is a living organism.

Just like bacteria, fungi, viruses and even parasitic animals live on and inside our body, the earth has all of those, plus plants, animals and humans that live on it. Are we essentially just cells on Gaia?

The earth seems to hit most of those earlier definitions of living. For many, the reproduction one is a hang-up as they imagine it closely to our terms. As if the earth is going to divide and split like a cell, and then a baby planet is suddenly following it around. But what if instead, like viruses, it's part of the life on earth that may spread to other planets.

Fungal spores can survive in space. Certain bacteria can too. And soon we humans may be colonizing other planets, spreading life. We've already sent bacteria through our galaxy. Could this not be looked at as the earth reproducing?

After all, a human doesn't pop out a fully formed human. A sperm cell meets the egg cell. And from those cells the organism grows. Couldn't life on other planets grow the same, starting with a cell, or the equivalent in planetary terms, a larger organism. If we terraform and populate Mars as Elon Musk aims for, over time the planet will be an alive ecosystem. In a sense, wouldn't the Earth just have reproduced?

"The Gaia hypothesis is undoubtedly a major step in the direction of a new animism, which is why it is so controversial…It involves a radical shift in point of view from the man-centered world of humanism to a recognition that we all depend on the providence of Gaia," writes Sheldrake. He then expands this idea beyond our planet. "The recognition of the earth as a living organism is a major step toward recognizing the wider life of the cosmos. If the earth is a living organism, what about the sun and the solar system as a whole? If the solar system is a kind of organism, what about the galaxy? Cosmology already portrays the entire universe as a kind of growing super-organism, born through the hatching of the cosmic egg."

There's that fractal pattern once again. Perhaps everything is alive. And that is the belief behind animism. That everything is animated with some sort of spiritual essence.

What about other things we definitely consider as non-living? Jagadis Chandra Bose, a Bengali polymath, wrote, "In pursuing investigations on the border region of physics and physiology, I was amazed to find boundary lines vanishing, and points of contact emerge between the realms of the Living and Non-Living. Metals are found to respond to stimuli; they are subject to fatigue, stimulated by certain drugs and 'killed' by poisons."

This is all mentioned just to point out that often in modern man the definition of life is looked at merely through our lens of how we live. While we may recognize other creatures as alive, the other issue is that we see everything in a hierarchical way. This is built into the standard scientific understanding of the world.

Everything we look at is through the lens of human perception, looking at what is similar or different to us. If something has a brain like us it is capable of some level of thought, though not as well as human thought.

The Western viewpoint is one of brain-centrism. Those with bigger and better brains are more alive than those that aren't. Of course, on top of this hierarchy are *Homo sapiens*, the wise man. Below us are the 'smarter' animals like elephants and dolphins that have language, exhibit emotion, and otherwise act like us humans in some regard. Then it is the rest of the mammals, followed by others, like birds. Lower down we go to reptiles and finally, those pesky insects.

With all of these we see there is some intelligence, but we call it instincts. We can see this is the triune brain theory which splits up the brain into:

1) the neocortex, the human brain.
2) the limbic system, the mammalian brain.
3) and the reptilian cortex, the basal ganglia.

While most neuroscientists look at this as a failed model, it has entered the mainstream as it's an easy way to talk about the brain.[5] The idea is that through evolution we've evolved these higher functioning brains, to arrive at the top.

However, there are even humans living and functioning essentially without brains! Hydrocephalus, also called "water on the brain," is a condition where the skull is filled with cerebrospinal fluid. While this typically leads to dysfunctional people, there are those that are normal or even excel with extreme hydrocephalus, while having "virtually no brain."[6]

Now, I won't say that the brain isn't important, at least for most of us, but this does raise some intriguing questions.

Still, this is how we tend to see evolution, and us at the pinnacle. Humans can think, mammals can feel, reptiles can react. But without the more evolved parts nothing is capable without the right brain. Except, that now we know that reptiles do appear to have emotions.[7] The more we look the more we find that all animals are not just mindless automaton like Descartes believed.

Stephen Walker, a neurological psychologist, stated, "All the fundamental parts of the vertebrate brain were present very early on, and can be observed in lampreys."

In 2012 experts in various fields of neuroscience gathered at The University of Cambridge and put together what is called *The Cambridge Declaration on Consciousness*. In it they stated, "The absence of a neocortex does not appear to preclude an organism from experiencing affective states. Convergent evidence indicates that non-human animals have the neuroanatomical, neurochemical, and neurophysiological substrates of conscious states along with the capacity to exhibit intentional behaviors. Consequently, the weight of evidence indicates that humans are not unique in possessing the neurological substrates that generate consciousness. Nonhuman animals, including all mammals and birds, and many other creatures, including octopuses, also possess these neurological substrates."[8]

In May, 2015, New Zealand was the first country to legally recognize animals as sentient beings with the Animal Welfare Amendment Act. France and Canada have passed similar acts.

What about plants? We can't find any brains there, so they can't be intelligent, right? Not so fast.

Charles Darwin himself, along with his son Francis, did experiments and hypothesized that the root-tips were brain-like structures in plants. They wrote, "It is hardly an exaggeration to say that the tip of the radicle thus endowed [with sensitivity] and having the power of directing the movements of the adjoining parts, acts like the brain of one of the lower animals; the brain being seated within the anterior end of the body, receiving impressions from the sense-organs, and directing the several movements."[9] This theory was discarded, only to be revived many years later.

As Buhner puts it, "The brain that we think of as a necessity for intelligence is only one possible form a neural network can take." Roots would be another option. Even the cell membrane in single-celled organisms functions as a neural network.

All the various beings out in nature are fully and completely alive. The roots of the plants and trees which can penetrate deep into the earth

256

depending on the species, or spread out large lateral distances, have the need to process information in order to survive and thrive.

Right along with this is the fungal or mycelial network. This has been called the 'original internet' or the 'wood wide web' because of how it passes information all across a natural landscape much like our own world wide web. This fungal mass is symbiotic along with the plant life. The plants feed the mycelium (taking up to one third of the food production) and the mycelium in turn break down the earth into usable minerals for the plant life, producing various chemicals plants need, and more.

And none of this would happen without bacteria. Just as we are covered in bacteria and other micro-organisms like viruses, so too is nature. This unseen world is everywhere and an important part of the ecology. In many cases, they're critically symbiotic just like our gut bacteria where both the host and the bacteria benefit.

As we saw in the chapter on Symbiosis, bacteria themselves have been shown to exhibit intelligence too. They move, they communicate, they cooperate. They basically build their own cities (biofilms) and even run electricity through them.[10] Research shows that even a unicellular slime mold can solve a maze reliably.[11]

A new field called plant neurobiology, is scoffed at by many because plants don't have neurons. Yet, plants do see, hear, smell, feel and taste. Plants do show behavior that indicates they have memory, and even think about the future.[12]

As an example of just one of the senses, Daniel Chamovitz writes in *What a Plant Knows*, "Plants perceive tactile sensation, and some of them actually 'feel' better than we do. Plants like the burr cucumber (*Sicyos angulatus*) are up to ten times more sensitive than we are when it comes to touch."

Another example; "Plants clearly have the ability to retain past events and to recall this information at a later period for integration into their development framework. Tobacco plants know the color of the last light they saw. Willow trees know if their neighbors have been attacked by caterpillars. These examples, and many more, illustrate a delayed response to a previous occurrence, which is a key component to memory."

And memory may not just be in the "individual" plant either. Research shows that a plant can alter its own DNA in response to stressors and then pass down this information to their offspring.[13] This sounds like self-directed evolution to me, not some random mutation followed by survival of the fittest.

Chamovitz concludes that whether plants are intelligent is a difficult answer to come up with, since intelligence can be defined in many different ways. "The question, I posit, should not be whether or not plants are *intelligent* – it will be ages before we all agree on what that term means; the question should be, 'Are plants aware?' and, in fact, they are."

But the Latin root of intelligence is *inter legere*, which means to choose. And Leslie Sieburth, a biologist at the University of Utah in Salt Lake City, puts it simply. "If intelligence is the capacity to acquire and apply knowledge, then, absolutely, plants are intelligent."

There's also *The Hidden Life of Trees*, by Peter Wohlleben, a book with a similar aim at showing the complexity of plant life. Wohlleben seems much more open to the idea that they are intelligent.

He shares how the forest is very much a social network. "Most individual trees of the same species growing in the same stand are connected to each other through their root systems. It appears that nutrient exchange and helping neighbors in times of need is the rule, and this leads to the conclusion that forests are superorganisms with interconnections much like ant colonies."

Trees communicate largely through scent. These chemicals may be dispersed in the air, but also sent through the tree roots and through fungal networks. Nor is it just chemicals, but also electrical impulses. And these impulses travel at one third of an inch per minute, a slow speed especially when compared to the quickness of our nervous system.[14]

While Chamovitz dismisses that plants can hear (just like other scientists dismissed every other sense in plants earlier), Wohlleben reports on experiments that show they can. Dr. Monica Gagliano showed that root tips would make a crackling sound at 220 hertz frequencies. Then when she played back this same frequency to other seedlings they would reorient themselves towards it.[15] We may not know how they hear, as they have no ears, but they do appear to.

Wohlleben writes, "The main reason we misunderstand trees,

however, is that they are so incredibly slow. Their childhood and youth last ten times as long as ours. Their complete life-span is at least five times as long as ours. Active movements such as unfurling leaves or growing new shoots take weeks or even months. And so it seems to us that trees are static beings, only slightly more active than rocks…It's hardly any wonder that many people see trees as nothing more than objects."

Many humans believe that mind is simply a by-product of the brain and nothing else. While there is no doubt that the brain is important (at least to us), the nervous system as a whole appears to be a more complex system than simply the brain. And the systems of plants act similar to our nervous system in many ways sending chemical and electrical messengers.

Michael Pollen says, "The line between plants and animals might be a little softer than we traditionally think of it as."

The more we look the more we find. Baluška and his colleagues wrote, "Not only have neuronal molecules been found in plants, but plant synapses are also present which use the same…processes for cell–cell communication as neuronal synapses...Root systems can identify self and non-self roots. Recent new views about consciousness and self-awareness, when considered as biological phenomena inseparable from adaptation and learning processes are compatible with the new neurobiologically oriented view of plants."[16]

Plant life appear to have every sense that we do, though slightly different, and they remember the past and plan for the future. They produce and communicate with both chemicals and electrical impulses. Not so different from you and I, are they?

So, if plants are aware, and have thoughts and feelings, does that not entail them to be treated in a certain way. Going beyond just animals, Ecuador put in its constitution, ratified in September 2008, the Rights of Nature. They state, "Nature, or Pacha Mama, where life is reproduced and occurs, has the right to integral respect for its existence and for the maintenance and regeneration of its life cycles, structure, functions and evolutionary processes."

While many would scoff at this idea, Buhner writes, "Extending equal value to plants—to treat them as human beings—is as laughable and inconceivable to most people now as it once was to extend equal value to women and slaves."

Nervous systems may be unique to animals in the forms that animals have. But, and this is a big but, it doesn't mean that other living things don't also have the means of sending and receiving signals.

We see that the cell membrane is not just a sack with which to carry everything inside but is the principal means by which cells communicate with other cells and the environment. This means that such things as bacteria and viruses are processing information and acting on it. They are living.

Buhner writes, "*Every* living organism *has* to have a means to perceive informational inflows in order to survive; *every* living organism possesses mechanisms to do so...Because all life-forms, irrespective of their nature, must, to survive, have a sense of *not me*, they all have a sense of self, they are in fact *self-aware*. Because all life-forms, irrespective of their nature, must, to survive, be able to analyze the nature of the *not me* that approaches them and, further, must be able to determine its intent, and further, be able to craft a response to that intent, all life-forms are, by definition, *intelligent*. Because all life-forms have to be able to determine the intent of the *not me* that approaches them, they also have to be able to determine *meaning*. In other words, all living organisms can not only process data, they also engage in a search for meaning, an analysis that runs much deeper than linear cause and effect. Thus, three capacities—self-awareness, intelligence, and the search for meaning—that have (erroneously) been ascribed as belonging *only* to human beings are in fact general conditions of every living organism."

That seems to be rock-solid logic to me. What about you?

And the cells themselves even within the human body appear to exhibit intelligent behavior too, independent from the brain. Brian Ford, in an article titled *"Are Cells Ingenious?,"* wrote, "Science has worshiped too heartily at the altar of molecular biology, and has ignored the astonishing complexity of single cells. They do not function like mere robots, but reveal themselves...as sentient and responsive entities...The human body is a coordinated system of cells living in a choreographed community for mutual benefit. We are nothing more than cell colonies, and we can only carry out tasks to which single cells point the way...The brain is currently viewed as fundamentally 'controlling' every aspect of the body's function. However, it is clear that most of the activity of cells is regulated without reference to this form of mediation."[17]

Life is not top-down command and control by the brain. While that is one aspect, just because that is how we do the majority of our thinking does not preclude many other ways.

Barbara McClintock, won the Nobel prize for her discovery of transposition or "jumping genes," the movement of DNA within organisms, with her lengthy study of corn. She wrote, "Every component of the organism is as much of an organism as every other part." We see the fractal pattern once again.

She also believes that it was the corn itself that led her to these discoveries. If cells and plants can communicate amongst themselves, is it possible to communicate with them too? When we understand that intelligence is not synonymous with having a brain, we can begin to tap into the intelligence of nature. We can communicate and how that is done is described next.

20
Heart Field and Heart Perception

"Speech or language [Nature] has none; but she creates tongues and hearts through which she feels and speaks."
– Johann Wolfgang von Goethe

"It has nothing to do with book knowing. It is heart knowing; this is a library of feelings."
– Bradford Keeney

A sk just about any ancient man or woman where the seat of their soul and intelligence was. The vast majority pointed to the heart. Only we, modern man, point to our head.

Is this because we are so much more advanced, or have we lost some ancient wisdom?

The 'gut brain,' and its symbiosis with the microbiome has already been addressed. It seems that this brain is 'intelligent' not just because of the human cells, but in a large part because of the bacteria that is present. So too, have we covered the fact that cells themselves exhibit their own awareness and reactions, independently of the central nervous system. It's not all top down control.

If the gut is the second 'brain' then the heart often makes up the third 'brain.' Once again, just in calling them this we see how brain-centric our culture is. Why don't we call the brain the second gut or heart instead? In this chapter, we'll be focused on the heart which recent research shows does far more than merely pump blood.

The heart generates an electromagnetic field significantly more powerful than the brain. The electrical component is sixty times larger in amplitude. The magnetic component is about 100 times stronger in the heart than in the brain.[1] These electromagnetic patterns are what are measured by an electrocardiogram (ECG) or a magnetocardiogram.

These electromagnetic fields have been found to have powerful ability to influence or entrain other fields. That means that one human's field can cause another's to sync up to it through touch or proximity.[2]

Based on these fields, brain waves then synchronize to heart beats, showing the hearts influence on the brain.[3] If the brain is the most important thing, why is it singing to the tune of the heart?

Heart rate variability (HRV) is a measurement of the time between beats in the heart. Contrary to popular opinion the heart is not supposed to beat like a clock. (A clue that it is not a machine.) Instead, higher variability between beats is a sign of health and leads to greater performance as it indicates that your heart's electrical activity is responsive to and with the nervous system. Typical effects of having greater HRV include less stress, less internal chatter, more emotional balance, greater mental clarity and focus.[4]

Remember that is not just our own heart, but the hearts around us can also cause these effects. One heart can synchronize to another. Perhaps this is the physics of empathy, as different emotional states change up HRV. It may very well be the science behind several methods of healing that are unconventional.

Note that the list of benefits of greater HRV is similar to the benefits of time nature, where a certain type of entrainment or synchronization also appears to take place.

We're taught, and many people still believe, that the heart pumps blood and little else. Like so much of our science that is accepted as self-evident, even this turns out to be false. The writers of an article titled *The Heart is Not a Pump* wrote, "The heart, an organ weighing about three hundred grams, is supposed to 'pump' some eight thousand liters of blood per day at rest and much more during activity, without fatigue. In terms of mechanical work this represents the lifting of approximately 100 pounds one mile high! In terms of capillary flow, the heart is performing an even more prodigious task of 'forcing' the blood with a viscosity five times greater than that of water through millions of capillaries with diameters often smaller than the red blood cells themselves! Clearly, such claims go beyond reason and imagination."[5] This is an impossible task if the heart was the only thing pumping.

The fact is that in a developing embryo the blood circulates before a heart exists. The blood, or whole circulatory system, pumps itself using a vortex action. The heart is not just a pump; it possesses other roles.

It produces hormones including atrial natriuretic factor (ANF), brain natriuretic peptide (BNP), adrenomedullin, endothelin-1 and more.[6] While these mostly act locally in the heart, they also interact with stress hormones, reproductive organs and the immune system. It was back in 1983 when the first of these was discovered that the heart was reclassified as part of the endocrine system.

The heart is also part of the nervous system. Dr. Dominique Surel writes, "Recent work in the relatively new field of neurocardiology has firmly established that the heart is a sensory organ and an information encoding and processing center, with an extensive intrinsic nervous system that's sufficiently sophisticated to qualify as a heart brain. Its circuitry enables it to learn, remember, and make functional decisions independent of the cranial brain. To everyone's surprise, the findings have demonstrated that the heart's intrinsic nervous system is a complex, self-organized system; its neuroplasticity, or ability to reorganize itself by forming new neural connections over both the short and long term, has been well demonstrated."

The heart sends more information to the brain, than in the other direction. This was investigated as far back as the late 1970s.[7] Once again, the brain doesn't run everything. Or as mathematician, physicist and theologian, Blaise Pascal put it, "The heart has reasons that reason cannot know."

The heart is a sensory organ. What that means is the heart senses like your eyes and your ears. It is used to reach out and feel something. Not in a tactile sense like you would with your hand, but instead to probe the deeper depth and meaning available, through the field it generates. It is through this that we can communicate with nature.

Indigenous people seem to have this ability. It is so-called developed people that appear to have lost it. Even so there are those who retain and use this sense.

Stephen Harrod Buhner writes extensively of this in *The Secret Teachings of Plants*. He wrote, "Many scientists have remarked with surprise that Luther Burbank, George Washington Carver, and even Nobel laureate Barbara McClintock all have said that it was the plants who told them what to do, who revealed their mysteries to them. The only requirement, they commented, was that they had to care for them, to treat them with respect, to have a feeling for the organism."

McClintock was mentioned in the last chapter. Many people may recognize the name of George Washington Carver for his notable results with peanuts, though, of course he did much else. Luther Burbank was capable of feeling which plants that he cultivated would, as they grew, best express themselves in the direction he was trying to reach. Helen Keller said of him, "He has the rarest of gifts, the receptive spirit of a child. Only a wise child can understand the language of flowers and trees."

If our entire nervous system is capable of picking up and sending signals, not just the brain, then here is how we may extend beyond the five senses and into what is commonly called sixth-sense territory. Everyone has had moments of knowing, that couldn't be explained through analytical thought. While many dismiss these as mere coincidences, the fact is that we don't understand everything about the various signaling mechanisms existing in the body.

Rollin McCraty, Ph.D., at the HeartMath Reseach Center, stated, "Overall, our data suggest that the heart and brain, together, are involved in receiving, processing, and decoding intuitive information. On the basis of these results and those of other research, it would thus appear that intuitive perception is a system-wide process in which both the heart and brain (and possibly other bodily systems) play a critical role."[8]

Buhner states it succinctly, "Analysis of information flow into the human body has shown that much of it impacts the heart first, flowing to the brain only after it has been perceived by the heart. What this means is that our *experience* of the world is routed first through our heart, which 'thinks' about the experience and then sends the data to the brain for further processing. When the heart receives information back from the brain about how to respond, the heart analyses it and decides whether or not the actions of the brain wants to take will be effective. The heart routinely engages in a neural dialogue with the brain and, in essence, the two decide together what actions to take."

The brain processes information after the heart has felt. And then that information can be passed back and forth. This is actually happening when you are deciding, and you think you should go one way but feel you should go another. Your brain and your heart disagree.

It is through the entraining fields of the heart that we can literally communicate with nature and with plants themselves. Plants do not have a brain like us. Thus, they do not think in the same way. They have no vocal cords; thus, they will not speak to you like another human would. It's not about mouths. Nor is it about ears. But they do have electromagnetic fields, which can be touched and can reach out. In fact, we are interacting with these fields all the time.

Explaining that synchronization doesn't just occur in humans, but in others too, Buhner writes, "When the electromagnetic fields of the two hearts come together, they also begin to oscillate or entrain to each other. But this phenomenon extends even further. When the heart's electromagnetic field and any other organism's electromagnetic field (whether it has a 'heart' or not) are in close proximity, the fields entrain or synchronize, and there is an extremely rapid and complex interchange of information."

The pervading idea of mechanistic science is that ancient cultures discovered the medicinal aspects of plants through trial and error. More often than not, when scientists investigate these ancient claims, they are vindicated by looking at the chemicals and interactions.

Yet all of the ancient people that are still around today, and those that were asked in years previous, said that it was the plants themselves that told people what to use for what in dreams and visions.

Take the case of the psychoactive brew ayuhuasca. This is a combination of a vine and the bark from other trees. Chemically, the visions and various psychedelic aspects of ayuhuasca occur because of the molecule dimethyltryptamine, or DMT, that is released. DMT, also called the "spirit molecule," is also theorized to be found endogenously inside of our bodies, produced in the pineal gland.[9]

Normally this chemical would simply break down in the stomach, because of mono amine oxidase, and nothing would occur. It is not orally active by itself. But when it is combined with a MAOI inhibitor, like is found in the ayuhuasca vine, *Banisteriopsis caapi*, it allows the DMT, found in chacrona, or *Psychotria viridis,* to be orally active.

When you consider that there are as many as 80,000 plants in the rainforest, is it really feasible to think that shamans mixed so many random plants together until they found this combination?

Buhner shares another viewpoint that shows how trial and error simply can't be the method of discovery. In the book *The Lost Language of Plants* he describes how an ancient man might have searched the forest for plants to stem blood loss from a wound, using trial and error, eventually finding that the amazing yarrow plant, *Achillea millefolium*, did so. Certainly, here trial and error could be a possibility. But Buhner goes on to the following example:

"Throughout the world, in addition to many other medicinal uses, artemisias are used to ward off negative influences, bad energy. As an example, Melvin Gilmore quotes a Dakota Indian of North America regarding Artemisia ludoviciana that it serves as a 'protection against maleficent powers; therefore, it was always proper to begin any ceremonial by using Artemisia in order to drive away evil influences.'

"So, here we have a man in the forest again, perhaps just walking along minding his own business, and he encounters negative influences, maleficent powers. He is quite afraid (as anyone would be) and begins looking for a plant to help. He holds yarrow up toward the negative influences but it fails to work. Grass, nothing. Marsh mallow, no. Cherry leaves—no effect. Panicking now, he rushes through the forest trying more and more plants, until, finally at the last minute, he grabs an Artemisia and holds it up toward the negative influence. The negative influence dissipates. Artemisia wards off negative influences. He shares the information and this use of Artemisia enters his people's cultural lore. By a similar process, it enters the knowledge base of all other cultures on Earth.

"For trial and error to be the method by which this plant information was gained (and not visions or dreams or talking plants), it must be assumed that negative influences, maleficent powers, exist. Most scientists

will not concede they exist, much less that they can be perceived, still less that a plant can ward them off. Yet throughout the world the vast majority of cultures identified this action of Artemisia uniformly."

When I read this passage, I laughed out loud. This cannot be explained rationally. It's a double bind that dismantles one aspect of the mechanical viewpoint of the world or another, forcing it all to come tumbling down.

Instead of dismissing natives and indigenous people across the world as ignorant and superstitious, why don't we instead seek to revisit this forgotten method of learning, the lost language of plants?

Do you see people that speak other languages than yours stupid? I know imperialist white men have done that for generations, but do you do so now? I hope not. Instead, I am sure you understand that solely because it is another language they speak, one that you don't understand, that communication is still occurring. And so it is with the language of plants.

Buhner writes extensively on the scientific theory behind how this can take place. In essence, it has to do with the cell's ability to respond to electromagnetism. "Living organisms amplify these meaningful electromagnetic waves and decode them in order to hear them (just as we do.) They then use the information and respond to the sender through their own uniquely fractalized electromagnetic communication. For all living organisms are transmitters as well as receivers; these communications always go both ways."

The heart comes in because, "A heart is, in fact, a large self-organized grouping of cells. Cells, operating individually at their own frequencies, can synchronize or *entrain* as they move into proximity with other cells...like heart cells, are so extensive and so closely coupled that they are supremely able to sense extremely weak electric fields at close to the theoretical limits of any system to do so. Fish use exactly this process in their bodies to produce their extremely sensitive electrical detection arrays...They can, in fact, perceive a change in an electrical field equivalent to one-millionth of a volt. Some fish have been found to be sensitive to fields as tiny as 25 billionths of a volt. This sensitivity is nearly refined enough for the fish to count individual electrons as they touch the surface of its skin."

Our ability to sense the meaning encoded within electromagnetic waves is a natural ability of all living things. It is part of the sensory encoding and decoding ability of living things; cells, bacteria, plants, animals and humans. With the right sort of focus these frequencies can be picked out, against the background noise, and amplified. This works in much the same way as a radio does. Or think of you listening to one specific conversation when dozens are going on in a busy room. Or that your eyes are focused on the words on this page rather than any of the environment around you.

"All organisms, in fact, possess mechanisms to 'fine tune' their internal electromagnetic dial in order to enhance the signals they receive. As the signal is fine-tuned, it gets stronger, and more and more background noise entrains to the signal, making it stronger still. This process is so powerful that a weak signal's strength can be increased ten thousand times," writes Buhner.

And yes, the heart as a sensory organ is not some fancy metaphor, but a scientific way of looking at it. He continues, "Alterations in heart function in response to external phenomena have the same kinds of effects on cortical functioning as do more classical sensory inputs, that is, visual, auditory, olfactory, tactile, and gustatory stimuli. The incoming sensory perceptions from the heart have the same ability to capture the attention and shift behavior as those five sensory mediums. When the heart is impacted by events in the external environment, information about those external events is encoded in various cardiac wave patterns (beating patterns, pressure waves in the blood, and so on) that are analogous to the different wave forms that come in from visual or auditory stimuli – light and sound waves...The heart wave's forms, experienced as emotions, also have embedded meaning and this meaning can be extracted from the emotional flow just as meaning is extracted from visual and auditory flow. Because we are trained to ignore these particular kinds of sensory cues and the information they contain, most people do not consciously utilize the heart as an organ of perception. Most of the information received is thus processed below conscious levels of cognition."

The sensory system of the heart is every bit as real and tangible as the sensory system of your sight, smell or your hearing. If you walked around with your eyes closed all the time, it wouldn't mean that sight didn't exist.

Just because we talk about only having five senses does not mean it's true.

Once again, I invite you to read *The Secret Teachings of Plants*, for far more detail. There Buhner covers in a book, what I'm trying to give justice to in a single chapter. You can also investigate further the research of the Institute of HeartMath. While they focus their work on humans it is lending lots of credence and data to these ideas, showing how it works and what occurs.

How to Communicate with Plants

"Stones have been known to move and trees to speak."
– Shakespeare

This is a big subject. It's like asking how do you communicate with humans? There is no one right way to do it, though we could all agree there are lots of wrong ways.

I still consider myself a novice in this practice. Conversational in the language, but with lots of errors. Not fully fluent and by no-means a native speaker. Still, here I'll be sharing what I have learned from my teachers, both human and plant, as well as my own personal experience.

Plant life exists on a different time scale then we do. They're not up and moving around, always busy, always doing stuff, like we are. To communicate with them requires a shift more onto their level. Sure, sometimes a plant will metaphorically yell at you, making its presence known strongly in something like an intense dream. But the majority of time, until those relationships are established, it's up to us to initiate the conversation. Until that time, most plants will be content to do plant things.

This practice is often called sitting with plants, because that is what you do. Find a plant and sit down near it. Get yourself comfortable. You certainly don't need to be in a full lotus position in order to do this. You can stand but typically you'll want to spend a fair amount of time, at the very least fifteen minutes. An hour is even better.

Think of a conversation with a stranger. If you only see them for a minute or two you can only have a surface level conversation. If it's a close friend you can go deep quickly, and so it is with plants too, once you know them.

When you visit someone's house you often will bring a gift. I've heard some say that they never visit anyone without some sort of offering. And so, it shall be with plants. For a long time, I didn't "get" offerings. It seemed wasteful to my Western mind. I sometimes engaged in the practice but more out of being told to do so, rather than feeling it. It wasn't until I traveled to Guatemala and spent time in Mayan ceremonies that I began to understand.

The way to communicate with nature, with the spirits, with the ancestors, is very much like communicating to other humans. We focus on the verbal part as that is primarily how we use language. But there is so much other communication going on between any two humans, including through the heart field.

An offering is a giving of yourself, a sign of respect, a recognition that it is not just the physical world involved. But acting in the physical world, we give something physical to connect.

Buhner writes, "The first step in learning to talk to plants is cultivating politeness...The first step is to respect our elders."

One of the standard offerings long used is tobacco. Another often used is alcohol. It seems the spirits like their drugs just like people do! (And another word for alcohol is spirits, which comes from alchemical traditions.) If you're not prepared with these ahead of time, you can also do something as simple as offering a stand or two of hair. Here you are literally giving of yourself.

It is interesting to think about this offering. If you put hair or tobacco on the ground, eventually it will be eaten up in decomposition. The web of life, mycelium and plant, the earth itself, will incorporate this "information" into itself. In this sense, the offering is something very real that does have lasting action. It may be subtle, but we are entering into the subtle realms.

Plants are largely under the influence of psychoactive drugs just as we are. While this might be surprising at first glance it really shouldn't be. We came from nature. Our nervous and chemical systems arose out of the same things from which everything else did. Our neurotransmitters like serotonin were transmitting across neurology before brains ever existed. Plus, all our drugs come from nature in the first place, or in the case of synthetic chemicals are often at least inspired by the real thing.

By giving an offering, you open up the channels for communication. These days when I'm traveling out in nature I carry a small pouch of tobacco with me.

The next step is to be present. Sitting with a plant is not a time to think about the past or the future. Sure, your mind will go there, in fact, the plant itself may send you there in a myriad of ways. But it is like meditation in the beginning. As your mind wanders, bring it back to your point of focus, the plant in front of you.

Introduce yourself to the plant. If they're going to open up and reveal themselves to you, they would like to know a little bit about you first. While you can think it, it is best to physically talk to the plant in the beginning. Tell them why you've come, who you are, about your offering and even what you might be seeking from them.

Then ask about the plant. Here is where there is a shift from the verbal into something deeper. Engage all of your senses. Start with those you're used to. Note the form, the color of the plant. Trace its leaves with your eyes. Reach out and feel the texture. Ask permission, then take a small piece. Smell it. Taste it. Use your five senses as an access point to the sixth.

Often in my introduction to a new plant I've never sat with, I will draw it in my notebook. When you draw, you look with more detailed eyes in order to be able to replicate its form.

Buhner writes, "As your body becomes more and more alive through the activation of your senses, *sensing* is what you do instead of thinking. Sensing takes the place of thinking. Awareness is focused through your senses, attentively noticing all that you sense. It has no time for thinking now. Your consciousness begins to move out of the brain, leaving the analytical mind behind. You being to find the world that our ancient ancestors knew so well."

Breathe with the plant. Every plant breathes in carbon dioxide and breathes out oxygen. We breathe in oxygen and breathe out carbon dioxide. We are symbionts in that way. Focus on your deep breathing and see/feel that breath enter and exit your lungs then travel to the plant, enter and exit their leaves, and back and forth. This is not just a thought experiment. If you're close enough this is literally happening with gaseous molecules! This intimate breathing can help establish the connection. Deep breathing gives you something to do while shifting you into a more meditative state, becoming more still, becoming more present.

Allow your eyes to defocus. Not a foveal view, but a spreading out your vision to take in the periphery. There is a difference in focusing intently with your eyes and taking it all in with a relaxed gaze. It's okay to start with the former during the intro of sitting with a plant, but you'll want to shift to the latter. Some like to close their eyes, but whether open or closed, this spread vision also serves to shift your state as well.

Dropping into an open and receptive state is required to "hear" the plants communicate back. Plants do not have vocal cords so don't expect a literal voice talking back. Depending on you, depending on the plant, the communication may come in various means through the heart. Remember that the information enters your heart first, before being routed to the brain.

The plant will communicate through your internal representations. Like a musical instrument, when you get into the right state, the plant may begin to play you.

You may see a picture or a movie. This could be a memory or something new imagined. Do not expect LSD-like visions. It is subtler than that. But that doesn't mean they're not visions. It's simply closer in nature to your regular thinking throughout the day.

A conversation from years ago, could pop into your head. Or a piece of music you love. Or one you hate. Words may come into your head with some sort of different quality to them than your normal thoughts. Notice the tone, the location, the rhythm.

And you will have feelings. This could be internal sensations, such as energy moving around. It can be emotional states that come and go. There may be times when you burst into tears or are elated in the most joyous spirits. Anger may rise. Or you may be feeling like you're tripping out, dude.

"Because of our long habituation in the linear mind and the things we have been taught about the livingness of the world, this is the hardest thing of all – to give reality to the feelings that flow into us from the world itself." Later, Buhner continues, "Most of us have been taught that feelings only come from within us…There will be one or more primary feelings: mad, sad, glad, or scared. Then a number of secondary feelings: a unique blending of the primary feelings into more subtle forms, like the million blending of colors from an artist's palette. These secondary feelings are encodes of more complex communications from plants…You are learning a new language now."

A smell, beyond the aroma of the plant may enter your nose. Or a taste fleeting across your mouth. You might get hot or cold. Or any number of other possibilities.

They say that each plant has a song and that the plant may teach you the song. And others have heard the same exact song upon comparison. I haven't personally experienced this, but I also can scarcely carry a tune.

All of these things can be consciously thought. Or the thoughts may just emerge from your unconscious as thoughts do throughout the day. But when you're sitting with a plant, and with some practice, you'll begin notice there is a difference between your thinking and this communication.

The immersive nature of a long-forgotten memory. The tone of words said. The *feeling* of the thing. The location of the thought (no they're not all inside your head but have locations in the space in and around us).

To understand and perceive these things also takes practice. I received a plenty in studying neuro-linguistic programming or NLP where a useful model of these perceptual qualities, or submodalities, exists. These are the characteristics of the pictures, sounds and feelings. Any meditation practice helps too, because this trains your "observer," that part of you that can observe your own thoughts. But you don't need that same training. Simply noticing what you notice you'll begin to notice these differences. The plants will teach you themselves.

Buhner writes, "As you develop your sensitivity, you can feel the plant begin to move toward you, respond to you, engage with you, entrain with your heart. You can tell, when you pay close attention, the moment when the two of you have established rapport."

Sitting with a plant for thirty minutes to an hour, your mind will

274

wander. You may start thinking about doing the laundry, or that you're hungry. That's okay. Just bring back your attention to the plant, to your breathing. Try asking a question again. Perhaps that hunger is coming about because the plant is used herbally to stimulate digestion. Or perhaps you just haven't eaten in a while. Through the communication, you can discover the difference.

One block that often occurs is thinking about yourself too much. This is an issue for many humans, me included. Even asking the plant to help you is a form of this. Ask the plant about itself. Ask what problems it is dealing with. Be curious and be concerned. Actually care.

Many times, when I'm sitting with plants I will have my notebook with me. Besides drawing the plant, I will note impressions, thoughts, and feelings that come. Since I get such great information from the plants, I like to be able to take notes. And I don't have a problem in sinking back into the state after writing something out.

But other times, and this may suit you better, you'll want nothing to distract your attention. Simply be with the plant completely. You can take notes later, codifying your thoughts and feelings into concrete form. If it is important enough, you will likely remember it.

Something else that is enjoyable is to sit with a plant you know nothing about, or just little bits and pieces like its common name. Do several sessions finding out what the plant reveals to you about itself. Only after you have engaged in this, you go online or in a book and read about the plant. Note how your own experience matches up with the knowledge of others.

My first experiences in plant sitting was with Oregon Grape during a workshop. I knew nothing about the plant. For me, and many others, it was our first interaction ever with it. Throughout our several sits over a few days we humans did not talk about the plant at all to each other as we were instructed. Yet when we shared our experiences of it at the end of our session there were many common threads throughout. A coincidence? I don't think so.

But don't expect yourself to have gleaned everything from a plant in a couple sessions. Do you know everything about a human after a few conversations?

After you have sat with a plant a number of times, look in a few books or online and find out the collective wisdom. Note where you match up and where you don't. Then with these things in mind, you can go back to the plant and with this book learning, and new perspectives may now be revealed to you as you ask new questions.

To talk to a plant, you don't just want to remain separate, but instead to become the plant. Walk, or should I say, stand there in its figurative shoes. It can be helpful to see yourself as sitting there with the plant, from the plants perspective were it to have eyes like you do. Floating out of your body to become the plant helps you to enter into its thoughts and feelings.

Buhner writes, "The meanings, the communications the plant emits, will eventually emerge within you in extremely elegant and sophisticated *gestalts* of understanding." A gestalt is an organized whole that is perceived as more than the sum of its parts. A gestalt means you'll understand something in lots of detail, in an instant, that could not be communicated in words as such. It may also mean it would be hard for you to translate into words too.

"You are refining not only your understanding of the plant, but your ability to perceive with the heart, to determine congruencies and subtle differences in meaning. You are making new muscles...The continual use of the heart as an organ of perception leads to refinement of the process until it becomes much more elegant and dependable than any scientific approach," states Buhner. This is a skill. As such, you must practice to become good at it.

Not all plants of the same species are the same. While there does seem to be an element of this where you're accessing the archetype of the plant spirit, there is also each plant as an individual. A new-growth, healthy plant is likely to communicate differently than one that is dying. Just like you wouldn't expect all humans to communicate the same, you shouldn't expect the plant world to either.

Finding plants in different stages of growth can be illuminating. Mullein in its first year where it is a basal rosette has a very different feel than its second year where it launches its flowering stalk, up to over seven feet tall. The area I live in Santa Cruz is rich in redwoods, though the vast majority of these were logged over a hundred years ago. What lives around is essentially the equivalent of children, one- to two-hundred-year-old trees. But there are a few old growths around. The first time sitting with one of these, to be described in a little bit, I could feel the depth of wisdom that wasn't present in the others.

Another interesting aspect can be found in sitting with wild plants, compared to those that are cultivated or gardened. Finding a plant in the wild, in its natural habitat, there seems to be different layers of information available. Here nature is the gardener, not human hands, thus you may discover a bit more about its nature. In the garden, you may learn a bit more about its relation to humankind.

Just like you have stronger connections with certain people, so it is with nature. Certain plants will resonate with you on a stronger level than others. Sitting with lemon balm was nice but sitting with wild rose was mind blowing. By working with a number of plants you'll come to find your plant allies. These are the plants that will help you grow as a human. And it's helpful to think of yourself as offering something back to the plants in return. When you begin this practice, pay attention to those signs or synchronicities in your life. Watch for certain plants showing up in your dreams. Notice if you hear or read about the same plant several times within a short period of time. When you're out in nature notice if a plant dramatically draws your attention. Sometimes it's almost as if they shout, "Hey you!"

As a practice, I would recommend sitting with a wide variety of plants. This will help to train your heart sense, to begin to learn the new alphabet, the single letters that you can begin to put into words, that is the language of plants. The contrast of what you pick up from different plants can help to show you the way. Just a single plant sit with a dozen different plants is a good way to start.

And once you find a plant that you resonate strongly with, spend multiple sessions with it. Go wide and then go deep. Nurture your relationship with this plant ally. Of course, if the plant is used herbally, consuming it is another aspect of that relationship.

The communication with plants exists on a non-local level. It is best to be present and there with the plant to get started. But once you have been with a plant a number of times you'll begin to internalize its message. It may come to you in dreams. Its presence can be felt anywhere and anytime you might need it. Sink into the feeling of the plant and your ally can be there with you even at a distance.

If a plant teaches you how to better handle your stress, when stress arrives, be with the plant internally and notice how that can help. If a different plant teaches you how to step into your power, feel its presence when you feel like shrinking away. If still another plant helps you to open your heart, like rose did for me, think of her before or during your loving communications with other humans.

Be forewarned, if you engage in this practice, the plants may ask something in return.

Not Just Plant Communication

"We can say that the earth has a vegetative soul, and that its flesh is the land, its bones are the structure of the rocks...its blood is the pools of water...its breathing and its pulse are the ebb and flow of the sea."
– Leonardo Da Vinci

Throughout this section I have referred to sitting with plants. But this process is not relegated to just that one kingdom. You can do the same with mushrooms, insects, animals and even other humans. The one issue with animals of all kinds is that they move, whereas the plants and mushrooms aren't going anywhere, not quickly anyway.

Using your heart perception in this way gives you access to a sense, completely forgotten by many of us. It gives us access to a new means of information, one very different than how most people interact with the world.

You can also do it with things that aren't "alive" in the classical sense. In the West, we've made our categories of what constitutes living and what does not. What about inert matter like rocks and water?

Virtually all ancient cultures were animists. That all was alive. While we may not be able to perceive that aliveness when we simply compare it to our own, alive and not alive is black and white thinking. Perhaps there is a spectrum.

Does the earth 'think' of the humans that live on it just like single bacterial cells in its body? Are we scarcely alive compared to the Earth?

Regardless of the aliveness of something, you can reach out and find the feeling of that thing through this same practice. If everything is energy as physics states, then it appears we can use this heart to reach out and touch it. This is something I engaged in for every chapter of this book. I sat with the sun. I sat with the moon. The stars, a fresh spring, the earth, the air, my internal bodily processes during a fast, during movement, with nature as a whole. It was this practice where parts of this book came from as it was revealed to me.

Describing one such occasion, Buhner writes, "I felt my spirit move and then some *Mountain* thing touched me, looked down from a mighty height, awakened from its contemplation, to see me, tiny, below. And it was old beyond knowing and has little to do with humans and its gaze rocked me as, for a second, I stood revealed. Then it returned to a contemplation of centuries, of millennia, living a kind of life that is as far beyond me as the stars are from the sun."

In a vision, I glimpsed into the mind of Gaia, and felt like my human neurology couldn't handle it. The human system is meant for human things, not planetary things, after all. I felt what it was like to be a single bacterium or a cell in her body. I've used this metaphor several times throughout this book, but in that moment, it was not a metaphor, it was something very real that I felt. The lasting impact of this event has changed me permanently.

In the next couple of chapters, I'll be sharing some of the stories and details gleaned from a plant, a tree and a mushroom. As you'll see these are quite different in nature, based on the plants themselves, and also what I aimed to learn.

Our whole culture has said that this sense does not exist. But when you begin to realize that it does and how to use it, it can open you up to a new world. I will finish up with one more quote from Rupert Sheldrake. "As soon as we allow ourselves to think of the world as alive, we recognize that a part of us knew this all along. It is like emerging from winter into spring."

21
Wild Rose's Love

"[Shamans] would simply say that everything is spirit and, if we are sensitive to this, it is quite possible for the spirit of a plant to enter and influence us, changing our energy and creating new possibilities for healing."
– Ross Heaven

"This healing from a plant reawakens in the human heart the capacity for deep feeling and connection with the natural world. It opens up an ancient world to those who are healed, a world they did not know existed. It stirs dying embers to flame."
– Stephen Harrod Buhner

What I am about to share with you is unconventional. It's a story of how the Wild Rose challenged me deeply and opened me into a new way of life. It's a story I haven't told to many people. Yet I feel it is important to share for two reasons. Number one, to share the experience of nature as living "sentient" entities. Secondly, as an example of helping heal the damaged masculine with the feminine. And thus, I am sharing it despite my inhibitions.

A couple years back I was involved in an herbalism training program at the School of Evolutionary Herbalism, under Sajah Popham. This program was multifaceted. One of the things included was the direct perception of plants.

In the previous chapter, I mentioned that in our first class, we worked with Oregon Grape. This was great, being my first experience and it was wonderful to see all the similarities in experience across the group. Back home I sat with a number of others to continue my training. But this did not prepare me for what was soon to come...

On the next session, we sat with Wild Rose.

This is the wild progenitor, from which all the thousands of varieties of cultivated roses you've seen, originally comes.

The rose is a feminine plant. Everyone knows that.

It personifies the feminine quality of beauty…and at the same time has a fierceness to it, as is embodied in the thorns.

It is considered powerful heart medicine. Yes, for the physical heart it does have some action with its antioxidant and anti-inflammatory qualities. But more predominately for the emotional and energetic heart.

In my first sit with rose I was overcome with shame. For whatever reason, I found myself unable to even look at the rose, my head hung low.

It was like she was showing me how closed off my heart had been.

Years of beating myself up mentally and emotionally, as well as the standard macho guy stuff of suppressing feelings. This was exacerbated by losing my mother to cancer. It's typical in this era for guys to armor up their hearts in this way.

By the end of that sit, the shame broke open to jubilation. Everything was majestic.

It was like she was showing me how good an open, fulfilled heart could be.

And this all was just the beginning. The next sit, was much of the same, showing other facets around the same area. Yet, it was in my final sit that weekend with the rose that the most profound experience occurred.

As I sat there with Rose the mosquitos hovered over me. After killing a few I knew that it was useless. Just that time of the year in the place we were at. There was a never-ending supply. So, I got up and moved.

And they still swarmed. I pulled both my arms into my t-shirt so they couldn't get to them. Yet, still they circled around. I could hear the constant "eeeeeeee" as they buzzed around my head. After a few more minutes I moved again, this time to a sunny spot, where I hoped there'd be less.

When I sat down in this new spot and connected with the Wild Rose she said to me, "You want connection to nature? Then allow the mosquitoes to feast on you."

A flash across my internal movie screen saw me sitting there, with my shirt off, covered in the insects, all feeding on me. I replied, "Hell, no."

The Rose replied in silence.

"You've got to be kidding me. I can't do that." More silence.

From my previous sits, I knew Wild Rose would challenge me. It already had. With that fierce feminine energy, she can be a bitch. But at the same time, it's what I needed. An internal struggle, heart and head, raged on.

I had to accept the challenge. There was no connection otherwise. I am reminded of oriental masters that would make a potential student wait on the doorsteps to prove their seriousness.

At least I had to try. Just then one mosquito landed on my shoulder. I watched as it pierced my skin with her proboscis. Focused on the moment, it heightened the feeling. Probably a minute passed. I watched its body become red and engorged with my blood, until it finally had enough and flew off.

That wasn't so bad. So, I moved back to my previous spot where there were more mosquitoes. They flew around me, a few landing and beginning to feast.

I attempted to welcome them. It wasn't easy. I flipped-flopped mentally, in one moment disgusted, in the next accepting. The several days previously that weekend I had taken glee in killing every mosquito that landed on me. Now I was giving sustenance willingly.

When one mosquito finished and flew off I said in an irritated voice "You're welcome," just like someone would say if no thanks was given. Then the Wild Rose said to me "No, you be thankful that they chose to feed on you."

So not only do I have to accept the bites but be thankful for them? As I sunk deeper into the state of gratitude I could begin to appreciate the mosquito. I thought about how much food from plants and animals I've eaten over the years. And how here, I had an opportunity to help give food and life. And it didn't cost me much, just a tiny pin prick of pain.

I almost felt like a mother breastfeeding her baby. (A very odd feeling to get in touch with as a man, I must say.)

The rose then said something that has stuck with me since that day and will for the rest of my life.

"When you can love a mosquito like a mother loves her baby, then you

will know unconditional love."

Before this time, my love had always been conditional. How deeply could I fall into this state? The rose continued to test me. A mosquito lands on my forehead. As it walks about its just too much and I blow it off with my breath. I see a bug crawling up my leg. Is that a tick? Come on! A mosquito is one thing, but a tick is another. I can't do it and I flick it off.

Finally, I decide I can handle the mosquitoes. I take off my shirt to bear more open skin and allow them to come and feed.

A short time later I hear the conch blow and it's time to go back. I thank the mosquitoes and the Rose for what they have shown me.

We then head into a drum journey, just like Native Americans do. It's an integration of the learnings from the plants and the course, a conclusion to our time together.

As I descend deeply into a vision I see my mother. I see the rose. It's both of them. And she presents back to me one-third of my heart.

For whatever reason, I already had one-third. Now this new part becomes integrated into me and I have two thirds. The journey is to still to continue, the final third to come in time.

All people have both the masculine and feminine in them, the yin and yang. To be a whole person, self-actualized, will mean healing and growing both sides.

And in that journey, you may find certain plant allies that help you to do so. Like the meeting with a mentor in the Hero's Journey we all face. (Actually, looking at it now, this whole experience with Wild Rose was its own Hero's Journey.)

Reflecting on this later I came across this passage from Buhner. "The feelings *are* the medicine. At this moment, the medicine is simply encoded in one particular form. If you forget this, lose sight of it, lose the feeling of it, go off in your mind someplace else, you are losing touch with the most essential thing. This is the one true thing that you have come to the plant to experience."

Taking the herbs is one method of gaining their help. Communicating with them may be even more powerful.

22
The Redwood Growth Strategy

"The redwoods, once seen, leave a mark or create a vision that stays with you always. No one has ever successfully painted or photographed a redwood tree. The feeling they produce is not transferable. From them comes silence and awe. It's not only their unbelievable stature, nor the color which seems to shift and vary under your eyes, no, they are not like any trees we know, they are ambassadors from another time."
— John Steinbeck

When working with the shaman, Sheryl Netzky, she tasked me with finding something in nature to work with that could help me grow my business. In my prior experience of working with plants, I wasn't after anything specific. Typically, it was to learn about the plant's medicinal aspects. Here I was seeking help with something else.

And I didn't decide on redwoods myself. As I walked through nature with this intention, they called out to me, saying they could help.

What follows is not a story or a single experience, like was shared above with Wild Rose. Instead it was reflections after several sits and, later, doing some online research regarding redwoods. (That's where all the quotes come from as well as the stats mentioned.) You'll see its very different in format.

Growth and Patience

"What can the redwoods tell us about ourselves? Well, I think they can tell us something about human time. The flickering, transitory quality of human time and the brevity of human life."
— Richard Preston

Redwood trees are among the fastest-growing trees on Earth. They can grow three to ten feet per year and reach their height generally within the first hundred years of their lives.

They're also among some of the oldest trees too, with a lifespan of over 2000 years. After that vertical growth, the rest of the growth is outward. From the tree base, branches grow outwards with quick speed. And if these aren't working out they'll die and often times fall off.

In business, this shows several qualities necessary. Grow quickly, prune quickly and, still, be patient. The faster a project can get going the quicker or not you can find if it is working out. If not, let it die or discard it. If it is, this growth will further fuel the tree's growth.

A lengthy time span must also be examined. To become "old-growth" takes many years. Ask; are the conditions right, is the planning right, in order to have this business last for a century?

Burls and Fairy Rings

Redwoods don't only grow by seeds. At the base burls will form. And if something happens to the main tree, these can then sprout new trees. Even if a tree falls over, new trees may sprout from its side.

From a cut base or damaged tree, often a ring of new trees will form. This is called a fairy ring.

In business, this is how one business can grow another. Utilizing the same strong root system these trees may even surpass the original in time. It shows how one business can support another, as in symbiosis.

That root can be likened to the main person behind the business, while the "trees" are the businesses themselves. Over time, different root systems may even infuse with each other. Thus, you may only have a few year old tree, but an ancient and well-established root system.

Rings in the Tree

As a tree grows it gets wider. The biggest redwoods are about 30 feet in diameter. The years can be counted as the rings inside the tree.

What is a "ring" to a business? These are the systems and the people involved. To grow the business requires adding both the right people and the right systems in place. This takes time, yet faster growth can be had if it is done intentionally.

Of course, they must be good systems and people. Growing in the wrong direction or with poor people and systems can take the tree, or business, off its base thus causing it to fall.

Under and Above

"Murmuring out of its myriad leaves
Down from its lofty top, rising two hundred feet high
Out of its stalwart trunk and limbs—out of its foot-thick bark
That chant of the seasons and time—chant, not of the past only, but the future.
— Walt Whitman

Despite their massive height, redwoods do not have the deepest roots. Generally, they only go down five to six feet, though they can span wide.

The roots are like the operations of a business, while the tree and branches above ground is the marketing. What can be seen from the outside, versus what can't be seen by the public. The marketing can grow massive, though this must be supported by strong roots. Without them the tree can go down in a strong wind storm.

Taking root in the right soil is like putting the right people and systems in place to support a big tree. While some people may skyrocket their success, it can be short lived as the base is not there to support it. This is not my way.

Strength and Weakness

Redwoods have thick bark which is antifungal and keeps insects at bay. They're even fire resistant, able to live on when a fire sweeps through, killing off everything else. However, this fire-resistant quality is also what led them to being logged almost to extinction, as the lumber is strong and maintains these qualities too.

Be careful that a strength doesn't become a weakness. Look at both

286

sides, the advantages and drawbacks, of any situation.

Wisdom Download

"A grove of giant redwood or sequoias should be kept just as we keep a great and beautiful cathedral."
— Theodore Roosevelt

Most of the redwoods around are merely children. With their potential lifespans, a hundred-year-old tree, the second growth, are teenagers at best in human terms! When you live millennia, you have the opportunity to learn a few things.

So, it was that when I sat with an old growth, it was like a wisdom download. With time comes experience and with experience comes seeing things more clearly. This occurred for me around two areas specifically:

1) The Biggest Leverage—being on the peak of a mountain I needed to clearly see the opportunities for the maximum leverage points within my business.

2) Saying NO—Everything I say yes to is stopping me from doing something else. Saying yes to too many things can put me into a state of overwhelm, where I'm more likely to shut down saying NO to everything.

As the redwood taught me about systems, I need to create and make habit a system of deciding to say yes or no. Also, instead of taking things on myself I need to more often say "Talk to so-and-so about that." Because I am entrepreneurial, and the ideas come every single day, I can at any time make a list of everything I'm doing and choose what to say NO too starting now.

Sitting with the old growth I realized I don't necessarily want to be driving the marketing. I like to do research, I like to be a thought-leader, I like to write and produce content. While I am grateful for the marketing knowledge I have, the more I can let that go into capable hands and systems, the happier and more effective I will be.

23
Sensory Stimulation with Artist's Conk

"The lover of nature is he whose inward and outwards senses are still truly adjusted to each other."
– Ralph Waldo Emerson

"Nature will bear the closest inspection. She invites us to lay our eye level with her smallest leaf, and take an insect view of its plain."
– Henry David Thoreau

The founder of Gestalt therapy, Fritz Perls, had an interesting saying. "Lose your mind and come to your senses." What did Perls mean by this? We've become too absorbed in thinking, in mental chatter, in what the Buddhists call the monkey mind.

By coming into your senses, that of sight, smell, touch, hearing, and taste, *(and feeling with the heart)* you become more present to the outside world. Doing so, you get out of that mental chatter.

While meditation is one way to do this, focusing on your breath, or a mantra, as is typically taught, nature may be an even better teacher of it. Your interactions with nature can be fully engaged through the senses.

Richard Louv writes, "By its broadest interpretation, nature-deficit disorder is an atrophied awareness, a diminished ability to find meaning in the life that surrounds us, whatever form it takes. This shrinkage of our lives has a direct impact on our physical, mental, and societal health. However, not only can nature-deficient disorder be reversed, but our lives can be vastly enriched through our relationship with nature, beginning with our senses."

Previously, we explored how plants have all the same senses we do. And that communication between human and plants occurs through a largely forgotten and denied sense. But even among the five basic senses, nature can help to expand these.

One day I was sitting with the artist's conk mushroom, *Ganoderma applanatum*. This fungus acquired its common name because the underside of it is white, and when pressed upon, leaves a permanent mark, thus it can be used like a canvas. It is in the same family as the more well-known reishi mushroom, *Ganoderma lucidum*.

I have found it, and several other mushrooms, to be amazing teachers. One of the lessons I received was to:

"Act as a baby, a child exploring its environment."

How do babies new to this world interact with it? They use their senses fully. Not yet at a stage where they can mentally chatter to themselves, their experience of the world is primary. More like other animals than like an adult human.

They look around. They listen to everything. They must touch everything. And not just with their hands. But everything goes up to their face, into their mouth engaging their sense of taste and smell.

Besides the gourmands around us, how much are our senses of taste and smell downplayed? Our palates are assaulted with the overpowering tastes of heavily processed foods, created by flavor chemists, stopping us from appreciating the subtler flavors present in many things.

Even whole categories of tastes, like bitterness, are simply relegated to being "bad" in our minds. Ditch the mental chatter around this and simply experience bitter for what it is and you may find your experience, and your palate, begins to shift.

How powerful is our sense of smell? For most of us it is scarcely used except in the cases of bad smells that offend us.

What was the last thing you can recall smelling? Was there anything today? Was it the stench of urine in an overused bathroom? A fart? Or was it when you literally stopped to smell the roses? Do you engage your sense of smell with your food, savoring the aroma before you even take a bite?

Did you know that the human nose can detect at least one trillion district scents?[1] We also have the ability to smell fear and happiness in the sweat of other humans.[2] We can engage in tracking by scent just like many other mammals do, if we put in the practice with awareness to do so.

Using our senses like a baby does is the best way to get started in our interactions with nature. Smell everything. In a damp forest, you'll note just how clean the air smells. It is far better that the chemicalized, disinfectant smell of a hospital. Smell the trees, the flowers, the blades of grass. Smell the water, the earth.

And taste it. Once again that fear of nature pervades. We're trained to be scared, that everything is poisonous. While there are a few poisonous things, even fewer are deadly. Most just cause mild discomfort.

Learning what is actually dangerous in the area you're in isn't all that difficult. In my area, I can identify poison oak, hemlock and death cap mushrooms (plus any lookalikes) and steer clear of those.

Besides this you can safely taste just about everything else. Leaves, bark, flowers, berries, even dirt. And note that I'm saying taste. Not eat handfuls of everything. If you tasted most of nature you'd find that most of it is inedible, but just because you put something in your mouth doesn't mean you need to swallow it either.

Become acquainted with bitterness, astringency, and the amazing tastes and smells of unique essential oils.

Doing so you'll come into far more complex and unique smells and tastes than you do in your daily life. The average person eats less than 20 different foods over a year. That's lack of variety. But one trip in nature could have you tasting much more than that.

I hope it goes without saying that I recommend doing this in "real" nature. That is where nature grows wildly without human intervention. At a city park, there's likely chemicals sprayed on the grass and around, and it is best to avoid tasting things. Here the danger isn't as much in nature but in how we poison it.

The taste of some leaves and flowers is absolutely incredible. Eat a few yarrow flowers and you just might be blown away by the multi-layered and intense flavor of it. I know I was the first time I did, and every time since. This expanded taste profile clues you into the fact that yarrow has many different medicinal properties.

Remember all that we discussed about bacteria? Here is an opportunity to reintroduce wild bacteria into your system. Perhaps in nature you'll find some symbiotic bacteria you ought to have but was wiped out of your system when you took antibiotics. Perhaps simply tasting a plant or the untainted dirt could be the best health supplement you ever took!

The best way to get to know nature is through your senses. Reading a book about nature, even this book, won't give you the primary experience that is needed in order to reap the benefits. It's a good start to give you ideas, to satisfy the monkey mind, but it is worse than worthless if it is never acted upon. Remember that health is about direct experience.

And remember that all your senses can be tuned up by going into nature while fasting. Buhner writes, "During fasting, the sensitivity of the body to the world around it increases substantially. Subtle perceptions long hidden under food, television, and daily life begin to be noticed again."

Back to the artist's conk. As I sat with it, it told me to *"Observe."* (Yes, sometimes the conversation is short and cryptic.) Sherlock Holmes told this same thing to Dr. Watson when explaining how he did what he did. "You have not observed. And yet you have seen."

And so, I did. I noticed details I had seen but never before observed. That the tree on which this mushroom grew was damaged, a large limb had partially cracked off, not far from where the conk was located. That the tree was a specific kind that grew in abundance in the forest, the California bay laurel.

After observing the mushroom and its environment for a while came the feeling that I had to get up, move around, and continue to observe. As I walked around the forest I could now observe which trees were the bay laurel and which ones were not. I know, it sounds stupidly simple, but this was an epiphany to me at the time.

I continued to walk and saw another damaged tree of this kind. I could see it from the distance. And I knew, from observation, that that tree would have artist's conks on it. Sure enough, when I approached and rounded the backside of it, I saw them there.

Nature, through the artist's conk, had taught me how to observe nature itself. It opened my eyes.

"Plant blindness" is a term coined by James Wandersee and Elizabeth Schussler to describe "the inability to see or notice the plants in one's own environment—leading to: (a) the inability to recognize the importance of plants in the biosphere, and in human affairs; (b) the inability to appreciate the aesthetic and unique biological features of the life forms belonging to the Plant Kingdom; and (c) the misguided, anthropocentric ranking of plants as inferior to animals, leading to the erroneous conclusion that they are unworthy of human consideration."[3]

As I've learned more from the plants and fungi, learned what can be used for food, for medicine, for making tools, and become more familiar with them, it is amazing how the richness of nature expands.

My next lesson from the conk had to do with listening to nature. With new ears, I could begin to hear the birds and insects as I had never heard them before.

"One of the single most important resources of the natural world is its voice–or natural soundscape," says musician Bernie Krause.

How far can our senses go? When taking a survival class our guide talked about his teacher. One story that stood out was that he could tell when a person was walking up a trail and would arrive in eight minutes to that spot where they stood. Based on what the birds chirped off in the distance he could tell not only of someone's presence but their location and direction too.

Our ability to sense nature can be quite powerful if we simply take the time to learn and practice. The great news is that nature itself will teach you.

Some blind humans have learned how to echo-locate like bats do.[4] While that may occur out of necessity, the fact is anyone could learn this ability.

Polynesians, and other peoples, have long been able to navigate open oceans, even when the sun and the stars were covered by clouds. This may occur because of tapping into the sense of magnetoreception, something every human has. Just for most of us, it lies dormant.

The whole five senses thing is just an old idea. Depending on what you call a sense we have between ten and thirty-three of them. Equilibrio-ception, thermoception, proprioception, nociception, interoception, and many more depending on how they may be sub-divided. In layman's terms these would be balance, temperature, joint position, pain, and awareness of various organs. In time, the currently accepted senses, such as electroreception, or the biological ability to perceive natural electrical stimuli, is likely to expand. The question is, how many are you really in touch with?

The abilities of our senses can go far beyond what we tend to use them for. But even our basic senses need help. The rise in myopia or nearsightedness was first thought to be genetic, then thought to be from spending too much time reading. However, the best research these days points to it simply from a lack of being outdoors.[5]

It seems that civilization leads to a deadening of these our senses. But, because of the complexity of nature, being out in it tends to enhance all the senses. The Bushmen of the Kalahari talk about a state of awakened perceptual awareness they call "second eyes, second ears."

In his books, Louv discusses that faith and spirituality may be likened to another sense. He writes, "It's hard to fathom how any kind of spiritual intelligence is possible without an appreciation for nature…The great work of the twenty-first century will be to reconnect to the natural world as a source of meaning." The connected sense you can get from being in nature is very similar to the connected sense often espoused in many religions, as well as new age spirituality. This is a sense that many people today seem to be lacking.

Whether you learn this from a mushroom or not, is up to you.

24

How to Approach Evolving Your Healthy Natural Lifestyle

"In a mechanistic world, nature worship makes no sense. There is no point in trying to form a personal relationship with blind mechanical processes or with blind chance. All that matters is to try and understand nature so that it can be controlled for human ends. By contrast, in a living world, nature contains living powers far greater than human powers. In the cosmic evolutionary process and in the evolution of life on earth, she is vastly more creative than man. She is the source of life, and she brings forth its myriad forms with inexhaustible creativity. She is all material processes; she is the cosmic flow of energy; she is in all physical fields; she is chance and merciless necessity. Indeed, if there is no God, she is everything."
– Rupert Sheldrake

"I like to think of nature as unlimited broadcasting stations, through which God speaks to us every day, every hour and every moment of our lives, if we will only tune in and remain so."
– George Washington Carver

Throughout these pages, we've covered lots of actionable information. But it does you no good if you don't actually put it into action. The common saying is "knowledge is power." Though it's not quite true. The truth is more along the lines of "applied knowledge is power."

There are two approaches to making any changes. Both are beneficial, though each has its own drawbacks. And one method or the other may be more uniquely suited to your personality. If you want to, you can also take both approaches simultaneously.

The first approach is the slow and steady approach. Think of the tortoise in the tale of the tortoise and the hare. From all the options presented in this book, pick one and only one thing. Perhaps that is to just get outdoors. Perhaps it is get light on your eyes first thing in the morning. Perhaps it is to find a local spring that you can go get water at. Perhaps its incorporating fasting. Whatever it is, you take this one change and work at it. "We cannot do everything at once, but we can do something at once," said former US president, Calvin Coolidge.

And you keep at it until it becomes habit, an integral part of your lifestyle. Here's the cool thing about what is covered in the book. Because they add to your health, in time you'll feel the results come from them. At that moment, you'll know that you can't go back. Returning to your old habits or lifestyle wouldn't make any sense.

I like to think of habits as gravity wells. While being regular in the setting or changing of a habit is important, once something is a habit, it's okay if you don't do it all the time. If it has truly become routine, even if you stopped doing it for a little while, at some point you'll think "What am I doing?" and you'll get right back to it. The gravity well has sucked you back in.

This approach is great because by making just one small step it is easy to focus on. In doing so it often gets done. However, the drawback is this approach can be a bit slow. Still, slow and steady can win the race.

It's important to look at your health and a natural lifestyle in the long term and the big picture, something that humans are notoriously bad at doing. If you did one small change like this each month, that would be twelve in a year, 120 in a decade. That's a lot of power for change!

The other way you can approach adding nature into your lifestyle is through massive action. Personally, this is the approach I like best. Go big or go home. Taking ten, twenty or close to everything mentioned in the book and start doing it all at once. Take something from every single section.

This is the hare approach. Careful that you don't burn out, or that it overwhelms you and, in the end, you simply return to your old ways. Realize that in the story the hare could have easily beat the tortoise if he hadn't been arrogant. That means done smartly, you can get massive results this way. Even so, recognize that with this approach the majority of things may not stick. Many will fall away. That's okay because you'll be left with a few things that do work.

If you're feeling the need for a change, this can be it. I like this approach because it can help people to reach a tipping point quicker. Isolating one change at a time is great for science, however our lives are not in a petri dish. If you want to make a change for your health, it is better to do twenty things in order to get the result. You won't necessarily know which one did it (plus it could be the combination of them that was the magic) but the more important thing is the result, isn't it?

And it does not require a whole lot of time either. If you can stack different steps into each other you can get more in less time.

When I made a commitment to make fresh spring water my main drinking water I didn't have too far to go. But, the spring took two hours to fill up five gallons. Instead of abandoning my plan, I would hike in the nearby woods. I would get grounded, do breathing exercises, and go sit with plants. (Most of the sits with the redwoods from the earlier chapter were during this time.) Plus, depending on what time I went the sun could be shining brightly too. I'd get several nature benefits all at once. Basically, to have fresh water, I had to spend time in nature. This is killing lots of birds with one stone. It's a chain of habits.

In fact, I was a little disappointed when the spring started flowing faster. It doesn't force the nature time like it used to. But like the stream formed from its flow, I adapted to this change.

Similarly, many of my workouts I do while barefoot, outside, breathing fresh air and getting sunlight. Or foraging for wild food will naturally take you through all these things.

Both of these approaches, the small steps and the massive change, can be combined. You can work at one small thing at a time, and occasionally take massive action too. Think of the daily action as a habitual change, whereas you might go spend a weekend in nature. The latter may not change your daily lifestyle, but you can pick up some internal changes from it.

Either way, it's an ongoing journey. You may think I must be perfect at all of this. But I am far from it. I had to start from scratch and it's been tough when I haven't had personal mentors in many aspects of this journey, besides those from nature itself. Slowly and surely, I have strived to get better in alignment with nature myself. It is, and will continue to be, an ongoing journey, for me and for everyone.

On that note, please share this book, or the messages of this book, with others. When your friends, your family, your community are engaged in these practices completing them is that much easier.

Ultimately, the aim of this book is to show how you can become powered by nature. How it is in your self-interest to do so. This selfishness can actually be a good thing, if it is properly aimed.

By doing so, you'll also come to support nature. That way we can make sure we don't destroy our planet, making it inhospitable to us and others, by using up all of the resources. While abundant resources are depletable.

In the end, we benefit. The earth benefits. All of life benefits.

Bibliography

1. Asprey, D. (2017). *Head Strong*. New York: HarperCollins.
2. Asprey, D. (2018). *The Bulletproof diet: Lose up to a pound a day, reclaim your energy and focus, and upgrade your life*. New York: Rodale.
3. Batmanghelidj, F. (2004). *Your bodys many cries for water*. Tagman Press.
4. Bawden-Smith, J. (2016). *In the dark*. Australia: Major Street Publishing.
5. Buhner, S. H. (2002). *The lost language of plants: The ecological importance of plant medicines to life on earth*. White River Junction, VT: Chelsea Green Pub.
6. Buhner, S. H. (2004). *The secret teachings of plants: The intelligence of the heart in the direct perception of nature*. Rochester, VT: Bear &.
7. Buhner, S. H. (2012). *Transformational power of fasting: The way to spiritual, physical, and emotional rejuvenation*. Rochester, VT: Healing Arts.
8. Buhner, S. H. (2014). *Plant intelligence and the imaginal realm: Beyond the doors of perception into the dreaming earth*. Rochester, VT: Bear & Company.
9. Chamovitz, D. (2017). *What a plant knows: A field guide to the senses*. New York: Scientific American/Farrar, Straus and Giroux.
10. Christopher, L. (2017). *Upgrade your breath*. Santa Cruz, CA: Legendary Strength
11. Christopher, L. (2015). *Upgrade your growth hormone*. Santa Cruz, CA: Legendary Strength
12. Christopher, L. (2016). *Upgrade your testosterone*. Santa Cruz, CA: Legendary Strength
13. Fung, J., & Moore, J. (2016). *The complete guide to fasting: Heal your body through intermittent, alternate-day, and extended fasting*. Las Vegas: Victory Belt Publishing.
14. Gedgaudas, N. T., & Perlmutter, D. (2018). *Primal fat burner: Going beyond the ketogenic diet to live longer, smarter and healthier*. London, England: Allen & Unwin.
15. Harari, Y. N. (2018). *Homo Deus: A brief history of tomorrow*. McClelland & Stewart.
16. Harari, Y. N. (2018). *Sapiens: A brief history of humankind*. New York: Harper Perennial.
17. Harris, R. F. (2018). *Rigor Mortis: How sloppy science creates worthless cures, crushes hope, and wastes billions*. New York: Basic Books.

18. Louv, R. (2013). *The nature principle: Reconnecting with life in a virtual age.* Chapel Hill, NC: Algonquin.
19. Louv, R. (2017). *Vitamin N: The essential guide to a nature-rich life.* London: Atlantic Books.
20. Montgomery, P. (2008). *Plant spirit healing: A guide to working with plant consciousness.* Rochester, VT: Bear & Co.
21. Ober, C., Sinatra, S. T., & Zucker, M. (2010). *Earthing: The most important health discovery ever?* Laguna Beach, CA: Basic Health Publications.
22. Perkins, J. M. (1999). *Psychonavigation: Techniques for travel beyond time.* Rochester, VT: Destiny Books.
23. Pollack, G. H. (2013). *The fourth phase of water: Beyond solid, liquid, and vapor.* Seattle: Ebner & Sons.
24. Pollan, M. (2006). *The omnivore's dilemma: A natural history of four meals.* New York: Penguin Press.
25. Price, W. A. (1948). *Nutrition and physical degeneration: A comparision of primitive and modern diets and their effects.* Los Angeles, CA: American Academy of Applied Nutrition.
26. Rampton, S., & Stauber, J. C. (2002). *Trust us, were experts!: How industry manipulates science and gambles with your future.* New York: Jeremy P. Tarcher/Putnam.
27. Robinson, J. (2014). *Eating on the wild side: The missing link to optimum health.* New York: Little, Brown and Company.
28. Shanahan, C., & Shanahan, L. (2018). *Deep nutrition: Why your genes need traditional food.* New York: Flatiron Books.
29. Sheldrake, R. (1994). *The rebirth of nature: The greening of science and God.* Rochester, VT: Park Street Press.
30. Sheldrake, R. (2012). *Science Set Free: Dispelling Dogma.* Random House.
31. Smith, R., & Lourie, B. (2009). *Slow Death by Rubber Duck: The Secret Danger of Everyday Things.* Canada: Knopf Random.
32. Stamets, P. (2002). *MycoMedicinals: An informational treatise on mushrooms.* Olympia: MycoMedia.
33. Teeguarden, R. (2000). *The ancient wisdom of the Chinese tonic herbs.* New York: Warner Books.
34. Teicholz, N. (2014). *The big fat surprise: Why butter, meat, and cheese belong in a healthy diet.* New York: Simon & Schuster.
35. Thomas, P., & Margulis, J. (2016). *The vaccine-friendly plan: Dr. Pauls safe and effective approach to immunity and health-from pregnancy through your childs teen years.* New York: Ballantine Books.
36. Welch, C. (2017). *Balance your hormones, balance your life.* S.l.: Motilal Banarsidass.

37. Wohlleben, P. (2018). *Hidden life of trees: What they feel, how they communicate - discoveries from a secret world*. S.l.: GREYSTONE BOOKS.
38. Wrangham, R. W. (2010). *Catching fire: How cooking made us human*. New York: Basic Books.
39. Yong, E. D. (2016). *I contain multitudes: The microbes within us and a grander view of life*. London: Vintage.

References

2 - My Health Journey

1. Morgan, G., Ward, R., & Barton, M. (2004). The contribution of cytotoxic chemotherapy to 5-year survival in adult malignancies. Clinical Oncology, 16(8), 549-560. https://www.ncbi.nlm.nih.gov/pubmed/15630849
2. Montagu, JD. Length of life in the ancient world: a controlled study. J R Soc Med. 1994 Jan; 87(1): 25–26. https://www.ncbi.nlm.nih.gov/pmc/articles/PMC1294277/
3. Hulsegge, G. et al. (2014). Todays adult generations are less healthy than their predecessors: generation shifts in metabolic risk factors: the Doetinchem Cohort Study. European Journal of Preventive Cardiology, 21(9), 1134-1144. http://journals.sagepub.com/doi/abs/10.1177/2047487313485512

3 - Principle Based Health

1. Sandeep J. Memory transference in organ transplant recipients. Journal of New Approaches to Medicine and Health. Volume 19, Issue 1, 24th April 2011. http://www.namahjournal.com/doc/Actual/Memory-transference-in-organ-transplant-recipients-vol-19-iss-1.html
2. Sender, R. (2016). Revised Estimates for the Number of Human and Bacteria Cells in the Body. PLOS Biology, 14(8). http://biorxiv.org/content/early/2016/01/06/036103
3. Zucca, M., & Savoia, D. (2010). The Antibiotic Resistance Crisis. Int J Biomed Sci., 2010 Jun; 6(2): 77–86. Retrieved from https://www.ncbi.nlm.nih.gov/pmc/articles/PMC3614743/
4. Gebauer, S. K., Chardigny, J., Jakobsen, M. U., Lamarche, B., Lock, A. L., Proctor, S. D., & Baer, D. J. (2011). Effects of Ruminant trans Fatty Acids on Cardiovascular Disease and Cancer: A Comprehensive Review of Epidemiological, Clinical, and Mechanistic Studies. Advances in Nutrition: An International Review Journal, 2(4), 332-354. doi:10.3945/an.111.000521 http://advances.nutrition.org/content/2/4/332.abstract
5. Auddy B, Hazra J, Mitra A, Abedon B, Ghosal S. A standardized Withania somnifera extract significantly reduces stress-related parameters in chronically stressed humans: A double-blind, randomized, placebo-controlled study. J Am Nutraceutical Assoc. 2008;11:50–6. https://www.researchgate.net/publication/242151370_A_Standardized_Withania_Somnifera_Extract_Significantly_Reduces_Stress-Related_Parameters_in_Chronically_Stressed_Humans_A_Double-Blind_Randomized_Placebo-Controlled_Study

4 - The Fall of Nature, The Rise of Scientism

1. Morris, Z. S., Wooding, S., & Grant, J. (2011). The answer is 17 years, what is the question: understanding time lags in translational research. Journal of the Royal Society of Medicine, 104(12), 510-520. https://www.ncbi.nlm.nih.gov/pmc/articles/PMC3241518/
2. Koonin, E. V. (2012). Does the central dogma still stand? Biology Direct, 7(1), 27. doi:10.1186/1745-6150-7-27 https://www.ncbi.nlm.nih.gov/pmc/articles/PMC3472225/
3. Garber, J. E., & Offit, K. (2005). Hereditary Cancer Predisposition Syndromes. Journal of Clinical Oncology, 23(2), 276-292. doi:10.1200/jco.2005.10.042 https://www.ncbi.nlm.nih.gov/pubmed/15637391
4. Gross CG. Neurogenesis in the adult brain: death of a dogma. Nat Rev Neurosci. 2000 Oct;1(1):67-73. https://www.ncbi.nlm.nih.gov/pubmed/11252770
5. Absinta, M., Ha, S., & Nair, G. (2017). Human and nonhuman primate meninges harbor lymphatic vessels that can be visualized noninvasively by MRI. ELife, 6. https://elifesciences.org/articles/29738
6. Flexner, Abraham (1910), Medical Education in the United States and Canada: A Report to the Carnegie Foundation for the Advancement of Teaching (PDF), Bulletin No. 4., New York City: The Carnegie Foundation for the Advancement of Teaching http://archive.carnegiefoundation.org/pdfs/elibrary/Carnegie_Flexner_Report.pdf
7. Duffy, T. The Flexner Report — 100 Years Later. Yale J Biol Med. 2011 Sep; 84(3): 269–276. https://www.ncbi.nlm.nih.gov/pmc/articles/PMC3178858/

8. Souza, R. (2015). Intake of saturated and trans unsaturated fatty acids and risk of all cause mortality, cardiovascular disease, and type 2 diabetes: systematic review and meta-analysis of observational studies. Bmj. doi:10.1136/bmj.h3978 http://www.bmj.com/content/351/bmj.h3978

9. Siri-Tarino, P. W. (2010). Meta-analysis of prospective cohort studies evaluating the association of saturated fat with cardiovascular disease. American Journal of Clinical Nutrition, 91(3), 535-546. doi:10.3945/ajcn.2009.27725
http://ajcn.nutrition.org/content/early/2010/01/13/ajcn.2009.27725.abstract

10. Smith, R. (1997). Peer review: reform or revolution? Bmj, 315(7111), 759-760.
https://www.ncbi.nlm.nih.gov/pmc/articles/PMC2127543/pdf/9345164.pdf

11. Wilk v. American Medical Association (U.S. District Court for the Northern District of Illinois - 671 F. Supp. 1465 - September 25, 1987). http://law.justia.com/cases/federal/district-courts/FSupp/671/1465/2595129/

12. United States of America v. GlaxoSmithKline LLC. (United States District Court for the Eastern District of Pennsylvania April 10, 1998). https://www.justice.gov/opa/pr/glaxosmithkline-plead-guilty-and-pay-3-billion-resolve-fraud-allegations-and-failure-report

13. Wolf, B., and Buckwalter, J. Randomized Surgical Trials and "Sham" Surgery: Relevance to Modern Orthopaedics and Minimally Invasive Surgery. Iowa Orthopedic Journal v.26; 2006
https://www.ncbi.nlm.nih.gov/pmc/articles/PMC1888585/

14. Gøtzsche PC. Our prescription drugs kill us in large numbers. Pol Arch Med Wewn. 2014;124(11):628-34. Epub 2014 Oct 30. https://www.ncbi.nlm.nih.gov/pubmed/25355584

15. Honors, M., Davenport, B. M., & Kinzig, K. P. (2009). Effects of consuming a high carbohydrate diet after eight weeks of exposure to a ketogenic diet. Nutrition & Metabolism, 6(1), 46.
https://nutritionandmetabolism.biomedcentral.com/articles/10.1186/1743-7075-6-46

16. Kundi, M. (2006). Causality and the Interpretation of Epidemiologic Evidence. Environmental Health Perspectives, 114(7), 969-974. https://www.ncbi.nlm.nih.gov/pmc/articles/PMC1513293/

17. Ioannidis, J.P. Why most published research findings are false. PLoS Med. 2005 Aug;2(8):e124.
https://www.ncbi.nlm.nih.gov/pubmed/16060722

18. Briffa, J. Aspartame and its effects on health. BMJ. 2005 Feb 5; 330(7486): 309–310.
https://www.ncbi.nlm.nih.gov/pmc/articles/PMC548217/

19. Lai, H. Industry Funding Bias and Conflict of Interest in Research on the Biological Effects of Exposure to Electromagnetic Radiation and Other Biomedical Research; The Funding Effect; Conflicts of Interest.
http://www.mainecoalitiontostopsmartmeters.org/wp-content/uploads/2013/04/EV18-Funding-Bias-Effects-4-8-13.-PUC-465.pdf

20. Krimsky, S., Rothenberg, L. S., Stott, P., & Kyle, G. (1996). Financial interests of authors in scientific journals: A pilot study of 14 publications. Science and Engineering Ethics, 2(4), 395-410.
https://link.springer.com/article/10.1007/BF02583927

21. Aviv, R. (2014, February 10). A Valuable Reputation. The New Yorker.
http://www.newyorker.com/magazine/2014/02/10/a-valuable-reputation

6 – Air

1. Hoek, G. et al. (2013). Long-term air pollution exposure and cardio- respiratory mortality: a review. Environmental Health, 12(1). https://www.ncbi.nlm.nih.gov/pmc/articles/PMC3679821/

2. Xu, X., Ha, S. U., & Basnet, R. (2016). A Review of Epidemiological Research on Adverse Neurological Effects of Exposure to Ambient Air Pollution. Frontiers in Public Health, 4.
https://www.ncbi.nlm.nih.gov/pmc/articles/PMC4974252/

3. Sunyer, J. et al. (2015). Association between Traffic-Related Air Pollution in Schools and Cognitive Development in Primary School Children: A Prospective Cohort Study. PLOS Medicine, 12(3).
https://www.ncbi.nlm.nih.gov/pmc/articles/PMC4348510/

4. Xu X, Sharma RK, et al. PM10 air pollution exposure during pregnancy and term low birth weight in Allegheny County, PA, 1994-2000. Int Arch Occup Environ Health (2010)
https://www.ncbi.nlm.nih.gov/pubmed/20496078

5. Vecoli, C., Pulignani, S., & Andreassi, M. (2016). Genetic and Epigenetic Mechanisms Linking Air Pollution and Congenital Heart Disease. Journal of Cardiovascular Development and Disease, 3(4), 32.
http://www.mdpi.com/2308-3425/3/4/32/pdf

6. Batterman, S., et al. (2014). Personal Exposure to Mixtures of Volatile Organic Compounds: Modeling and Further Analysis of the RIOPA Data. Res Rep Health Eff Inst., 181, 3–63. https://www.ncbi.nlm.nih.gov/pmc/articles/PMC4577247/

7. Lu, C., Lin, J., & Chen, Y. (2015). Building-Related Symptoms among Office Employees Associated with Indoor Carbon Dioxide and Total Volatile Organic Compounds. International Journal of Environmental Research and Public Health, 12(6), 5833-5845. https://www.ncbi.nlm.nih.gov/pmc/articles/PMC4483674/

8. Rudel, R. A., Brody, J. G., Spengler, J. D., Vallarino, J., Geno, P. W., Sun, G., & Yau, A. (2001). Identification of Selected Hormonally Active Agents and Animal Mammary Carcinogens in Commercial and Residential Air and Dust Samples. Journal of the Air & Waste Management Association, 51(4), 499-513. https://www.ncbi.nlm.nih.gov/pubmed/11321907

9. Bennett, J., & Inamdar, A. (2015). Are Some Fungal Volatile Organic Compounds (VOCs) Mycotoxins? Toxins, 7(9), 3785-3804. https://www.ncbi.nlm.nih.gov/pmc/articles/PMC4591661/

10. Khan, A. H., & Karuppayil, S. M. (2012). Fungal pollution of indoor environments and its management. Saudi Journal of Biological Sciences, 19(4), 405-426. https://www.ncbi.nlm.nih.gov/pmc/articles/PMC3730554/

11. Onen S.H., et al. (1994) Prevention and treatment of sleep disorders through regulation of sleeping habits. Presse Med. 1994 Mar 12;23(10):485-9. https://www.ncbi.nlm.nih.gov/pubmed/8022726

12. Tsunetsugu, Y., Park, B., & Miyazaki, Y. (2009). Trends in research related to "Shinrin-yoku" (taking in the forest atmosphere or forest bathing) in Japan. Environmental Health and Preventive Medicine Environ Health Prev Med, 27-37. http://www.ncbi.nlm.nih.gov/pubmed/19585091

13. Cho, K. S., Lim, Y. et al. (2017). Terpenes from Forests and Human Health. Toxicological Research, 33(2), 97-106. https://www.ncbi.nlm.nih.gov/pubmed/28443180

14. BC Wolverton, WL Douglas, K Bounds (July 1989). A study of interior landscape plants for indoor air pollution abatement (Report). NASA. NASA-TM-108061. http://ntrs.nasa.gov/archive/nasa/casi.ntrs.nasa.gov/19930073077.pdf

15. Christoph Richter, "Phytonzidforschung—ein Beitrag zur Ressourcenfrage" ("Phytoncide research—a contribution to resource questions"), Hercynia N.F. 24(1) 1987

16. Claudio, L. (2011). Planting Healthier Indoor Air. Environmental Health Perspectives, 119(10). https://www.ncbi.nlm.nih.gov/pmc/articles/PMC3230460/

17. Meattle, K. (n.d.). How to grow fresh air. Retrieved May 16, 2017, from https://www.ted.com/talks/kamal_meattle_on_how_to_grow_your_own_fresh_air/

18. Central Pollution Control Board, Ministry of Environment & Forests. (2008) Epidemiological Study on Effect of Air Pollution on Human Health (Adults) in Delhi. Environment Health Series http://cpcb.nic.in/upload/NewItems/NewItem_161_Adult.pdf

19. Valentino, F. L., Leuenberger, M., Uglietti, C., & Sturm, P. (2008). Measurements and trend analysis of O2, CO2 and δ13C of CO2 from the high altitude research station Junfgraujoch, Switzerland — A comparison with the observations from the remote site Puy de Dôme, France. Science of The Total Environment, 391(2-3), 203-210. https://www.ncbi.nlm.nih.gov/pubmed/18023848

20. Kox, M. (2014). Voluntary activation of the sympathetic nervous system and attenuation of the innate immune response in humans. Proceedings of the National Academy of Sciences, 111(20), 7379-7384. https://www.ncbi.nlm.nih.gov/pmc/articles/PMC4034215/

21. Sampanthavivat M. et al. (2012) Hyperbaric oxygen in the treatment of childhood autism: a randomised controlled trial. Diving Hyperb Med. 2012 Sep;42(3):128-33. https://www.ncbi.nlm.nih.gov/pubmed/22987458

22. Mcdonagh, M. S. (n.d.). Hyperbaric Oxygen Therapy for Brain Injury, Cerebral Palsy, and Stroke: Evidence Report/Technology Assessment, Number 85. PsycEXTRA Dataset. https://www.ncbi.nlm.nih.gov/books/NBK11904/

23. Daruwalla J & Christophi C. (2006) Hyperbaric oxygen therapy for malignancy: a review. World J Surg. 2006 Dec;30(12):2112-31. https://www.ncbi.nlm.nih.gov/pubmed/17102915

24. Heiden, M. G., Cantley, L. C., & Thompson, C. B. (2009). Understanding the Warburg Effect: The Metabolic Requirements of Cell Proliferation. Science, 324(5930), 1029-1033. https://www.ncbi.nlm.nih.gov/pubmed/19460998

25. Wyon, D. P. (2004). The effects of indoor air quality on performance and productivity. Indoor Air, 14(S7), 92-101. https://www.ncbi.nlm.nih.gov/pubmed/15330777

7 - Water

1. Thomas, M. P. (2010). Calcium and Magnesium in Drinking-water: Public Health Significance. International Journal of Environmental Studies, 67(4), 612-613. http://apps.who.int/iris/bitstream/10665/43836/1/9789241563550_eng.pdf

2. Benton, D., Jenkins, K. T., Watkins, H. T., & Young, H. A. (2016). Minor degree of hypohydration adversely influences cognition: a mediator analysis. American Journal of Clinical Nutrition, 104(3), 603-612. https://www.ncbi.nlm.nih.gov/pubmed/27510536

3. Murray B. Hydration and physical performance. J Am Coll Nutr. 2007 Oct; 26(5 Suppl):542S-548S. https://www.ncbi.nlm.nih.gov/pubmed/17921463

4. Manz, F., & Wentz, A. (2005). The Importance of Good Hydration for the Prevention of Chronic Diseases. Nutrition Reviews, 63. https://www.ncbi.nlm.nih.gov/pubmed/16028566/

5. Barry Popkin, Kristen D'Anci, and Irwin Rosenberg. Water, Hydration and Health. Nutr Rev. 2010 Aug; 68(8): 439–458. https://www.ncbi.nlm.nih.gov/pmc/articles/PMC2908954/

6. Oliver, B. G., & Cosgrove, E. G. (1975). Metal Concentrations in the Sewage, Effluents, and Sludges of Some Southern Ontario Wastewater Treatment Plants. Environmental Letters, 9(1), 75-90. https://www.ncbi.nlm.nih.gov/pubmed/1183416

7. Bove, F., Shim, Y., & Zeitz, P. (2002). Drinking Water Contaminants and Adverse Pregnancy Outcomes: A Review. Environmental Health Perspectives, 110(S1), 61-74. https://www.ncbi.nlm.nih.gov/pubmed/11834464

8. Committee on Fluoride in Drinking Water, National Research Council. Fluoride in Drinking Water. (2006). http://www.actionpa.org/fluoride/nrc/NRC-2006.pdf

9. Grandjean, P., & Landrigan, P. J. (2014). Neurobehavioural effects of developmental toxicity. The Lancet Neurology, 13(3), 330-338. http://www.thelancet.com/journals/laneur/article/PIIS1474-4422(13)70278-3/abstract

10. Zarse, K. et al. (2011): Low-dose lithium uptake promotes longevity in humans and metazoans.. In: Eur J Nutr 50(5):387-389; https://www.ncbi.nlm.nih.gov/pubmed/21301855

11. Watkins, K., & Josling, P. (spring 2010). A pilot study to determine the impact of transdermal magnesium treatment on serum levels and whole body CaMg ratios . The Nutrition Practitioner. Retrieved from http://www.cnelm.com/NutritionPractitioner/Issues/Issue_11_1/Articles/7%20Transdermal%20Mg%20revised2.pdf

12. Tomasino, D. New Technology Provides Scientific Evidence of Water's Capacity to Store

13. and Amplify Weak Electromagnetic and Subtle Energy Fields. HeartMath Research Center. https://www.heartmath.org/research/research-library/energetics/new-technology-provides-scientific-evidence-of-waters-capacity/

14. Chun Z. Yang, et al. Most Plastic Products Release Estrogenic Chemicals: A Potential Health Problem That Can Be Solved. Environ Health Perspect. 2011 Jul 1; 119(7): 989–996. https://www.ncbi.nlm.nih.gov/pmc/articles/PMC3222987/

8 - Movement

1. Jorgens, D.M. et al. Deep nuclear invaginations are linked to cytoskeletal filaments - integrated bioimaging of epithelial cells in 3D culture. J Cell Sci. 2017 Jan 1;130(1):177-189. https://www.ncbi.nlm.nih.gov/pubmed/27505896

2. Okeefe, J. H., Vogel, R., Lavie, C. J., & Cordain, L. (2010). Achieving Hunter-gatherer Fitness in the 21st Century: Back to the Future. The American Journal of Medicine, 123(12), 1082-1086. https://www.ncbi.nlm.nih.gov/pubmed/20843503

3. Neville Owen, et al. Too Much Sitting: The Population-Health Science of Sedentary Behavior. Exerc Sport Sci Rev. 2010 Jul; 38(3): 105–113. https://www.ncbi.nlm.nih.gov/pmc/articles/PMC3404815/

4. Hewes, G. W. (1955). World Distribution of Certain Postural Habits. American Anthropologist, 57(2), 231-244. http://onlinelibrary.wiley.com/doi/10.1525/aa.1955.57.2.02a00040/pdf

5. Brito, L. B. et al. (2012). Ability to sit and rise from the floor as a predictor of all-cause mortality. European Journal of Preventive Cardiology, 21(7), 892-898. https://www.ncbi.nlm.nih.gov/pubmed/23242910

6. Lee, S. J., & Hidler, J. (2008). Biomechanics of overground vs. treadmill walking in healthy individuals. Journal of Applied Physiology, 104(3), 747-755. https://www.ncbi.nlm.nih.gov/pubmed/18048582

7. Yabe, Y., & Taga, G. (2010). Influence of experience of treadmill exercise on visual perception while on a treadmill. Japanese Psychological Research, 52(2), 67-77. https://www.researchgate.net/publication/229725029_Influence_of_experience_of_treadmill_exercise_on_visual_perception_while_on_a_treadmill

8. Ramos, J. S., Dalleck, L. C., Tjonna, A. E., Beetham, K. S., & Coombes, J. S. (2015). The Impact of High-Intensity Interval Training Versus Moderate-Intensity Continuous Training on Vascular Function: a Systematic Review and Meta-Analysis. Sports Medicine, 45(5), 679-692 https://www.ncbi.nlm.nih.gov/pubmed/25771785

9. Catrine Tudor-Locke, et al. How many steps/day are enough? for adults. International Journal of Behavioral Nutrition and Physical Activity 2011. 8:79 https://ijbnpa.biomedcentral.com/articles/10.1186/1479-5868-8-79

10. Beddhu, S., et al. (2015). Light-Intensity Physical Activities and Mortality in the United States General Population and CKD Subpopulation. Clinical Journal of the American Society of Nephrology, 10(7), 1145-1153. https://www.ncbi.nlm.nih.gov/pubmed/25931456

11. Erickson K.I. et al. Exercise training increases size of hippocampus and improves memory. Proc Natl Acad Sci U S A. 2011 Feb 15;108(7):3017-22. https://www.ncbi.nlm.nih.gov/pubmed/21282661

12. Olszewski WL, Engeset A, Sokolowski J. Lymph flow and protein in the normal male leg during lying, getting up, and walking. Lymphology. 1977 Sep;10(3):178-83. https://www.ncbi.nlm.nih.gov/pubmed/563502

13. Humphrey, J. D. (2007). Vascular Adaptation and Mechanical Homeostasis at Tissue, Cellular, and Sub-cellular Levels. Cell Biochemistry and Biophysics, 50(2), 53-78. https://www.ncbi.nlm.nih.gov/pubmed/18209957

14. Rossi, W. A., D.P.M. (1999, March). Why Shoes Make "Normal" Gait Impossible. Podiatry Management, 50-61. https://nwfootankle.com/files/rossiWhyShoesMakeNormalGaitImpossible.pdf

15. Sakakibara, R. et al. Influence of Body Position on Defecation in Humans. Lower Urinary Tract Symptoms. Volume 2, Issue 1, April 2010, Pages 16–21. http://onlinelibrary.wiley.com/doi/10.1111/j.1757-5672.2009.00057.x/abstract

16. Mooventhan, A., & Nivethitha, L. (2014). Scientific evidence-based effects of hydrotherapy on various systems of the body. North American Journal of Medical Sciences, 6(5), 199. https://www.ncbi.nlm.nih.gov/pmc/articles/PMC4049052/

17. Li, J. et al. (2015). Health Effects from Swimming Training in Chlorinated Pools and the Corresponding Metabolic Stress Pathways. Plos One, 10(3). https://www.ncbi.nlm.nih.gov/pmc/articles/PMC4351252/

18. Venkataraman VV, Kraft TS, Dominy NJ. Tree climbing and human evolution. Proc Natl Acad Sci U S A. 2013 Jan 22;110(4):1237-42. https://www.ncbi.nlm.nih.gov/pubmed/23277565

19. Tetley, M. (2000). Instinctive sleeping and resting postures: an anthropological and zoological approach to treatment of low back and joint pain. Bmj, 321(7276), 1616-1618. https://www.ncbi.nlm.nih.gov/pmc/articles/PMC1119282/

20. Rogerson, M., & Barton, J. (2015). Effects of the Visual Exercise Environments on Cognitive Directed Attention, Energy Expenditure and Perceived Exertion. International Journal of Environmental Research and Public Health, 12(7), 7321-7336. https://www.ncbi.nlm.nih.gov/pmc/articles/PMC4515658/

21. Duncan, M. (2014). The Effect of Green Exercise on Blood Pressure, Heart Rate and Mood State in Primary School Children. International Journal of Environmental Research and Public Health, 11(4), 3678-3688. https://www.ncbi.nlm.nih.gov/pmc/articles/PMC4025002/

22. Joly, L. (2011). Exercise, nature and socially interactive based initiatives improve mood and self-esteem in the clinical population. Primary Health Care, 21(7), 15-15. https://www.ncbi.nlm.nih.gov/pubmed/22616429

9 - Sun

1. Legates, T. A., Fernandez, D. C., & Hattar, S. (2014). Light as a central modulator of circadian rhythms, sleep and affect. Nature Reviews Neuroscience, 15(7), 443-454. https://www.ncbi.nlm.nih.gov/pubmed/24917305

2. Kecklund, G., & Axelsson, J. (2016). Health consequences of shift work and insufficient sleep. *British Medical Journal.*

3. Xu, C., Zhang, J., Mihai, D. M., & Washington, I. (2013). Light-harvesting chlorophyll pigments enable mammalian mitochondria to capture photonic energy and produce ATP. Journal of Cell Science, 127(2), 388-399. https://www.ncbi.nlm.nih.gov/pubmed/24198392

4. Mead, M. N. (2008). Benefits of Sunlight: A Bright Spot for Human Health. Environmental Health Perspectives, 116(4). https://www.ncbi.nlm.nih.gov/pmc/articles/PMC2290997/

5. Kolata, G. (2004, July 20). I BEG TO DIFFER; A Dermatologist Who's Not Afraid to Sit on the Beach. New York Times. Retrieved from http://www.nytimes.com/2004/07/20/health/i-beg-to-differ-a-dermatologist-who-s-not-afraid-to-sit-on-the-beach.html

6. Fang S, Sui D, Wang Y, et al. Association of vitamin d levels with outcome in patients with melanoma after adjustment for C-reactive protein J Clin Oncol.

7. Lindqvist, P. G., Epstein, E., Nielsen, K., Landin-Olsson, M., Ingvar, C., & Olsson, H. (2016). Avoidance of sun exposure as a risk factor for major causes of death: a competing risk analysis of the Melanoma in Southern Sweden cohort. Journal of Internal Medicine, 280(4), 375-387. https://www.ncbi.nlm.nih.gov/pubmed/26992108

8. Krause, M. et al. (2012). Sunscreens: are they beneficial for health? An overview of endocrine disrupting properties of UV-filters. International Journal of Andrology, 35(3), 424-436. https://www.ncbi.nlm.nih.gov/pubmed/22612478

9. Sies, H., & Stahl, W. (2004). Nutritional Protection Against Skin Damage From Sunlight. Annual Review of Nutrition, 24(1), 173-200. https://www.ncbi.nlm.nih.gov/pubmed/15189118

10. Patra, V., Byrne, S. N., & Wolf, P. (2016). The Skin Microbiome: Is It Affected by UV-induced Immune Suppression? Frontiers in Microbiology, 7. https://www.ncbi.nlm.nih.gov/pmc/articles/PMC4979252/

11. Sunyecz, J. (2008). The use of calcium and vitamin D in the management of osteoporosis. Therapeutics and Clinical Risk Management, Volume 4, 827-836. https://www.ncbi.nlm.nih.gov/pmc/articles/PMC2621390/

12. Thacher, T. D., & Clarke, B. L. (n.d.). Vitamin D Insufficiency. SciVee. https://www.ncbi.nlm.nih.gov/pmc/articles/PMC3012634/

13. Bjelakovic, G., et al. (2011). Vitamin D supplementation for prevention of mortality in adults. Cochrane Database of Systematic Reviews. https://www.ncbi.nlm.nih.gov/pubmed/21735411

14. Ramagopalan, S. V., Heger, A., et al. (2010). A ChIP-seq defined genome-wide map of vitamin D receptor binding: Associations with disease and evolution. Genome Research, 20(10), 1352-1360. https://www.ncbi.nlm.nih.gov/pubmed/20736230

15. Seneff, S., Davidson, R. M., Lauritzen, A., Samsel, A., & Wainwright, G. (2015). A novel hypothesis for atherosclerosis as a cholesterol sulfate deficiency syndrome. Theoretical Biology and Medical Modelling, 12(1). https://www.ncbi.nlm.nih.gov/pmc/articles/PMC4456713/

16. Fell, G., Robinson, K., Mao, J., Woolf, C., & Fisher, D. (2014). Skin β-Endorphin Mediates Addiction to UV Light. Cell, 157(7), 1527-1534. http://www.cell.com/cell/abstract/S0092-8674(14)00611-4

17. Rouzaud, F., Kadekaro, A. L., Abdel-Malek, Z. A., & Hearing, V. J. (2005). MC1R and the response of melanocytes to ultraviolet radiation. Mutation Research/Fundamental and Molecular Mechanisms of Mutagenesis, 571(1-2), 133-152. https://www.ncbi.nlm.nih.gov/pubmed/15748644

18. Agar, N., & Young, A. R. (2005). Melanogenesis: a photoprotective response to DNA damage? Mutation Research/Fundamental and Molecular Mechanisms of Mutagenesis, 571(1-2), 121-132. Retrieved from https://www.ncbi.nlm.nih.gov/pubmed/15748643

19. Pavlovic, S., Liezmann, C., et al. (2010). Substance P Is a Key Mediator of Stress-Induced Protection from Allergic Sensitization via Modified Antigen Presentation. The Journal of Immunology, 186(2), 848-855. http://www.jimmunol.org/content/186/2/848.full

20. Legat, F. J., Griesbacher, T., et al. (2002). Repeated subinflammatory ultraviolet B irradiation increases substance P and calcitonin gene-related peptide content and augments mustard oil-induced neurogenic inflammation in the skin of rats. Neuroscience Letters, 329(3), 309-313. http://www.sciencedirect.com/science/article/pii/S0304394002004287

21. Liu, D., Fernandez, B. O., et al. (2014). UVA Irradiation of Human Skin Vasodilates Arterial Vasculature and Lowers Blood Pressure Independently of Nitric Oxide Synthase. Journal of Investigative Dermatology, 134(7), 1839-1846. https://www.ncbi.nlm.nih.gov/pubmed/24445737

22. Rana, S., Byrne, S. N., Macdonald, L. J., Chan, C. Y., & Halliday, G. M. (2008). Ultraviolet B Suppresses Immunity by Inhibiting Effector and Memory T Cells. The American Journal of Pathology, 172(4), 993-1004. https://www.ncbi.nlm.nih.gov/pubmed/18292235

23. Lehrer, R. I., & Ganz, T. (2002). Cathelicidins: a family of endogenous antimicrobial peptides. Current Opinion in Hematology, 9(1), 18-22. https://www.ncbi.nlm.nih.gov/pmc/articles/PMC3487008/

24. Grant, W. B. (2014). Solar Ultraviolet Irradiance and Cancer Incidence and Mortality. Sunlight, Vitamin D and Skin Cancer, 52-62. https://www.ncbi.nlm.nih.gov/labs/articles/25207360/

25. Redberg, R. F. (2015). Health Benefits of Sauna Bathing. JAMA Internal Medicine, 175(4), 548. http://jamanetwork.com/journals/jamainternalmedicine/article-abstract/2130717

26. Wurtman, R. J. (1975). The Effects of Light on the Human Body. Scientific American, 233(1), 68-77. http://web.mit.edu/dick/www/pdf/286.pdf

27. Hagenau, T., Vest, R., et al. (2008). Global vitamin D levels in relation to age, gender, skin pigmentation and latitude: an ecologic meta-regression analysis. Osteoporosis International, 20(1), 133-140. https://www.ncbi.nlm.nih.gov/pubmed/18458986.

28. Helmer AC, Jensen CH: Vitamin D precursors removed from the skin by washing. Studies Inst Divi Thomae 1937, 1:207-216.

29. Luxwolda, M. F., Kuipers, R. S., Kema, I. P., Dijck-Brouwer, D. A., & Muskiet, F. A. (2012). Traditionally living populations in East Africa have a mean serum 25-hydroxyvitamin D concentration of 115 nmol/l. British Journal of Nutrition, 108(09), 1557-1561. https://www.ncbi.nlm.nih.gov/pubmed/22264449

30. Hollis, B. W., Wagner, C. L., Drezner, M. K., & Binkley, N. C. (2007). Circulating vitamin D3 and 25-hydroxyvitamin D in humans: An important tool to define adequate nutritional vitamin D status. The Journal of Steroid Biochemistry and Molecular Biology, 103(3-5), 631-634. https://www.ncbi.nlm.nih.gov/pubmed/17218096/.

31. Myerson, A., & Neustadt, R. (1939). Influence Of Ultraviolet Irradiation Upon Excretion Of Sex Hormones In The Male1 1. Endocrinology, 25(1), 7-12.

10 - Light and the Moon

1. Broussard, J., & Brady, M. J. (2010). The impact of sleep disturbances on adipocyte function and lipid metabolism. Best Practice & Research Clinical Endocrinology & Metabolism, 24(5), 763-773. https://www.ncbi.nlm.nih.gov/pmc/articles/PMC3031100/

2. Mead, M. N. (2008). Benefits of Sunlight: A Bright Spot for Human Health. Environmental Health Perspectives, 116(4). https://www.ncbi.nlm.nih.gov/pmc/articles/PMC2290997/

3. Ferraro, J., & Steger, R. (1990). Diurnal variations in brain serotonin are driven by the photic cycle and are not circadian in nature. Brain Research, 512(1), 121-124. https://www.ncbi.nlm.nih.gov/pubmed/2337799/

4. Lambert, G. (2002). Effect of sunlight and season on serotonin turnover in the brain. The Lancet, 360(9348), 1840-1842. http://www.sciencedirect.com/science/article/pii/S0140673602117375

5. Blask, D. E. (2009). Melatonin, sleep disturbance and cancer risk. Sleep Medicine Reviews, 13(4), 257-264. http://www.sciencedirect.com/science/article/pii/S1087079208000786

6. Wurtman, R. J. (1975). The Effects of Light on the Human Body. Scientific American, 233(1), 68-77. http://web.mit.edu/dick/www/pdf/286.pdf

7. Tomany SC, Cruickshanks KJ, Klein R, et al. The Beaver Dam Eye Study: sunlight and the 10-year incidence of age-related maculopathy. Arch Ophthalmol. 2004;122:750–757 https://www.ncbi.nlm.nih.gov/pubmed/15136324

8. Kloog, I., Haim, A., Stevens, R. G., Barchana, M., & Portnov, B. A. (2008). Light at Night Co-distributes with Incident Breast but not Lung Cancer in the Female Population of Israel. Chronobiology International, 25(1), 65-81. https://www.ncbi.nlm.nih.gov/pubmed/18293150

9. Bella, G. D., Mascia, F., Gualano, L., & Bella, L. D. (2013). Melatonin Anticancer Effects: Review. International Journal of Molecular Sciences, 14(2), 2410-2430. https://www.ncbi.nlm.nih.gov/pmc/articles/PMC3587994/

10. Albreiki, M. S., Middleton, B., & Hampton, S. M. (2017). A single night light exposure acutely alters hormonal and metabolic responses in healthy participants. Endocrine Connections, 6(2), 100-110. https://www.ncbi.nlm.nih.gov/m/pubmed/28270559/

11. Algvere PV, Marshall J, Seregard S. Age-related maculopathy and the impact of blue light hazard. Acta Ophthalmology. 2006 Feb;84(1):4-15 https://www.ncbi.nlm.nih.gov/pubmed/16445433

12. Kuse, Y. et al. (2014). Damage of photoreceptor-derived cells in culture induced by light emitting diode-derived blue light. Scientific Reports, 4(1). https://www.ncbi.nlm.nih.gov/pmc/articles/PMC4048889/

13. G. Tosini, I. Ferguson, and K. Tsubota. Effects of blue light on the circadian system and eye physiology. Molecular Vision 2016; 22: 61–72. https://www.ncbi.nlm.nih.gov/pmc/articles/PMC4734149/

14. Velex-Montoya, R. et al. Current knowledge and trends in age-related macular degeneration: genetics, epidemiology, and prevention. Retina. 2014 Mar;34(3):423-41. https://www.ncbi.nlm.nih.gov/pubmed/24285245

15. Godley, B. F., et al. (2005). Blue Light Induces Mitochondrial DNA Damage and Free Radical Production in Epithelial Cells. Journal of Biological Chemistry, 280(22), 21061-21066. https://www.ncbi.nlm.nih.gov/pubmed/15797866

16. Cissé, Y. M., Russart, K. L., & Nelson, R. J. (2017). Parental Exposure to Dim Light at Night Prior to Mating Alters Offspring Adaptive Immunity. Scientific Reports, 7, 45497. https://www.nature.com/articles/srep45497

17. Cheung, I. N., Zee, P. C., Shalman, D., Malkani, R. G., Kang, J., & Reid, K. J. (2016). Morning and Evening Blue-Enriched Light Exposure Alters Metabolic Function in Normal Weight Adults. Plos One, 11(5). http://journals.plos.org/plosone/article?id=10.1371/journal.pone.0155601

18. Zimecki M. The lunar cycle: effects on human and animal behavior and physiology. Postepy Hig Med Dosw (Online). 2006;60:1-7. https://www.ncbi.nlm.nih.gov/pubmed/16407788

19. Alina Iosif & Bruce Ballon. Bad Moon Rising: the persistent belief in lunar connections to madness. CMAJ. 2005 Dec 6; 173(12): 1498–1500. https://www.ncbi.nlm.nih.gov/pmc/articles/PMC1316181/

20. Melrose, S. (2015). Seasonal Affective Disorder: An Overview of Assessment and Treatment Approaches. Depression Research and Treatment, 2015, 1-6. https://www.ncbi.nlm.nih.gov/pmc/articles/PMC4673349/

21. Charmane I. Eastman, et al. Bright Light Treatment of Winter Depression A Placebo-Controlled Trial. Arch Gen Psychiatry. 1998;55(10):883-889. http://jamanetwork.com/journals/jamapsychiatry/fullarticle/204290

11 - Earthing

1. Barnett, L. (2005). Keep in touch: The importance of touch in infant development. Infant Observation, 8(2), 115-123. http://www.tandfonline.com/doi/abs/10.1080/13698030500171530

2. G. Chevalier, K. Mori & J. Oschman. The effect of earthing (grounding) on human physiology. Europeon Biology and Bioelctromagnetics. Jan 31, 2006; 600-621 http://162.214.7.219/~earthio0/wp-content/uploads/2016/07/Effects-of-Earthing-on-Human-Physiology-Part-1.pdf

3. Chevalier, G., Sinatra, S. T., Oschman, J. L., Sokal, K., & Sokal, P. (2012). Earthing: Health Implications of Reconnecting the Human Body to the Earths Surface Electrons. Journal of Environmental and Public Health, 2012, 1-8. https://www.hindawi.com/journals/jeph/2012/291541/

4. Oschman, J., Chevalier, G., & Brown, R. (2015). The effects of grounding (earthing) on inflammation, the immune response, wound healing, and prevention and treatment of chronic inflammatory and autoimmune diseases. Journal of Inflammation Research, 83. https://www.dovepress.com/articles.php?article_id=21001

5. Chevalier, G., Brown, R., & Hill, M. (2015). Grounding after moderate eccentric contractions reduces muscle damage. Open Access Journal of Sports Medicine, 305. https://www.dovepress.com/articles.php?article_id=23771

6. Ghaly, M., & Teplitz, D. (2004). The Biologic Effects of Grounding the Human Body During Sleep as Measured by Cortisol Levels and Subjective Reporting of Sleep, Pain, and Stress. The Journal of Alternative and Complementary Medicine, 10(5), 767-776. http://162.214.7.219/~earthio0/wp-content/uploads/2016/07/Cortisol-Study.pdf

7. Brown, R., & Chevalier, G. (2015). Grounding the Human Body during Yoga Exercise with a Grounded Yoga Mat Reduces Blood Viscosity. Open Journal of Preventive Medicine, 05(04), 159-168. http://www.scirp.org/Journal/PaperInformation.aspx?PaperID=55445#.VSa19_nF_7A

8. Chevalier, G., Sinatra, S. T., Oschman, J. L., & Delany, R. M. (2013). Earthing (Grounding) the Human Body Reduces Blood Viscosity—a Major Factor in Cardiovascular Disease. The Journal of Alternative and Complementary Medicine, 19(2), 102-110. http://online.liebertpub.com/doi/pdfplus/10.1089/acm.2011.0820

9. Sokal, K., & Sokal, P. (2011). Earthing the Human Body Influences Physiologic Processes. The Journal of Alternative and Complementary Medicine, 17(4), 301-308. http://162.214.7.219/~earthio0/wp-content/uploads/2016/07/Sokal-and-Sokal-2011-Physiologic-processes.pdf

10. Adams, J. A. (2014). Effect of mobile telephones on sperm quality: A systematic review and meta-analysis. Environment International, 70, 106-112. https://www.ncbi.nlm.nih.gov/pubmed/24927498

11. Chen, C., Ma, X., Zhong, M., & Yu, Z. (2010). Extremely low-frequency electromagnetic fields exposure and female breast cancer risk: a meta-analysis based on 24,338 cases and 60,628 controls. Breast Cancer Research and Treatment, 123(2), 569-576. https://www.ncbi.nlm.nih.gov/pubmed/24984538

12. Blank, M., & Goodman, R. M. (2012). Electromagnetic fields and health: DNA-based dosimetry. Electromagnetic Biology and Medicine, 31(4), 243-249. https://www.ncbi.nlm.nih.gov/pubmed/22676645

13. Environmental Health Trust. NIH National Toxicology Program Cell Phone Radiofrequency Radiation Study. https://ehtrust.org/cell-phone-radiofrequency-radiation-study/

14. Pall, M. L. (2013). Electromagnetic fields actviaactivation of voltage-gated calcium channels to produce beneficial or adverse effects. Journal of Cellular and Molecular Medicine, 17(8), 958-965. https://www.ncbi.nlm.nih.gov/pmc/articles/PMC3780531/

15. Brown, R. (2016). Effects of Grounding on Body Voltage and Current in the Presence of Electromagnetic Fields. The Journal of Alternative and Complementary Medicine. http://162.214.7.219/~earthio0/wp-content/uploads/2016/06/Effects-of-Grounding-on-Body-Voltage-and-Current-in-the-Presence-of-Electromagnetic-Fields-2016.pdf

16. G. Chevalier & S. Sinatra. Emotional Stress, Heart Rate Variability, Grounding, and Improved Autonomic Tone: Clinical Applications. Integrative Medicine Jun/Jul 2011. http://162.214.7.219/~earthio0/wp-content/uploads/2016/07/Emotional-stress-study.pdf

17. Chevalier, G. (2015). The Effect Of Grounding The Human Body On Mood1. Psychological Reports, 116(2), 534-543. http://journals.sagepub.com/doi/abs/10.2466/06.PR0.116k21w5

18. Sokal P. & Sokal, K. The neuromodulative role of earthing. Medical Hypotheses, November 2011, Pages 824-826. http://www.sciencedirect.com/science/article/pii/S0306987711003641

19. R. Gifford. The Consequences of Living in High-Rise Buildings. Architectural Science Review 50(1):2-17 March 2007. https://www.researchgate.net/publication/233490985

12 - Food

1. Abbott, S. K., Else, P. L., Atkins, T. A., & Hulbert, A. (2012). Fatty acid composition of membrane bilayers: Importance of diet polyunsaturated fat balance. Biochimica et Biophysica Acta (BBA) - Biomembranes, 1818(5), 1309-1317. http://www.sciencedirect.com/science/article/pii/S0005273612000156

2. Cameron-Smith, D., Albert, B. B., & Cutfield, W. S. (2015). Fishing for answers: is oxidation of fish oil supplements a problem? Journal of Nutritional Science, 4. https://www.ncbi.nlm.nih.gov/pmc/articles/PMC4681158/

3. Hollon, J., et al. (2015). Effect of Gliadin on Permeability of Intestinal Biopsy Explants from Celiac Disease Patients and Patients with Non-Celiac Gluten Sensitivity. Nutrients, 7(3), 1565-1576. https://www.ncbi.nlm.nih.gov/pmc/articles/PMC4377866/

4. Stockman, J. (2009). The Spread of Obesity in a Large Social Network over 32 Years. Yearbook of Pediatrics, 2009, 464-466. http://www.nejm.org/doi/full/10.1056/NEJMsa066082#t=article

5. Kulovitz, M. G., et al. (2014). Potential role of meal frequency as a strategy for weight loss and health in overweight or obese adults. Nutrition, 30(4), 386-392. https://www.ncbi.nlm.nih.gov/pubmed/24268866

6. Claus, S. P., Guillou, H., & Ellero-Simatos, S. (2016). The gut microbiota: a major player in the toxicity of environmental pollutants? Npj Biofilms and Microbiomes, 2, 16003. https://www.nature.com/articles/npjbiofilms20163

7. Randolf, L. F. Effects of an Atomic Bomb Explosion on Corn Seeds (US Navy, Naval Medical Research Section, Joint Task Force One). http://www.dtic.mil/dtic/tr/fulltext/u2/473888.pdf

8. Seneff, S., & Samsel, A. (2015). Glyphosate, pathways to modern diseases III: Manganese, neurological diseases, and associated pathologies. Surgical Neurology International, 6(1), 45. https://www.ncbi.nlm.nih.gov/pmc/articles/PMC4392553/

9. Herrmann K.M. & Weaver L.M. THE SHIKIMATE PATHWAY. Annu Rev Plant Physiol Plant Mol Biol. 1999 Jun;50:473-503. https://www.ncbi.nlm.nih.gov/pubmed/15012217

10. Kleter, G. A., Peijnenburg, A. A., & Aarts, H. J. (2005). Health Considerations Regarding Horizontal Transfer of Microbial Transgenes Present in Genetically Modified Crops. Journal of Biomedicine and Biotechnology, 2005(4), 326-352. https://www.ncbi.nlm.nih.gov/pmc/articles/PMC1364539/

11. Cassidy, E. (Mar 2015). Feeding the World Without GMOs. Environmental Working Group http://cdn3.ewg.org/sites/default/files/EWG%20Feeding%20the%20World%20Without%20GMOs%20 2015.pdf?_ga=1.177273068.899249347.1427809392

12. Heinemann, J. A. (Aug. 28, 2012). Evaluation of risks from creation of novel RNA molecules in genetically engineered wheat plants and recommendations for risk assessment (Tech.). Centre for Integrated Research in Biosafety. University of Canterbury. http://safefoodfoundation.org/wp-content/uploads/2012/09/Heinemann-Expert-Scientific-Opinion.pdf

13. Kaneko, J. J., & Ralston, N. V. (2007). Selenium and Mercury in Pelagic Fish in the Central North Pacific Near Hawaii. Biological Trace Element Research, 119(3), 242-254. https://www.ncbi.nlm.nih.gov/pubmed/17916947

14. Chattopadhyay, M. K. (2014). Use of antibiotics as feed additives: a burning question. Frontiers in Microbiology, 5. https://www.ncbi.nlm.nih.gov/pmc/articles/PMC4078264/

15. Lammers, B., Heinrichs, A., & Kensinger, R. (1999). The Effects of Accelerated Growth Rates and Estrogen Implants in Prepubertal Holstein Heifers on Growth, Feed Efficiency, and Blood Parameters. Journal of Dairy Science, 82(8), 1746-1752. http://www.journalofdairyscience.org/article/S0022-0302(99)75405-6/abstract

16. Karsten, H., Patterson, P., Stout, R., & Crews, G. (2010). Vitamins A, E and fatty acid composition of the eggs of caged hens and pastured hens. Renewable Agriculture and Food Systems, 25(01), 45-54. https://www.cambridge.org/core/journals/renewable-agriculture-and-food-systems/article/vitamins-a-e-and-fatty-acid-composition-of-the-eggs-of-caged-hens-and-pastured-hens/552BA04E5A9E3CD7E49E405B339ECA32

17. Kumar, V., Sinha, A. K., Makkar, H. P., & Becker, K. (2010). Dietary roles of phytate and phytase in human nutrition: A review. Food Chemistry, 120(4), 945-959. http://www.sciencedirect.com/science/article/pii/S0308814609013624

18. Anderson JT, Grande F, Keys A. Hydrogenated fats in the diet and lipids in the serum of man. J Nutr. 1961 Dec;75:388-94. https://www.ncbi.nlm.nih.gov/pubmed/13861251

19. Djoussé, L., & Gaziano, J. M. (2009). Dietary cholesterol and coronary artery disease: A systematic review. Current Atherosclerosis Reports, 11(6), 418-422. https://www.ncbi.nlm.nih.gov/pubmed/19852882

20. Siri-Tarino PW, Sun Q, Hu FB, & Krauss RM. Meta-analysis of prospective cohort studies evaluating the association of saturated fat with cardiovascular disease. Am J Clin Nutr. 2010 Oct;92(4):759-65. https://www.ncbi.nlm.nih.gov/pubmed/20685950

21. Yamagishi, K., et al. (2010). Dietary intake of saturated fatty acids and mortality from cardiovascular disease in Japanese: the Japan Collaborative Cohort Study for Evaluation of Cancer Risk (JACC) Study. American Journal of Clinical Nutrition, 92(4), 759-765. https://www.ncbi.nlm.nih.gov/pubmed/20685950

22. Okuyama, H., Kobayashi, J., and Watanabe, S. (1997) Dietary fatty acids ii The n-6/n-3 balance and chronic, elderly diseases. Excess linoleic acid and relative n-3 deficiency syndrome seen in Japan. Prog. Lipid Res. 353409457. https://www.ncbi.nlm.nih.gov/pubmed/9246358

23. Nichols, P., Glencross, B., Petrie, J., & Singh, S. (2014). Readily Available Sources of Long-Chain Omega-3 Oils: Is Farmed Australian Seafood a Better Source of the Good Oil than Wild-Caught Seafood? Nutrients, 6(3), 1063-1079. https://www.ncbi.nlm.nih.gov/pmc/articles/PMC3967178/

24. Kotani S, Sakaguchi E, Warashina S, et al. "Dietary supplementation of arachidonic and docosahexaenoic acids improves cognitive function." Neuroscience Research. 2006. https://www.ncbi.nlm.nih.gov/labs/articles/16905216/

25. Daley CA, Abbott A, Doyle PS, et al. "A review of fatty acid profiles and antioxidant content in grass-fed and grain-fed beef." Nutr J. 2010; 9: 10. https://www.ncbi.nlm.nih.gov/pubmed/20219103

26. Fox C, Ramsoomair D, Carter C. Magnesium: its proven and potential clinical significance. South Med J. 2001 Dec;94(12):1195-201. https://www.ncbi.nlm.nih.gov/pubmed/11811859

27. Piovesan, D., Profiti, G., Martelli, P. L., & Casadio, R. (2012). The human "magnesome": detecting magnesium binding sites on human proteins. BMC Bioinformatics, 13(Suppl 14). https://www.ncbi.nlm.nih.gov/pmc/articles/PMC3439678/

28. Naghii, M. R., et al. (2011). Comparative effects of daily and weekly boron supplementation on plasma steroid hormones and proinflammatory cytokines. Journal of Trace Elements in Medicine and Biology, 25(1), 54-58. https://www.ncbi.nlm.nih.gov/pubmed/21129941

29. Chitturi, R. et al. (2015). A review on role of essential trace elements in health and disease. Journal of Dr. NTR University of Health Sciences, 4(2), 75. http://www.jdrntruhs.org/article.asp?issn=2277-8632;year=2015;volume=4;issue=2;spage=75;epage=85;aulast=Prashanth

30. Milton K (1987) "Primate diets and gut morphology: implications for hominid evolution." In: Food and Evolution: Toward a Theory of Food Habits, eds. Harris M, Ross EB; Temple University Press, Philadelphia, pp. 93-115.

31. Aiello, L. C., & Wheeler, P. (1995). The Expensive-Tissue Hypothesis: The Brain and the Digestive System in Human and Primate Evolution. Current Anthropology, 36(2), 199-221. https://www.jstor.org/stable/2744104

32. Wang, Yiqun, Campbell, TC., et al. "Fish consumption, blood docosahexaenoic acid and chronic diseases in Chinese rural populations." Comparative Biochemistry and Physiology Part A: Molecular & Integrative Physiology 136.1 (2003): 127-40. http://www.sciencedirect.com/science/article/pii/S1095643303000163

33. Humane Reearch Council. Study of Current and Former Vegetarians and Vegans. Print. December 2014. https://faunalytics.org/wp-content/uploads/2015/06/Faunalytics_Current-Former-Vegetarians_Full-Report.pdf

34. Beckett JL, Oltjen JW. Estimation of the water requirement for beef production in the United States. J Anim Sci. 1993 Apr;71(4):818-26. https://www.ncbi.nlm.nih.gov/pubmed/8478283

35. Teague, W. R. (2016). The role of ruminants in reducing agricultures carbon footprint in North America. Journal of Soil and Water Conservation, 71(2), 156-164. http://www.jswconline.org/content/71/2/156.full.pdf+html

36. Rennard, B. O., Ertl, R. F., Gossman, G. L., Robbins, R. A., & Rennard, S. I. (2000). Chicken Soup Inhibits Neutrophil Chemotaxis In Vitro. Chest, 118(4), 1150-1157. http://journal.publications.chestnet.org/article.aspx?articleid=1079188

37. Conzatti A., et al. Clinical and molecular evidence of the consumption of broccoli, glucoraphanin and sulforaphane in humans. Nutr Hosp. 2014 Nov 30;31(2):559-69 https://www.ncbi.nlm.nih.gov/pubmed/25617536

38. N. Nagata, et al. Glucoraphanin Ameliorates Obesity and Insulin Resistance Through Adipose Tissue Browning and Reduction of Metabolic Endotoxemia in Mice. Diabetes, 2017. http://diabetes.diabetesjournals.org/content/early/2017/02/12/db16-0662

13 - Fast and Feast

1. Stewart, W. K., & Fleming, L. W. (1973). Features of a successful therapeutic fast of 382 days duration. Postgraduate Medical Journal, 49(569), 203-209. https://www.ncbi.nlm.nih.gov/pmc/articles/PMC2495396/

2. Hartman, A. L., & Stafstrom, C. E. (2013). Harnessing the power of metabolism for seizure prevention: Focus on dietary treatments. Epilepsy & Behavior, 26(3), 266-272. https://www.ncbi.nlm.nih.gov/pmc/articles/PMC3562425/

3. Paoli, A., Rubini, A., Volek, J. S., & Grimaldi, K. A. (2014). Beyond weight loss: a review of the therapeutic uses of very-low-carbohydrate (ketogenic) diets. European Journal of Clinical Nutrition, 68(5), 641-641. https://www.ncbi.nlm.nih.gov/pmc/articles/PMC3826507/

4. Zhang, Y. et al. (2013). Ketosis Proportionately Spares Glucose Utilization in Brain. Journal of Cerebral Blood Flow & Metabolism, 33(8), 1307-1311. https://www.ncbi.nlm.nih.gov/pmc/articles/PMC3734783/

5. Barr SB and Wright JC.Postprandial energy expenditure in whole-food and processed-food meals: implications for daily energy expenditure. Food Nutr Res. 2010 Jul 2;54. https://www.ncbi.nlm.nih.gov/pubmed/20613890

6. Dimaraki, E. V., & Jaffe, C. A. (2006). Role of endogenous ghrelin in growth hormone secretion, appetite regulation and metabolism. Reviews in Endocrine and Metabolic Disorders, 7(4), 237-249. http://www.ncbi.nlm.nih.gov/pubmed/17195943

7. Horne, B., Muhlestein, J. et al. (2013). Randomized cross-over trial of short-term water-only fasting: Metabolic and cardiovascular consequences. Nutrition, Metabolism and Cardiovascular Diseases, 23(11), 1050-1057. https://www.ncbi.nlm.nih.gov/pubmed/23220077

8.   Ho, K. Y. et al. (1988). Fasting enhances growth hormone secretion and amplifies the complex rhythms of growth hormone secretion in man. Journal of Clinical Investigation, 81(4), 968-975. http://www.ncbi.nlm.nih.gov/pmc/articles/PMC329619/

9.   C. Morris, D. Aeschbach, and F. Scheer. Circadian System, Sleep and Endocrinology. Mol Cell Endocrinol. 2012 Feb 5; 349(1): 91–104. https://www.ncbi.nlm.nih.gov/pmc/articles/PMC3242827/

10. Lammers, L. A. (2017). Effect of Short-Term Fasting on Systemic Cytochrome P450-Mediated Drug Metabolism in Healthy Subjects: A Randomized, Controlled, Crossover Study Using a Cocktail Approach. Clinical Pharmacokinetics. https://www.ncbi.nlm.nih.gov/pubmed/28229374

11. Longo, V., & Mattson, M. (2014). Fasting: Molecular Mechanisms and Clinical Applications. Cell Metabolism, 19(2), 181-192. https://www.ncbi.nlm.nih.gov/pmc/articles/PMC3946160/

12. Alirezaei, M. (2010). Short-term fasting induces profound neuronal autophagy. Autophagy, 6(6), 702-710. https://www.ncbi.nlm.nih.gov/pmc/articles/PMC3106288/

13. Choi, I. (2016). A Diet Mimicking Fasting Promotes Regeneration and Reduces Autoimmunity and Multiple Sclerosis Symptoms. Cell Reports, 15(10), 2136-2146. https://www.ncbi.nlm.nih.gov/pubmed/27239035

14. García-Prat, L., Muñoz-Cánoves, P., & Martínez-Vicente, M. (2017). Monitoring Autophagy in Muscle Stem Cells. Methods in Molecular Biology Muscle Stem Cells, 255-280. https://www.ncbi.nlm.nih.gov/pubmed/28247355

15. Cheng, C., et al. (2016). Prolonged Fasting Reduces IGF-1/PKA to Promote Hematopoietic-Stem-Cell-Based Regeneration and Reverse Immunosuppression. Cell Stem Cell, 18(2), 291-292. https://www.ncbi.nlm.nih.gov/pmc/articles/PMC4102383/

16. Petrovski, G., & Das, D. K. (2010). Does autophagy take a front seat in lifespan extension? Journal of Cellular and Molecular Medicine, 14(11), 2543-2551. https://www.ncbi.nlm.nih.gov/pmc/articles/PMC4373474/

17. Laplante, M., & Sabatini, D. (2012). mTOR Signaling in Growth Control and Disease. Cell, 149(2), 274-293. https://www.ncbi.nlm.nih.gov/pmc/articles/PMC3331679/

18. Duncan, R.E. et al. Regulation of Lipolysis in Adipocytes. Annu Rev Nutr. 2007; 27: 79–101. https://www.ncbi.nlm.nih.gov/pmc/articles/PMC2885771/

19. Horne, B., Muhlestein, J., & Anderson, J. L. (2015). Health effects of intermittent fasting: hormesis or harm? A systematic review. American Journal of Clinical Nutrition, 102(2), 464-470. https://www.ncbi.nlm.nih.gov/pubmed/26135345

20. Oarada, M. (2011). Refeeding with a high-protein diet after a 48 h fast causes acute hepatocellular injury in mice. British Journal of Nutrition, 107(10), 1435-1444. https://www.ncbi.nlm.nih.gov/pubmed/21902856

21. Pickett, K. E. (2001). Multilevel analyses of neighbourhood socioeconomic context and health outcomes: a critical review. Journal of Epidemiology & Community Health, 55(2), 111-122. http://jech.bmj.com/content/55/2/111.short

14 - Herbalism

1.   Trojanowska A. [Lettuce, lactuca sp., as a medicinal plant in polish publications of the 19th century]. Kwart Hist Nauki Tech. 2005;50(3-4):123-34.   https://www.ncbi.nlm.nih.gov/pubmed/17153150

2.   Barnes J, Anderson LA, Phillipson JD. St John's wort (Hypericum perforatum L.): a review of its chemistry, pharmacology and clinical properties. J Pharm Pharmacol. 2001 May;53(5):583-600. https://www.ncbi.nlm.nih.gov/pubmed/11370698

3.   Tian, J. (2014). Antidepressant-like activity of adhyperforin, a novel constituent of Hypericum perforatum L. Scientific Reports, 4(1). https://www.ncbi.nlm.nih.gov/pubmed/25005489

4.   Rasoanaivo, P., Wright, C. W., Willcox, M. L., & Gilbert, B. (2011). Whole plant extracts versus single compounds for the treatment of malaria: synergy and positive interactions. Malaria Journal, 10(Suppl 1). https://www.ncbi.nlm.nih.gov/pmc/articles/PMC3059462/

5.   Veeresham, C. (2012). Natural products derived from plants as a source of drugs. Journal of Advanced Pharmaceutical Technology & Research, 3(4), 200. https://www.ncbi.nlm.nih.gov/pmc/articles/PMC3560124/

6.   Environmental Working Group. "Greening" Hospitals: An Analysis of Pollution Prevention in America's Top Hospitals.   June 1998 http://static.ewg.org/reports/1998/GreeningHospitals.pdf

7. Rupeshkumar, M., et al. (2016). Ganoderma lucidum: A Review with Special Emphasis on the Treatment of Various Cancer. Journal of Applied Pharmacy, 8(4). https://www.omicsonline.org/open-access/ganoderma-lucidum-a-review-with-special-emphasis-on-the-treatment-of-various-cancer-1920-4159-1000228.php?aid=81128

8. Patel, S., & Goyal, A. (2011). Recent developments in mushrooms as anti-cancer therapeutics: a review. 3 Biotech, 2(1), 1-15. https://www.ncbi.nlm.nih.gov/pmc/articles/PMC3339609/

9. University of Minnesota. (2006, October 23). Discovery About Evolution Of Fungi Has Implications For Humans. ScienceDaily. www.sciencedaily.com/releases/2006/10/061021115712.htm

10. Socala, K., et al. (2015). Evaluation of Anticonvulsant, Antidepressant-, and Anxiolytic-like Effects of an Aqueous Extract from Cultured Mycelia of the Lingzhi or Reishi Medicinal Mushroom Ganoderma lucidum (Higher Basidiomycetes) in Mice. International Journal of Medicinal Mushrooms, 17(3), 209-218. http://www.dl.begellhouse.com/journals/708ae68d64b17c52,7b35b5ed6bb0a817,2c53560e0cbb691f.html

11. Jia-Shi Zhu, Georges M. Halpern, and Kenneth Jones. The Scientific Rediscovery of an Ancient Chinese Herbal Medicine: Cordyceps sinensis Part I. The Journal of Alternative and Complementary Medicine. February 2008, 4(3): 289-303. http://online.liebertpub.com/doi/abs/10.1089/acm.1998.4.3-289

12. Mori, K. et al. (2008). Nerve Growth Factor-Inducing Activity of Hericium erinaceus in 1321N1 Human Astrocytoma Cells. Biological & Pharmaceutical Bulletin, 31(9), 1727-1732. https://www.ncbi.nlm.nih.gov/pubmed/18758067

13. Brekhman II, Dardymov IV, 1969. New substances of plant origin which increase nonspecific resistance. Ann Rev Pharmacol 9: 419-30 https://www.ncbi.nlm.nih.gov/pubmed/4892434

14. Panossian, A., Wikman, G., & Wagner, H. (1999). Plant adaptogens III. Earlier and more recent aspects and concepts on their mode of action. Phytomedicine, 6(4), 287-300. http://www.scicompdf.se/rosenrot/panossian_1999.pdf

15. Panossian, A., & Wagner, H. (2005). Stimulating effect of adaptogens: an overview with particular reference to their efficacy following single dose administration. Phytotherapy Research, 19(10), 819-838. https://www.ncbi.nlm.nih.gov/pubmed/16261511

16. G. (2010). Chamomile: A herbal medicine of the past with a bright future (Review). Molecular Medicine Reports, 3(6). https://www.ncbi.nlm.nih.gov/pmc/articles/PMC2995283/

17. Gohil, K., Patel, J., & Gajjar, A. (2010). Pharmacological review on Centella asiatica: A potential herbal cure-all. Indian Journal of Pharmaceutical Sciences, 72(5), 546. https://www.ncbi.nlm.nih.gov/pmc/articles/PMC3116297/

18. Elsas, S. et al. (2010). Passiflora incarnata L. (Passionflower) extracts elicit GABA currents in hippocampal neurons in vitro, and show anxiogenic and anticonvulsant effects in vivo, varying with extraction method. Phytomedicine, 17(12), 940-949. https://www.ncbi.nlm.nih.gov/pmc/articles/PMC2941540/

19. Karabín, M., Hudcová, T., Jelínek, L., & Dostálek, P. (2016). Biologically Active Compounds from Hops and Prospects for Their Use. Comprehensive Reviews in Food Science and Food Safety, 15(3), 542-567. http://onlinelibrary.wiley.com/doi/10.1111/1541-4337.12201/pdf

20. Hingorani, L., Patel, S., & Ebersole, B. (2012). Sustained cognitive effects and safety of HPLC-standardized Bacopa Monnieri extract: A randomized, placebo controlled clinical trial. Planta Medica, 78(11). https://www.thieme-connect.com/products/ejournals/abstract/10.1055/s-0032-1320681

21. Šaden-Krehula, M., Tajić, M., & Kolbah, D. (1971). Testosterone, epitestosterone and androstenedione in the pollen of scotch pineP. silvestris L. Experientia, 27(1), 108-109. http://www.ncbi.nlm.nih.gov/pubmed/5549221

22. Travison TG., et al. A population-level decline in serum testosterone levels in American men. J Clin Endocrinol Metab. 2007 Jan;92(1):196-202. https://www.ncbi.nlm.nih.gov/pubmed/17062768

23. Levine, H., et al. (2017). Temporal trends in sperm count: a systematic review and meta-regression analysis. Human Reproduction Update, 1-14. https://academic.oup.com/DocumentLibrary/humupd/PR/dmx022_final.pdf

24. Henkel, R. R. (2013). Tongkat Ali as a Potential Herbal Supplement for Physically Active Male and Female Seniors-A Pilot Study. Phytotherapy Research, 28(4), 544-550. https://www.ncbi.nlm.nih.gov/pubmed/23754792

25. Alok, S. et al. (2013). Plant profile, phytochemistry and pharmacology of Asparagus racemosus (Shatavari): A review. Asian Pacific Journal of Tropical Disease, 3(3), 242-251. https://www.ncbi.nlm.nih.gov/pmc/articles/PMC4027291/
Rotblatt, M.D. Dong Quai: A Review. AHC Media. August 1999; Volume 1: 65-69. https://www.ahcmedia.com/articles/42506-dong-quai-a-review

26. Krebs, T. S., & Johansen, P. (2013). Psychedelics and Mental Health: A Population Study. PLoS ONE, 8(8). http://journals.plos.org/plosone/article?id=10.1371/journal.pone.0063972

27. Walsh, R. (1982). Psychedelics and Psychological Well-Being. Journal of Humanistic Psychology, 22(3), 22-32. http://journals.sagepub.com/doi/abs/10.1177/0022167882223004

28. Emerson, A., Ponté, L., Jerome, L., & Doblin, R. (2014). History and Future of the Multidisciplinary Association for Psychedelic Studies (MAPS). Journal of Psychoactive Drugs, 46(1), 27-36. https://www.ncbi.nlm.nih.gov/pubmed/24830183

29. Grob, C. S., et al. Pilot Study of Psilocybin Treatment for Anxiety in Patients With Advanced-Stage Cancer Arch Gen Psychiatry. 2011;68(1):71-78 http://jamanetwork.com/journals/jamapsychiatry/fullarticle/210962

15 - Symbiosis

1. Dukowicz, A., Lacy, B., Levine, G. Small Intestinal Bacterial Overgrowth: A Comprehensive Review. Gastroenterol Hepatol (N Y). 2007 Feb; 3(2): 112–122. https://www.ncbi.nlm.nih.gov/pmc/articles/PMC3099351/

2. Sender, R., Fuchs, S., & Milo, R. (2016). Revised estimates for the number of human and bacteria cells in the body. https://www.ncbi.nlm.nih.gov/pmc/articles/PMC4991899/

3. Jiménez, E. (2008). Is meconium from healthy newborns actually sterile? Research in Microbiology, 159(3), 187-193. https://www.ncbi.nlm.nih.gov/pubmed/18281199

4. Fierer, N., Hamady, M., Lauber, C. L., & Knight, R. (2008). The influence of sex, handedness, and washing on the diversity of hand surface bacteria. Proceedings of the National Academy of Sciences, 105(46), 17994-17999. https://www.ncbi.nlm.nih.gov/pubmed/19004758

5. Cui, L., Morris, A., & Ghedin, E. (2013). The human mycobiome in health and disease. Genome Medicine, 5(7), 63. https://www.ncbi.nlm.nih.gov/pmc/articles/PMC3978422/

6. Virgin, H. (2014). The Virome in Mammalian Physiology and Disease. Cell, 157(1), 142-150. https://www.ncbi.nlm.nih.gov/pmc/articles/PMC3977141/

7. Hanage WP, Fraser C, Spratt BG. Fuzzy species among recombinogenic bacteria. BMC Biol. 2005 Mar 7;3:6. https://www.ncbi.nlm.nih.gov/pubmed/15752428

8. Windsor, D. A. (1995). Equal Rights for Parasites. Conservation Biology, 9(1), 1-2. http://onlinelibrary.wiley.com/doi/10.1046/j.1523-1739.1995.09010001.x/pdf

9. Lukeš, J. et al. (2014). (Self-) infections with parasites: re-interpretations for the present. Trends in Parasitology, 30(8), 377-385. http://www.cell.com/article/S1471-4922(14)00108-1/abstract

10. Rook, G. A. (2013). Regulation of the immune system by biodiversity from the natural environment: An ecosystem service essential to health. Proceedings of the National Academy of Sciences, 110(46), 18360-18367. https://www.ncbi.nlm.nih.gov/pubmed/24154724

11. Mcdade, T. W., Rutherford, J., Adair, L., & Kuzawa, C. W. (2009). Early origins of inflammation: microbial exposures in infancy predict lower levels of C-reactive protein in adulthood. Proceedings of the Royal Society B: Biological Sciences, 277(1684), 1129-1137. http://rspb.royalsocietypublishing.org/content/early/2009/12/08/rspb.2009.1795

12. Rook, G. A. (2013). Microbial Exposures and Other Early Childhood Influences on the Subsequent Function of the Immune System. Primates, Pathogens, and Evolution, 331-362. https://www.ncbi.nlm.nih.gov/pubmed/24732404

13. Rooks, M. G., & Garrett, W. S. (2016). Gut microbiota, metabolites and host immunity. Nature Reviews Immunology, 16(6), 341-352. https://www.nature.com/nri/journal/v16/n6/box/nri.2016.42_BX2.html

14. Sagan, Lynn (1967). "On the origin of mitosing cells". Journal of Theoretical Biology. 14 (3): 225–274. https://www.ncbi.nlm.nih.gov/pubmed/11541392

15. Neu, J., & Rushing, J. (2011). Cesarean Versus Vaginal Delivery: Long-term Infant Outcomes and the Hygiene Hypothesis. Clinics in Perinatology, 38(2), 321-331. https://www.ncbi.nlm.nih.gov/pmc/articles/PMC3110651/

16. Mueller, N. T., et al. (2015). The infant microbiome development: mom matters. Trends in Molecular Medicine, 21(2), 109-117. https://www.ncbi.nlm.nih.gov/pmc/articles/PMC4464665/

17. German, JB; Lebrilla, CB; Mills, DA. "Human milk oligosaccharides: evolution, structures and bioselectivity as substrates for intestinal bacteria". Nestle Nutr Workshop Ser Pediatr Program. 62: 205–22. https://www.ncbi.nlm.nih.gov/pmc/articles/PMC4348064/

18. Breast Cancer and Breastfeeding: Collaborative Reanalysis of Individual Data from 47 Epidemiological Studies in 30 Countries, Including 50 302 Women With Breast Cancer and 96 973 Women Without the Disease. (2003). Obstetrical & Gynecological Survey, 58(2), 94-95. https://www.ncbi.nlm.nih.gov/pubmed/12133652

19. Global, Regional, and National Levels of Maternal Mortality, 1990–2015. (2017). Obstetrical & Gynecological Survey, 72(1), 11-13. http://www.thelancet.com/pdfs/journals/lancet/PIIS0140-6736(16)31470-2.pdf

20. David. L.A. et al. Diet rapidly and reproducibly alters the human gut microbiome. Nature 505, 559–563 (23 January 2014) https://www.nature.com/nature/journal/v505/n7484/full/nature12820.html

21. Almada, C. N., et al. (2016). Paraprobiotics: Evidences on their ability to modify biological responses, inactivation methods and perspectives on their application in foods. Trends in Food Science & Technology, 58, 96-114. http://www.sciencedirect.com/science/article/pii/S0924224416302412

22. Claus, S. P., Guillou, H., & Ellero-Simatos, S. (2016). The gut microbiota: a major player in the toxicity of environmental pollutants? Npj Biofilms and Microbiomes, 2(1). https://www.nature.com/articles/npjbiofilms20163

23. Suez J, et al. 2014. Artificial sweeteners induce glucose intolerance by altering the gut microbiota. Nature Oct; 9;514(7521):181-6. https://www.ncbi.nlm.nih.gov/pubmed/25231862

24. Cho I, Blaser MJ. 2012. The human microbiome: at the interface of health and disease. Nat Rev Genet, Mar 13;13(4):260-70. https://www.ncbi.nlm.nih.gov/pmc/articles/PMC3418802/

25. Vijay-Kumar, M. et al. Metabolic syndrome and altered gut microbiota in mice lacking Toll-like receptor 5. Science. 2010 Apr 9;328(5975):228-31. https://www.ncbi.nlm.nih.gov/pubmed/20203013

26. Walters, W. A., Xu, Z., & Knight, R. (2014). Meta-analyses of human gut microbes associated with obesity and IBD. FEBS Letters, 588(22), 4223-4233. https://www.ncbi.nlm.nih.gov/pmc/articles/PMC5050012/

27. Espín, J. C., González-Sarrías, A., & Tomás-Barberán, F. A. (2017). The gut microbiota: A key factor in the therapeutic effects of (poly)phenols. Biochemical Pharmacology. https://www.ncbi.nlm.nih.gov/pubmed/28483461

28. Sonnenburg, E. D., Smits, S. A., Tikhonov, M., Higginbottom, S. K., Wingreen, N. S., & Sonnenburg, J. L. (2016). Diet-induced extinctions in the gut microbiota compound over generations. Nature, 529(7585), 212-215. http://www.nature.com/nature/journal/v529/n7585/full/nature16504.html

29. Boulangé CL., et al. Impact of the gut microbiota on inflammation, obesity, and metabolic disease. Genome Med. 2016; 8: 42. https://www.ncbi.nlm.nih.gov/pmc/articles/PMC4839080/

30. Bollinger, R. R., Barbas, A. S., Bush, E. L., Lin, S. S., & Parker, W. (2007). Biofilms in the large bowel suggest an apparent function of the human vermiform appendix. Journal of Theoretical Biology, 249(4), 826-831. https://www.ncbi.nlm.nih.gov/pubmed/17936308

31. Cryan, J. F., & Dinan, T. G. (2012). Mind-altering microorganisms: the impact of the gut microbiota on brain and behaviour. Nature Reviews Neuroscience, 13(10), 701-712. https://www.ncbi.nlm.nih.gov/pubmed/22968153

32. Canani, R. B. (2011). Potential beneficial effects of butyrate in intestinal and extraintestinal diseases. World Journal of Gastroenterology, 17(12), 1519. https://www.ncbi.nlm.nih.gov/pmc/articles/PMC3070119/

33. Dinan, T. G., Stanton, C., & Cryan, J. F. (2013). Psychobiotics: A Novel Class of Psychotropic. Biological Psychiatry, 74(10), 720-726. http://www.biologicalpsychiatryjournal.com/article/S0006-3223(13)00408-3/fulltext

34. Yano, JM., et al. Indigenous bacteria from the gut microbiota regulate host serotonin biosynthesis. Cell. 2015 Apr 9; 161(2): 264–276. https://www.ncbi.nlm.nih.gov/pmc/articles/PMC4393509/

35. Jacob, E. B., Becker, I., Shapira, Y., & Levine, H. (2004). Bacterial linguistic communication and social intelligence. Trends in Microbiology, 12(8), 366-372. https://www.ncbi.nlm.nih.gov/pubmed/15276612

36. Shapiro, J. (2007). Bacteria are small but not stupid: cognition, natural genetic engineering and socio-bacteriology. Studies in History and Philosophy of Science Part C: Studies in History and Philosophy of Biological and Biomedical Sciences, 38(4), 807-819. https://www.ncbi.nlm.nih.gov/pubmed/18053935

37.   Summers, R. W. et al. (2005). Trichuris suis therapy in Crohns disease. Gut, 54(1), 87-90.
      https://www.ncbi.nlm.nih.gov/pmc/articles/PMC1774382/
38.   Thoemmes, M. S., Fergus, D. J., Urban, J., Trautwein, M., & Dunn, R. R. (2014). Ubiquity and
      Diversity of Human-Associated Demodex Mites. PLoS ONE, 9(8).
      http://journals.plos.org/plosone/article?id=10.1371/journal.pone.0106265
39.   Chen, Y. E., & Tsao, H. (2013). The skin microbiome: Current perspectives and future challenges.
      Journal of the American Academy of Dermatology, 69(1).
      https://www.ncbi.nlm.nih.gov/pmc/articles/PMC3686918/
40.   Vom Saal FS; et al. (2007). "Chapel Hill bisphenol A expert panel consensus statement: integration of
      mechanisms, effects in animals and potential to impact human health at current levels of exposure".
      Reprod Toxicol. 24 (2): 131–8. https://assets.documentcloud.org/documents/1010781/2007-
      0801bpaconsensus.pdf
41.   Obregon-Tito, A. J. et al. (2015). Subsistence strategies in traditional societies distinguish gut
      microbiomes. Nature Communications, 6, 6505. https://www.nature.com/articles/ncomms7505

16 - Fear of Nature

1.   Pacheco, O., et al. Zika Virus Disease in Colombia — Preliminary Report. New England Journal of
      Medicine, 2016. http://www.nejm.org/doi/10.1056/NEJMoa1604037
2.   Muangphrom, P., Seki, H., Fukushima, E. O., & Muranaka, T. (2016). Artemisinin-based antimalarial
      research: Application of biotechnology to the production of artemisinin, its mode of action, and the
      mechanism of resistance of Plasmodium parasites. Journal of Natural Medicines J Nat Med, 70(3), 318-
      334. https://www.ncbi.nlm.nih.gov/pubmed/27250562
3.   Ang HH, Chan KL, Mak JW. In vitro antimalarial activity of quassinoids from Eurycoma longifolia
      against Malaysian chloroquine-resistant Plasmodium falciparum isolates. Planta Med. 1995;61(2):177–
      178. https://www.ncbi.nlm.nih.gov/pubmed/7753926
4.   Mohd Ridzuan, Sow A, Noor Rain A, Mohd Ilham A, Zakiah I. Eurycoma longifolia extract-artemisinin
      combination: parasitemia suppression of Plasmodium yoelii-infected mice. Trop Biomed. 2007
      Jun;24(1):111-8 https://www.ncbi.nlm.nih.gov/pubmed/17568384

17 - Disconnect to Reconnect

1.   Atchley, R. A., Strayer, D. L., & Atchley, P. (2012). Creativity in the Wild: Improving Creative
      Reasoning through Immersion in Natural Settings. PLoS ONE, 7(12).
      https://www.ncbi.nlm.nih.gov/pmc/articles/PMC3520840/

18 - Spending Time in Nature

1.   Park, B. J. et al. (2009). The physiological effects of Shinrin-yoku (taking in the forest atmosphere or
      forest bathing): evidence from field experiments in 24 forests across Japan. Environmental Health and
      Preventive Medicine, 15(1), 18-26. https://www.ncbi.nlm.nih.gov/pubmed/19568835
2.   Li, Q. (2009). Effect of forest bathing trips on human immune function. Environmental Health and
      Preventive Medicine, 15(1), 9-17. https://www.ncbi.nlm.nih.gov/pmc/articles/PMC2793341/
3.   Bell, J. F., Wilson, J. S., & Liu, G. C. (2008). Neighborhood Greenness and 2-Year Changes in Body
      Mass Index of Children and Youth. American Journal of Preventive Medicine, 35(6), 547-553.
      https://www.ncbi.nlm.nih.gov/pubmed/19000844
4.   Ulrich, R. (1984). View through a window may influence recovery from surgery. Science, 224(4647),
      420-421. https://www.ncbi.nlm.nih.gov/pubmed/6143402
5.   Maller, C. et al. Healthy parks, healthy people. Deakin University and Parks Victoria. March 2008.
      https://www.deakin.edu.au/__data/assets/pdf_file/0016/310750/HPHP-2nd-Edition.pdf
6.   Berman MG, Jonides J, Kaplan S. The cognitive benefits of interacting with nature. Psychol Sci. 2008
      Dec;19(12):1207-12. https://www.ncbi.nlm.nih.gov/pubmed/19121124
7.   Lewis, M. H. (2004). Environmental complexity and central nervous system development and function.
      Mental Retardation and Developmental Disabilities Research Reviews, 10(2), 91-95.
      http://onlinelibrary.wiley.com/doi/10.1002/mrdd.20017/abstract

8. Barton, J., & Pretty, J. (2010). What is the Best Dose of Nature and Green Exercise for Improving Mental Health? A Multi-Study Analysis. Environmental Science & Technology, 44(10), 3947-3955. http://pubs.acs.org/doi/abs/10.1021/es903183r

9. Gullone, E. (2000). The Biophilia Hypothesis and Life in the 21st Century: Increasing Mental Health or Increasing Pathology? Journal of Happiness Studies, 1(3), 293-322. https://link.springer.com/article/10.1023%2FA%3A1010043827986?LI=true

10. Davis, J. Psychological Benefits of Nature Experiences: An Outline of Research and Theory. Naropa University and School of Lost Borders. July 2004. http://www.soulcraft.co/essays/psychological_benefits_of_nature_experiences.pdf

11. Wuthnow, R. Peak Experiences: Some Empirical Tests. (1978). Journal of Humanistic Psychology, 18(3), 59-76. http://journals.sagepub.com/doi/abs/10.1177/002216787801800307

19 - The Life and Intelligence of Nature

1. Healy, K., et al. A recent study in Animal Behavior reveals that body mass and metabolic rate determine how animals of different species perceive time. Animal Behaviour 86: 4, October 2013, Pages 685–696. http://www.sciencedirect.com/science/article/pii/S0003347213003060

2. Mitton, Jeffry B. & Grant, Michael C. 1996. Genetic Variation and the Natural History of Quaking Aspen. BioScience 46, 1, 25-31. http://www.jstor.org/stable/1312652?seq=1#page_scan_tab_contents

3. Schulz, F., et al. Giant viruses with an expanded complement of translation system components. Science 07 Apr 2017: Vol. 356, Issue 6333, pp. 82-85. http://science.sciencemag.org/content/356/6333/82

4. J. E. Lovelock (1972). "Gaia as seen through the atmosphere". Atmospheric Environment. 6 (8): 579–580. http://www.sciencedirect.com/science/article/pii/0004698172900765

5. Kiverstein, J., & Miller, M. (2015). The embodied brain: towards a radical embodied cognitive neuroscience. Frontiers in Human Neuroscience, 9, 237. http://journal.frontiersin.org/article/10.3389/fnhum.2015.00237/full

6. Roger Lewin (12 December 1980). "Is Your Brain Really Necessary?". Science. 210 (4475): 1232–1234. https://www.ncbi.nlm.nih.gov/pubmed/7434023

7. Warwick, C., et al. (2013). Assessing reptile welfare using behavioural criteria. In Practice, 35(3), 123-131. http://inpractice.bmj.com/content/35/3/123

8. Low, P. The Cambridge Declaration on Consciousness. July 7, 2012. The University of Cambridge. http://fcmconference.org/img/CambridgeDeclarationOnConsciousness.pdf

9. Baluška, F., Mancuso, S., Volkmann, D., & Barlow, P. (2009). The 'root-brain' hypothesis of Charles and Francis Darwin. Plant Signaling & Behavior, 4(12), 1121-1127. https://www.ncbi.nlm.nih.gov/pubmed/20514226

10. Humphries, J., et al. Species-Independent Attraction to Biofilms through Electrical Signaling. Cell. Vol. 168, Issues 1-2, p200–209. Jan 2017. http://www.cell.com/cell/fulltext/S0092-8674(16)31728-7

11. Nakagaki, T. (2001). Smart behavior of true slime mold in a labyrinth. Research in Microbiology, 152(9), 767-770. https://www.ncbi.nlm.nih.gov/pubmed/11763236

12. Brenner, E. D. (2006). Plant neurobiology: an integrated view of plant signaling. Trends in Plant Science, 11(8), 413-419. https://www.ncbi.nlm.nih.gov/pubmed/16843034

13. Molinier, J, Ries, G., Zipfel, C. & Hohn, B. Transgeneration memory of stress in plants. Nature 442, 1046-1049 (31 August 2006) https://www.nature.com/nature/journal/v442/n7106/full/nature05022.html

14. Anhauser, M. The Silent Scream of the Lima Bean. Max Planck Research, April 2007. https://www.mpg.de/942876/W001_Biology-Medicine_060_065.pdf

15. Gagliano, M., Mancuso, S., & Robert, D. (2012). Towards understanding plant bioacoustics. Trends in Plant Science, 17(6), 323-325. http://www.sciencedirect.com/science/article/pii/S1360138512000544

16. Baluška, F., Volkmann, D., Hlavacka, A., Mancuso, S., & Barlow, P. W. (n.d.). Neurobiological View of Plants and Their Body Plan. Communication in Plants, 19-35. https://www.researchgate.net/publication/265100277_Proof_2_Neurobiological_View_of_Plants_and_Their_Body_Plan

17. Ford, Brian J. (2004). "Are Cells Ingenious?" Microscope. 52 (3/4): 135–144. http://www.brianjford.com/04-12-ingens.pdf

20 - Heart Field and Heart Perception

1. Mccraty, R. (2014). The Energetic Heart: Bioelectromagnetic Interactions Within and Between People. The Neuropsychotherapist, 6(1), 22-43. https://www.heartmath.org/research/research-library/energetics/energetic-heart-bioelectromagnetic-communication-within-and-between-people/
2. McCraty, R., Atkinson, M., et al. The Electricity of Touch: Detection and Measurement of Cardiac Energy Exchange Between People. Karl H. Pribram, ed. Brain and Values: Is a Biological Science of Values Possible. Mahwah, NJ: Lawrence Erlbaum Associates, Publishers, 1998: 359-379. https://www.heartmath.org/research/research-library/energetics/electricity-of-touch/
3. Kim, D., Lee, K., Kim, J., Whang, M., & Kang, S. W. (2013). Dynamic correlations between heart and brain rhythm during Autogenic meditation. Frontiers in Human Neuroscience, 7. https://www.ncbi.nlm.nih.gov/pmc/articles/PMC3728977/
4. Mccraty, R., & Tomasino, D. (n.d.). Heart Rhythm Coherence Feedback: A New Tool for Stress Reduction, Rehabilitation, and Performance Enhancement. PsycEXTRA Dataset. https://www.heartmath.org/research/research-library/clinical/heart-rhythm-coherence-feedback/
5. Marinelli R., Furst, B., van der Goe H., McGinn A., Marinelli W. The Heart is Not a Pump: A Refutation of the Pressure Propulsion Premise of Heart Function. Frontier Perspectives, 1995, 5: 15-24. http://www.rsarchive.org/RelArtic/Marinelli/
6. Ogawa, T., & Bold, A. J. (2014). The heart as an endocrine organ. Endocrine Connections, 3(2). https://www.ncbi.nlm.nih.gov/pmc/articles/PMC3987289/
7. Lacey, B. C., & Lacey, J. I. (1978). Two-way communication between the heart and the brain: Significance of time within the cardiac cycle. American Psychologist, 33(2), 99-113. https://www.ncbi.nlm.nih.gov/pubmed/637402
8. Mccraty, R., Atkinson, M., & Bradley, R. T. (2004). Electrophysiological Evidence of Intuition: Part 2. A System-Wide Process? The Journal of Alternative and Complementary Medicine, 10(2), 325-336. https://www.heartmath.org/research/research-library/intuition/electrophysiological-evidence-of-intuition-part-2/
9. Barker SA, Borjigin J, Lomnicka I, Strassman R. "LC/MS/MS analysis of the endogenous dimethyltryptamine hallucinogens, their precursors, and major metabolites in rat pineal gland microdialysate". Biomed Chromatogr. 27 (12): 1690–1700. https://www.ncbi.nlm.nih.gov/pubmed/23881860

23 - Sensory Stimulation with Artist's Conk

1. Bushdid, C., Magnasco, M. O., Vosshall, L. B., & Keller, A. (2014). Humans Can Discriminate More than 1 Trillion Olfactory Stimuli. Science, 343(6177), 1370-1372. http://vosshall.rockefeller.edu/assets/file/BushdidScience2014.pdf
2. Chen D., Haviland-Jones J. (2000). Human olfactory communication of emotion. Perceptual & Motor Skills, 91, 771–781. http://journals.sagepub.com/doi/10.2466/pms.2000.91.3.771
3. Wandersee, J.S. & Schussler, E.E. Toward a Theory of Plant Blindness. Plant Science Bulletin 47:1 (2001) http://www.botany.org/bsa/psb/2001/psb47-1.html
4. Milne, J. L., Goodale, M. A., & Thaler, L. (2014). The role of head movements in the discrimination of 2-D shape by blind echolocation experts. Attention, Perception, & Psychophysics, 76(6), 1828-1837. https://www.ncbi.nlm.nih.gov/pubmed/24874262
5. Dolgin, E. (2015). The myopia boom. Nature, 519(7543), 276-278. https://www.nature.com/news/the-myopia-boom-1.17120

Index

About the Author

Born without genetic gifts, a weak and scrawny Logan Christopher sought out the best training information in his pursuit of super strength, mind power and radiant health. Nowadays, he's known for his famous feats of pulling an 8,800 lb. firetruck by his hair, juggling flaming kettlebells, and supporting half a ton in the wrestler's bridge. Called the "Physical Culture Renaissance Man" his typical workouts might include backflips, freestanding handstand pushups, tearing phonebooks in half, bending steel, deadlifting a heavy barbell, or lifting rocks overhead.

Far from being all brawn and no brain Logan has sought optimal performance with mental training and sports psychology which he has explored in depth, becoming an NLP Trainer, certified hypnotist, EFT practitioner and more. That's also how he got started in the field of health and nutrition which inevitably led to Chinese, Ayurvedic and Western herbalism.

His personal philosophy is to bring together the best movement skill, health information, and mental training to achieve peak performance. He is the author of many books and video programs to help people increase their strength, skills, health and mental performance. Discover how you too can become super strong, both mentally and physically, at www.LegendaryStrength.com and find the superior herbs to support all aspects of your performance at www.LostEmpireHerbs.com.

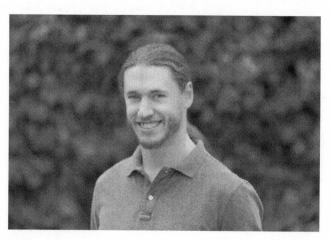